EXPERT GUIDE TO
PAIN MANAGEMENT

D1512116

OTHER TITLES IN THE ACP EXPERT GUIDES SERIES

ALLERGY AND IMMUNOLOGY
Edited by Raymond G. Slavin and Robert E. Reisman

INFECTIOUS DISEASES
Edited by James S. Tan

ONCOLOGY
Edited by Jacob D. Bitran

OTOLARYNGOLOGY
Edited by Karen H. Calhoun
Associate Editors: David E. Eibling and Mark K. Wax

RHEUMATOLOGY
Edited by Arthur M.F. Yee and Stephen A. Paget

For a catalogue of publications available from ACP, contact:

Customer Service Center
American College of Physicians
190 N. Independence Mall West
Philadelphia, PA 19106-1572
215-351-2600
800-523-1546, ext. 2600

Visit our Web site at www.acponline.org

EXPERT GUIDE TO

PAIN MANAGEMENT

Bill McCarberg, MD

University of California, San Diego
and
Kaiser Permanente

Steven D. Passik, PhD

Memorial Sloan–Kettering Cancer Center

AMERICAN COLLEGE OF PHYSICIANS

PHILADELPHIA

Clinical Consultant: David R. Goldmann, MD, FACP
Manager, Book Publishing: Diane McCabe
Developmental Editor: Victoria Hoenigke
Production Supervisor: Allan S. Kleinberg
Senior Production Editor: Karen C. Nolan
Interior Design: Kate Nichols
Cover Design: Elizabeth Swartz
Index: Nelle Garrecht

Manufactured in the United States of America
Printed by Versa Press
Composition by UB Communications

Library of Congress Cataloging-in-Publication Data

Expert guide to pain management / [edited by] Bill H. McCarberg, Steven D. Passik.
    p. ; cm – (ACP expert guides series)
    Includes bibliographical references and index.
    ISBN 1-930513-61-5
. 1. Pain—Treatment. 2. Analgesia. I. Title: Pain management. II. McCarberg, Bill H.
    III. Passik, Steven D. IV. Series.
    [DNLM: 1. Pain—therapy. 2. Chronic Disease—therapy. WL 704 E959 2005]
    RB127.E967 2005
    616'.04—dc22

                                                                                    2005043633

The authors and publisher have exerted every effort to ensure that drug selection and dosage set forth in this book are in accordance with recommendations and practice at the time of publication. In view of ongoing research, occasional changes in government regulations, and the constant flow of information relating to drug therapy and drug reactions, the reader is urged to check the package insert for each drug for any change in indications and dosage and for additional warnings and precautions. This care is particularly important when the recommended agent is a new or infrequently used drug.

05 06 07 08 09 / 10 9 8 7 6 5 4 3 2 1

Contributors

Mary Baluss, JD
Director, Pain Law Initiative
Washington, DC

Stanley J. Bigos, MD
Professor of Orthopedic Surgery
 and Environmental Health
University of Washington School
 of Medicine
Director, Spine Research Clinic
Seattle, Washington

Daniel Brookoff, MD, PhD
Methodist Pain Clinic
Methodist Central Hospital
Memphis, Tennessee

Daniel B. Carr, MD
Lecturer
Departments of Anesthesia and
 Pharmacology
New England Medical Center
Boston, Massachusetts

Daniel J. Clauw, MD
Assistant Dean for Clinical and
 Translational Research
Professor of Internal Medicine
Director of Chronic Pain and
 Fatigue Center
Director of Center for Advancement
 of Clinical Research
University of Michigan Medical School
Ann Arbor, Michigan

Antoine B. Douaihy, MD
Assistant Professor
Department of Psychiatry
University of Pittsburgh School of
 Medicine
Medical Director, Addiction
 Medicine Services
Western Psychiatric Institute and
 Clinic
Pittsburgh, Pennsylvania

Robert H. Dworkin, PhD
Department of Anesthesiology
University of Rochester School of
 Medicine and Dentistry
Rochester, New York

Scott M. Fishman, MD
Division of Pain Medicine
Department of Anesthesiology and
 Pain Medicine
University of California, Davis
Sacramento, California

Maureen A. Flannery, MD
Department of Family Practice
University of Kentucky College of
 Medicine
Lexington, Kentucky

Mark P. Jensen, PhD
Professor
Department of Rehabilitation
 Medicine
University of Washington
Seattle, Washington

Roger J. Jou, MD
Department of Psychiatry
Western Psychiatric Institute and
 Clinic
University of Pittsburgh School of
 Medicine
Pittsburgh, Pennsylvania

Kenneth L. Kirsh, PhD
Symptom Management and
 Palliative Care Program
Markey Cancer Center
University of Kentucky
Lexington, Kentucky

Bill McCarberg, MD
Assistant Clinical Professor–Voluntary
University of California, San Diego
Founder, Chronic Pain Management
  Program
Kaiser Permanente
San Diego, California

Jane E. McKee, MSN, ARNP
Clinicians Network for Counseling
  and Psychotherapy
Portland, Oregon

Ewan McNicol, MS
Clinical Pharmacist
Pharmacy Department
Tufts–New England Medical Center
Boston, Massachusetts

Gagan Mahajan, MD
Division of Pain Medicine
Department of Anesthesiology and
  Pain Medicine
University of California, Davis
Sacramento, California

Alec B. O'Connor, MD
General Medicine Unit
Department of Medicine
University of Rochester School of
  Medicine and Dentistry
Rochester, New York

Steven D. Passik, PhD
Associate Attending Psychologist
Memorial Sloan–Kettering Cancer
  Center
New York, New York

Russell K. Portenoy, MD
Chairman, Department of Pain
  Medicine and Palliative Care
Beth Israel Medical Center
Professor of Neurology and
  Anesthesiology
Albert Einstein College of Medicine
New York, New York

James P. Robinson, MD, PhD
Associate Professor and
  Rehabilitation Physician
UWMC Roosevelt Pain Center
University of Washington
Seattle, Washington

Joel R. Saper, MD, FACP, FAAN
Michigan Head Pain and
  Neurological Institute
Ann Arbor, Michigan

Dennis C. Turk, PhD
John and Emma Bonica Professor
  of Anesthesiology and Pain
  Research
Department of Anesthesiology
University of Washington
Seattle, Washington

Lana Wania-Galicia, MD
Division of Pain Medicine
Department of Anesthesiology and
  Pain Medicine
University of California, Davis
Sacramento, California

Foreword

C hronic pain is highly prevalent and extraordinarily complex. Population-based surveys suggest that approximately one third of Americans experience frequent or persistent pain, and that one third of those who have pain report a significant impact on function or quality of life. Pain may be associated with progressive or static injury to virtually any tissue, or occur in the absence of an explanatory lesion. Pain may or may not be accompanied by physical impairments, or by disturbances in mood or social functioning. Some patients are highly disabled by their pain, whereas others function well.

Although clinicians continue to rely on useful classifications such as *nociceptive pain* and *neuropathic pain,* these distinctions are an extreme simplification of the many inter-related processes—biomedical and psychological—that may sustain chronic pain in predisposed individuals. Chronic pain is, in fact, many diseases. Scientists and clinicians are only now beginning to define, classify, and analyze its complex mechanisms.

At the same time, however, the commonalities across populations with chronic pain are too relevant clinically to be ignored. From the broadest perspective, these commonalities may be understood as justifying the view that chronic pain is, overall, an illness. Its manifestations necessarily vary, but the potential for complex linkages between the sensory experience of pain and the adverse effects on every domain of human functioning is shared by all. This understanding of pain as illness is one the foundations of the modern approach to pain management.

The magnitude and complexity of chronic pain challenge every level of the health care system. To provide competent pain assessment and management to the millions who need help, physicians must make the study of pain a component of best practice in all primary care settings *and* pain specialists must have a broad representation throughout the United States.

Unfortunately, there is substantial documentation that a best-practice approach is not the standard of care for most patients, and access to specialists is very limited. This reality, combined with studies that demonstrate clear under-treatment in those populations characterized by an evidence-based consensus about optimal care (such as those with cancer pain), highlights the importance of chronic pain as a major public health problem. The annual cost in the United States of chronic pain in terms of direct medical expenditures, informal costs, and lost productivity has been estimated at $100 billion.

To acknowledge that there is considerable distance to travel before every patient can access the best pain care possible should not lead one to pessimism or despair. The past four decades have witnessed astonishing advances in both the science and practice of pain management. This volume joins an ever-growing number of books, journals, and other sources of information that document these advances and educate the health care giver about pain and its management. Although the medical culture has moved in fits and starts, the general direction is toward recognition of the need for more research and more care related to pain.

Progress, therefore, will be made, but it is likely to come slowly and haltingly. The treatment of pain can be controversial, such as the role of chronic opioid therapy for noncancer pain, and the debate often reaches into the area of public policy. Nonetheless, the advances in research and the increasing number of consensus views within the professional community provide the means to help many patients. Surely a time is not too distant when every patient will be able to access competent care for the potentially devastating illness of chronic pain.

Bill McCarberg, MD
Steven D. Passik, PhD
Russell K. Portenoy, MD

Contents

1

■   ■   ■

Chronic Pain as Disease: The Pathophysiology of Disordered Pain

Daniel Brookoff, MD, PhD

*When pain is chronic, it not only involves the painful area,
it involves the entire being.*

MICHEL DE MONTAIGNE

The treatment of pain has been of concern to patients and their physicians for thousands of years. In that time, there have been many different conceptual models of pain. At certain times, pain was thought to be an emotion. At other times, it was thought to be a pathogen. Aristotle taught that pain was not a sense but rather an affective state, "a passion of the soul". Descartes wrote that pain was indeed a physical sensation traveling to our minds via delicate threads. Through all that time, and even more so today, effective treatments for pain have been available to sufferers, but these treatments have frequently been withheld, more often for philosophical than for medical reasons.

The aim of this chapter is to present a model for the physiology of normal pain, which is not a disease, and a model for the pathophysiology of chronic pain, which is a group of legitimate medical disorders worthy of medical treatment. Although life is full of physical *pain*, life does not have to be full of physical *suffering*. As Hippocrates taught us, it is the suffering individual that physicians must face, not just his pain. My hope is that these models will be a guide as we carry out the duty with which the Hippocratic physicians charged us: the alleviation of suffering (1).

A Brief History of Chronic Pain

More than 4000 years ago, Chinese physicians described a balance of vital energy, the *ch'i,* which flowed through the organs and vital structures

1

through a network of bodily conduits called meridians. Disease and pain were thought to be due to an imbalance of two opposing forces, yin and yang, related to obstructions (deficiencies) or outpourings (excesses) in the circulation of the *ch'i*. This view linked pathology of the visceral organs with dysfunction of somatic structures and abnormal sensations throughout the body such as chronic pain, giving rise to medical treatments designed to restore balance. Among these were the first effective treatments for chronic pain, including the precursors to many of the medications and techniques that we use today (2).

The Hippocratic physicians did not see chronic pain as a mere symptom that was unworthy of treatment as many physicians do today. Without the concept of "underlying disease", pain was not viewed as an alarm or a sentinel or a prodrome of illness – it was regarded as the illness itself. Hippocratic physicians had not yet conceived of the positive value of pain. The Hippocratics taught that pain predisposed a part of the body to attract and invoke disease. Their observation that artificially induced pain was sharper than naturally occurring pain led to their use of painful remedies such as blistering agents, rubifactents, and moxibustion, a traditional Chinese therapy which consisted of burning a fabric or vegetable material on the skin in order to create a diversionary point (1). In addition to painful therapies, the physicians of antiquity were familiar with the use of narcotic plants such as mandrake, henbane (*Hyoscyamus niger*), nightshade, and opium poppies (3). In the first century AD, Dioscorides described the formulation of a strong pain medication in *De materia medica*. The juice of the plant *Papaverum nigrum* was dried in the sun and then kneaded into small cakes, which he termed *opium*.

During the Middle Ages, a link was established between pain and the concept of divine punishment. Pain relief came to be opposed on religious grounds. Pain and illness were seen as a necessary apprenticeship to the full functioning of the human spirit (4). Chronic pain and suffering took on a redemptive value. Church literature discussed how suffering brought the individual closer to Christ. How could this belief be reconciled with a surgical operation that was intended to eliminate or alleviate pain? The surgery itself must be painful. This led to an antipathy towards anesthesia and to a contention that "those operations in which sedatives have been used with the aim of sparing the sick some pain have been less successful" (4). Postoperative pain was seen both as a sign that healing was underway and a necessary suffering for the good of the soul.

With the onset of the Age of Enlightenment, western medicine began to appreciate the usefulness and value of pain outside of a religious context. Pain was seen as a warning or alarm, diverting the individual from harmful lifestyles. Pain also took on a diagnostic value. Distinguishing between the various types of pain led to better diagnoses of the underlying pathology.

The 17th century saw a divergence between physicians who promoted "natural healing" and those who aggressively promoted the interventional "art of medicine". The former included British physicians such as Thomas Sydenham ("The English Hippocrates") who drew attention to observing "the course of nature" in illness. Sydenham felt that it was important to treat pain. He revived and publicized the use of opium-containing compounds that were held in disrepute by other physicians. Sydenham wrote that "so necessary an instrument is opium in the hand of a skillful man that medicine would be a cripple without it" (5). He was among the first modern physicians to discuss dosing analgesics for children. To Sydenham goes the credit for popularizing the use of analgesics and developing the formulation for laudanum (opium tincture) (Table 1-1).

In 18th century England, surgery – associated with manual, physical labor – was considered a skilled craft rather than a profession. Surgeons were considered separate from, and subordinate to, the physicians, those who had studied the Art of Healing at university (hence the distinction between the gentleman "Doctor" and the surgical "Mister"). In the newly independent United States, however, some in the medical profession began to bridle against British tradition and urged for a re-thinking of the medical hierarchy. Eventually, the status of surgeons in the United States was elevated to that of physicians and, indeed, came to be considered heroic.

A major advocate of this change was "The Father of American Medicine," Benjamin Rush, one of the founders of America's first medical school. Whereas his predecessors had sought to balance "depletive therapies" (e.g., bloodletting, purging, emetics, mercury) with "restorative treatments" or "tonics" (e.g., chinchona, opium, alcohol), Rush eschewed the tonics and championed the universal deployment of harsh depletive remedies and their "heroic administration" in massive doses (6). Rush's teachings dominated American academic medicine well into the 1830s and reverberate to this day. Rush maintained that without the heroic intervention of the Medical Art most illnesses would naturally worsen, terminating in death (6). The first duty of the physician was "heroic action to fight disease". In opposition to the Hippocratic credo of "Do no harm" – which at that time had been altered to "*First of all,* do no harm" (7) – Rush regarded the physician who killed his patient through overdosing as merely zealous whereas the physician who allowed a patient to die through insufficiently vigorous therapy was both a murderer and a quack (8).

Table 1-1   Sydenham's Recipe for Laudanum

- *Sherry:* 1 pint
- *Opium:* 2 ounces
- *Saffron:* 1 ounce
- *Cinnamon:* 1 ounce powdered
- *Clove:* 1 ounce powdered

Mix and simmer over a vapor bath for 2 to 3 days until the tincture has the proper consistency.

From Latham RG, ed. The Works of Thomas Sydenham. London: The Thomas Sydenham Society; 1848.

A Modern – and Ancient – View of Chronic Pain

In light of recent advances in our understanding of anatomy and physiology, the present time may be propitious for revisiting the concept of yin and yang. We can now regard pain as an expression of the function of a very complex and delicately balanced *nociceptive system*. When this system functions properly it protects us from injury, promotes healing, protects us from further trauma, and sustains life. In this way, it is analogous to the other balanced healing systems that keep us alive, such as the coagulation system.

Looking at how our understanding of the coagulation system has evolved over the past one hundred years gives us a useful model for how physicians can gradually grasp the complexities of important physiological regulatory mechanism. For hundreds of years we knew only about the procoagulant parts of the coagulation system. As recently as 30 years ago, teaching about the coagulation system meant teaching about the coagulation cascade. The fact that liquid blood coagulated in response to injury was thought of as a miracle. Later we began to understand that the real miracle was that blood was not clotting all the time. Eventually, we understood that there was a complex counterbalancing anti-coagulation system that was activated as soon as coagulation was triggered. Because of the relationship between these counterbalancing systems, coagulation could be localized in time and place, maintaining a meaningful relationship to trauma and promoting survival. When coagulation and anticoagulation maintain this balance we are healthy. When this balance is disrupted, we have a group of diseases collectively termed the *coagulopathies,* clinically expressed as destructive clotting-related events ranging from thromboembolism to hemorrhage. When faced with a patient with a coagulopathy, we do not institute treatment aimed at obliterating clotting, we seek to restore the balance and promote healthful coagulation.

In the nociceptive system, generators of pain are similarly balanced by a complex antinociceptive system that allows pain to perform its life-sustaining functions while maintaining its topographical and temporal relationship to the inciting injury. These functions include alarming us to injuries; developing transient hypersensitivities, which protect the injured areas from further damage; linking to memories, which teach us to avoid future injury; and activating natural pain relievers, so that we can continue functioning as the injury heals. When the pain system functions effectively it promotes life. When pain becomes disconnected from its original meaning due to an imbalance of its nociceptive and antinociceptive functions, it becomes a disease—chronic pain—that diminishes life. *Chronic pain is pain that has lost its purpose.*

A comparison of the physiology of normal pain and the pathophysiology of chronic pain reveals important neurochemical differences that support the contention that chronic pain is indeed a medical disorder. Or rather, like the coagulopathies, chronic pain is a group of medical disorders with identifiable pathophysiologies that should guide us to rational treatments. Ultimately, these treatments will not merely suppress pain but restore balance, promote function, and alleviate suffering.

Many western words for pain come from the Latin root *doles,* which is an objective word that can have an inanimate object, such as *caput doles,* which translates to "My head feels pain" or "I have a headache". In distinction, the Latin root for suffering, *suffere,* means "to bear, endure, or allow". It is a verb which requires an active subject (e.g., a person). In modern parlance, we are back to Hippocrates when we take this to mean "Pain happens to a body; suffering happens to a person."

"What Does the Pain Feel Like?"

The understanding that there are different types of pain and that attention to these differences can help guide medical treatment goes back to antiquity. The Hippocratics taught that the patient had an obligation to disclose and describe his pain. It was the patient's duty to relate accurately what he had experienced, and the physician's duty to listen (1). In the early classifications of pain, when the imbalance of humours was seen as a more important generator of disease than the dysfunction of organs, details about the type and intensity of the pain prevailed over location. Books on diagnostics focused on the semiotics of illness and encouraged attention to the minutiae of descriptions because "the mode of the pain indicates the judgement which should be made about the illness" (9).

For example, differentiation of various types of "inflammation of the chest" allowed physicians to distinguish between different conditions (and their different outcomes). "The pain is tearing and superficial and increases with movements of the arms or trunk in inflammation of the chest wall. Pain is lancinating in pleurisy, it is deeper and often gravitative in peripneumonia; it is more general, more widely prevalent and duller in catarrh" (9). Today, patients in chronic pain are still often asked "What does the pain feel like?" but lack of verbal skills and language limitations may limit the response. As Virginia Woolf wrote, "The merest schoolgirl, when she falls in love, has Shakespeare or Keats to speak her mind for her; but let a sufferer try to describe a pain in his head to a doctor and language at once runs dry" (10).

Galen was one of the first to conceptualize the physiology of nociception when he described pain as a response to events that occurred outside the body. There were, he wrote, three necessary conditions for the perception of pain: an organ to receive an outside impression, a connecting passageway, and an organizational center to transform the sensation into a conscious perception (11). With the development of the field of pathological anatomy, the identity of the affected area or the damaged organ assumed increasing importance. However, post-mortem examinations often found no trace of damage, and such pain was often termed *functional* rather than *structural*.

Different Types of Pain and Their Causes

We can recollect that we suffered but in no way remember the particular quality of the pain which we suffered.

HERMANN BOERHAAVE (12)

A current basis for discriminating between different types of pain depends on its physiological generator of the pain. Injury to peripheral tissues such as skin, muscle, or fascia gives rise to *somatic* pain. Pain generated by visceral tissues is not always related to injury and gives rise to sensations that can be distinctly identified as *visceral* pain. Injury, stimulation, or regrowth of nerves can give rise to various forms of *neuropathic* pain, which is often characterized by dysesthetic sensations such as burning, painful numbness, or electrical sensations with lancinations. Recognition that these generators give rise to different sensory experiences reinforces the Hippocratic exhortation to listen to our patients' descriptions of pain.

Somatic Pain

For most physicians the model of "normal pain" is that of pain linked temporally and topographically to injury to superficial connective tissue. Most of the acute pain that we experience in our lifetime is somatic, pain related to minor trauma to skin, muscle, or fascia. As already mentioned, this type of pain has several functions. It acts as an alarm that is localized in time and place. Its most intense component has a fast onset after the injury, and it is typically dampened long before the injury heals. The injured area is left with a persistent hypersensitivity that protects against trauma and promotes healing. The pain is also rapidly integrated into memory, which further helps to prevent repeated injuries. For example, children with attention deficit or learning disorders, which frequently involve problems with memory, are found to be at risk for repeat injuries even though they can sense pain adequately (13). Timely relief of the pain is another function of the nociceptive system that is just as important to normal function as is the ability to sense pain (14). While the memory of injuries is typically profound and evocative, recalling the injury generally does not involve re-experiencing the sensation of pain. Under normal circumstances, we are supposed to remember and learn from our pain, but we are not supposed to keep re-living it.

The Process of Inflammation

Even minor disruption of tissue causes the release of chemical mediators from lysosomes and cell membranes, giving rise to a chemically cascading inflammatory reaction which triggers electrical signals in sensory nerves that carry the message of pain to the brain (15). Because of the self-augmenting nature of this inflammatory reaction, an intense pain signal can be rapidly generated by a minor injury. The analogy I use when describing this to patients is that of smoke alarms, which we program to give off the loudest blare with the first hint of smoke (i.e., the signal is out of proportion to the stimulus).

The chemical reactions that link the release of cellular elements to pain have much in common with other cascading healing processes such as coagulation and wound healing. They even share some of the same mediators such as the serine protease kallikreins, which cleave high and low molecular weight kinninogens to form the kinins, the peptides bradykinin and kallidin. Bradykinin, which works through the activation of specific B_1 and B_2 receptors, is one of the most important chemical mediators of acute pain. Activation of B_2 receptors stimulates excitatory currents in specific populations of sensory neurons called *nociceptors,* which carry the electrical signal of pain to the dorsal horn of the spinal cord (Fig. 1-1). Post-activation hyperpolarization limits the ability of these nociceptors to fire repetitively, and the initial excitatory effects of bradykinin are transient due to this rapid desensitization. This can account for the short-lived "intensely sharp" element of acute somatic pain. Activation of B_1 receptors on mast cells and macrophages provokes the elaboration of other inflammatory mediators, such as cytokines, histamine, and nitric oxide, and amplifies the inflammatory reaction. Activation of B_1 receptors on vascular cells causes increases in vascular permeability (16).

Injuries to cells will also cause release of a group of cell membrane phospholipids, collectively known as *eicosanoids,* which are metabolized by the arachadonic acid pathway to prostaglandins and thromboxanes or via the lipooxygenase pathway to leukotrienes (LT-D_4 and LT-B_4) and slow-reacting substances, all of which are potent mediators of inflammation (17). Activation of the enzyme phopholipase A, which is stimulated by bradykinin acting through the B_1 receptor on inflammatory cells, triggers the arachadonic acid pathway, resulting in the production of prostaglandins, prominently PG-I_2 but also PG-D_2, PG-E_1, and PG-E_2. These prostaglandins do not primarily evoke a pain impulse, but they modify B_2 receptors on sensory neurons and sensitize nociceptor terminals to mechanical and thermal stimuli, setting up persistent hypersensitivity of the injured area (hyperalgesia) and the perception of pain in response to mechanical or thermal stimuli that were not painful in the uninjured state (allodynia) These delayed excitatory effects of bradykinin are specifically inhibited by cyclooxygenase inhibitors (18).

Another mediator of delayed-onset pain is leukotriene LT-B_4, which exerts its effects through its action as a chemoattractant for leukocytes which, in turn, release a factor called 8R,15S-diHETE; the last acts as a specific receptor on afferent nerves that is distinct from the prostaglandin receptor (19). Still other mediators of inflammation, including adenosine and mast-cell activators,

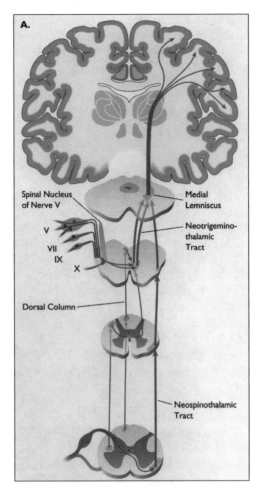

Figure 1-1   Different spinal tracts transmit different types of pain. There are several ascending tracts through which a pain signal can be transmitted to the brain. The two main sets of ascending pathways are the lateral system (panel *A*) and the medial system (panel *B, facing page*).

The lateral system is composed of long thick fibers and is most closely associated with somatic pain. This system transmits information about the onset of an injury and its precise location, intensity, and duration. Signals in these tracts are generally most intense at the onset of an injury. The fibers in the lateral system connect to areas of the brain that can quickly generate a response aimed at preventing further damage.

Fibers in the lateral system can be facilitated or inhibited by endogenous hormones or neurotransmitters, medications, or other neuronal inputs. These neuronal inputs can be generated in peripheral tissue (e.g., a child rubbing a scraped knee after a painful fall) or from within the central nervous system (e.g., by an implanted neurostimulator). The function of the lateral system can also be influenced by the behavioral or cognitive state of the individual. For example, a phenomenon called *stress-induced analgesia* can allow an individual to "ignore" intense acute pain due to a severe injury and take action which would normally be considered heroic or even impossible, such as bearing weight on a fractured

(Cont'd on facing page)

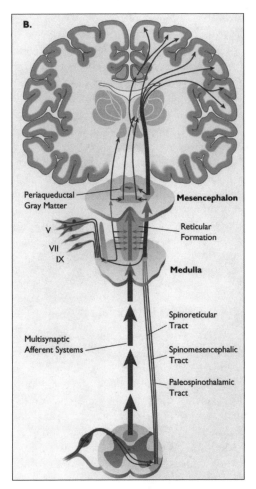

leg. The "meaning" of the injury can determine whether the patient will experience this type of analgesia. This may explain why people can more frequently perform "painful" heroic acts in order to rescue individuals with whom they have a close relationship, such as a relative or friend, than a person with whom they do not have an emotional connection.

The medial system is composed of phylogenetically older fibers that transmit impulses more slowly. This system collects inputs from a more widespread group of neurons transmitting pain signals from an area of tissue (e.g., in a visceral organ) and is less involved with localization of an impulse. This may explain why visceral pain is generally less responsive to neurostimulation than somatic pain. Medial pathways determine the level of general arousal due to an injury and transmit tonic information to the brain about the persistence of the injury.

The pain pathways are classically considered "crossed pathways" (i.e., the destruction of a segment of the spinothalamic tract yields contralateral analgesia in the dermatomes below the level of the transection), but there are actually both crossed and uncrossed fibers. Connections between the two systems exist that can explain why certain injuries that would be expected to generate signals associated with somatic pain can, under certain circumstances, "jump the track" and generate signals that would give rise to an experience more closely associated with visceral pain.

come from the lysosomal contents of injured cells. Adenosine activates the A_2 receptor on nociceptors. Activation of mast cells leads to the release of platelet-activating factors which in turn leads to the release of serotonin. Serotonin enhances the response of nociceptors to bradykinin and directly activates 5-HT3 and 5-HT1A receptors on nociceptive afferents (20).

Persistent inflammation can also lead to local tissue acidosis, which contributes to pain and hyperalgesia through the generation of protons. Protons selectively activate nociceptors and sensitize nociceptors to mechanical stimuli. Leukocytes, which are attracted by inflammatory mediators and by signals generated by peripheral nerves, elaborate interleukins that promote further inflammation. Interleukin-1 (IL-1) stimulates the activity of phospholipase-C, which promotes the production of prostaglandin-E. Interleukin-8 (IL-8) produces sympathetic-dependent hyperalgesia that is independent of the action of prostaglandins (21). Specific inflammatory factors may be related to specific disease states. For example, certain cancers (e.g., prostate tumors) can elaborate high concentrations of endothelin-1, which can primarily activate populations of afferent nerves causing severe pain (22).

A Role for Nerves in Peripheral Inflammation

Pain-transmitting nerve cells, specifically non-myelinated C fibers and small-caliber myelinated A-delta fibers, appear to play a dual role in translating trauma into pain. Not only do these cells carry electrical signals from the periphery to the spinal cord, they also secrete inflammatory mediators. In response to stimulation of their distal endings by kinins, these nerves release pro-inflammatory chemicals such as calcitonin-gene related peptide (CGRP) and substance P, both of which promote inflammation and which, with prolonged secretion, can promote the growth of pain nerves, possibly contributing to chronic pain states (23). This efferent function for nociceptive nerves was first suggested over 70 years ago when it was ascertained that these peripheral fibers mediated the "flare reaction" surrounding acute cutaneous injuries that did not require a connection to the spinal cord (24).

It has long been noted that cutaneous nerves generally contain more than four times the number of small non-myelinated pain fibers than larger myelinated tactile fibers (25), even though electrical activity concerning tactile stimulation is much more frequent than sensory transmissions related to pain. This suggests that the effect or other functions of these nerves may be as important as their afferent function. These peripheral fibers may play an important role in the efferent control of healing by regulating blood flow and vascular permeability in peripheral tissues, maintaining integrity of skin and controlling certain immunological functions such as emigration of leukocytes (26).

If inflammation persists, factors that promote nerve growth may be released, prolonging inflammation and setting the stage for the establishment of chronic pain. The source of these nerve growth factors can be immune cells (mast cells, macrophages, lymphocytes), fibroblasts, or Schwann cells in inflammed tissue. In skin, the main source of nerve growth factors are basal keratinocytes. Peripheral concentrations of nerve growth factors are increased in models of chronic inflammation such as the human synovium in arthritis (27) or the bladder wall in interstitial cystitis (28).

Peripheral Hyperalgesia and Allodynia

Peripheral inflammation will not only give rise to acute pain, it will also induce hyperalgesia and allodynia. As already mentioned, hyperalgesia is a sensitized state in which a mildly painful stimulus will cause exaggerated pain, and allodynia describes a state where a normally non-noxious stimulus such as light touch or movement will be perceived as painful. An example of the latter occurs when an area of skin has suffered a burn. Not only will that area of skin hurt, but a normally non-painful stimulus such as light touch will also be painful. Interleukin-1 is important in the initiation of hyperalgesia (29). The release of nerve growth factors such as substance P-activating NK-1 receptors on inflammatory cells is often important for the maintenance of the allodynic state, which is often a feature of chronic pain. Sympathetic activation and release of norepinephrine can also produce hyperalgesia but only in the presence of tissue injury. In these cases, norepinephrine may potentiate pain by stimulating the production of prostaglandins and activating phospholipase C (30).

Chemosensitive afferent nerves may become so sensitized by persistent pain that a low-intensity stimulus will provoke hyperalgesia. In certain syndromes, unremittant pain signals may activate usually quiet mechanosensitive afferent nerves ("silent afferents") that are present in synovial tissue and in all viscous organs (31). Once activated, even slight movement or minimal deformity of surrounding tissues can generate pain. This type of allodynia is common in chronic degenerative arthritis, low back pain, and severe irritable bowel syndrome (IBS) and other chronically painful conditions.

In addition to causing local pain at the site of an injury, bradykinin can act in the brain and spinal cord to cause global hyperalgesia. This may account for the diffuse myalgias that often accompany infections and other inflammatory states. In animal models, this can be induced by intracerebral injection of bacterial lipopolysaccharides, which globally enhance nociceptive transmission, amplifying all pains. Lipopolysaccharides are thought to act by inducing immune cells to secrete interleukin-1-beta, resulting in the stimulation of vagal afferents via the tractus solitarius that connects to descending pathways from the raphe magnus that synapse with the descending spinal cord tracts that cause diffuse hyperalgesia (15).

Maintaining the Balance: Natural Anti-Inflammatories

As with other balanced chemical reactions in the body, tissue trauma results in the release of a mix of agonists and antagonists of inflammation.

Angiotensin-converting enzyme and other peptidases inactivate bradykinin and other kinins. Another natural anti-inflammatory compound is beta-endorphin, which is released by peripheral leukocytes. Through their action on opiate receptors on nerve fibers, endorphins inhibit the release of pro-inflammatory mediators (such as substance P from peripheral sensory nerve endings), reducing peripheral vasodilatation. Opioid receptors are up-regulated on cutaneous nerves in inflamed tissue, though this can be undermined by nerve damage (e.g., ligation of the sciatic nerve). Corticotropin-releasing factor (CRF), a major secretagogue for opioid peptides from leukocytes and in the pituitary, is locally produced in inflamed tissue. Corticosteroids inhibit phospholipase A_2, preventing the generation of arachidonic acid (32). IL-1 elaborated by immune cells, usually thought of as a potent mediator of inflammation from immune cells, can do the same. Locally applied IL-1 and CRF produce antinociceptive effects in inflamed but not non-inflamed tissues (33).

Visceral Pain

In 1628, an English nobleman and his son went hunting with Charles I. The boy was thrown from his horse and injured his chest, tearing open his rib cage and exposing his heart and lungs. The king summoned his physician, William Harvey, who probed the exposed viscera with his dagger and noted that the boy, though fully conscious, could not detect the pricking or pinching of his heart and lungs. Harvey concluded that these organs were insensate (34).Visceral tissue will release inflammatory mediators in response to injury, but the pain response differs from that in somatic tissue.

The viscera do not have the same protective apparatus signaling tissue damage as do connective tissues. For example, there are no specific nociceptors found in the heart and bradykinin does not elicit pain when injected into the coronary arteries or pericardial sac (35). Most visceral organs are invested with high-threshold afferents, which are triggered by intense contractions of the hollow viscus. The nerves that carry these signals are large-diameter myelinated fibers that synapse with the posterior columns of the spinal cord, a pattern of input which parallels that for proprioception from the limbs and the trunk (36). Prolonged stimulation or injury leads to a unique form of peripheral sensitization that is dependent on activation and recruitment of silent nociceptors which respond mostly to mechanical stimuli and may eventually become activated by normal functioning.

These two sets of nerves, high-threshold contraction receptors and intensity-coding silent afferents, can generate pain in the absence of injury or abnormal mechanical activity, as is the case in IBS, where normal GI activity becomes painful. Different organs are invested with a unique palette of receptors that respond to stretch, pressure, and inflammatory chemicals (37). Some visceral organs (e.g., the esophagus) do have nerves with specific receptors for bradykinin. In addition, bradykinin released from injured viscera can trigger vagal impulses (38).

Typically, pain emanating from the viscera is diffuse and poorly localized. This reflects differences in innervation between somatic and visceral tissue. Somatic fibers are precisely located at the spinal cord and the brain, whereas afferent viscerosensory fibers overlap each other and converge at several levels within the central nervous system. Because of this pattern of innervation, visceral injury is often accompanied by motor and autonomic reflexes, and these may be the major generators of the perceived pain related to visceral injury. Of the afferents fibers that innervate the viscera, C-fibers and A-delta fibers make up less than 30% compared with over 80% in skin and connective tissue (39). Nearly 80% of visceral afferents are silent mechanosensitive afferents. Although specific areas of the skin and connective tissue are neurologically mapped to single areas of the spinal cord, much of the viscera, such as the gut, have dual sensory circuits, with splanchnic nerves innervating the entire gut projecting to the thoracolumbar spine and vagal afferents from the proximal gut to the sigmoid colon. The close overlap of the brain centers concerned with processing visceral afferent information, autonomic function, and arousal accounts for the distinct reflexive and affective components of visceral pain. This results in a higher degree of visceral-autonomic intergration in visceral pain, and the recruitment of endocrine function by the time sensation becomes conscious, usually via stimulation of the vagal fibers, over 85% of which are afferent (40).

Visceral Pain versus Somatic Pain

The differences in somatic and visceral neural architecture invest somatic and visceral pains with different meanings. This has been well-expressed by Al-Chaer and colleagues (41):

> Somatosensory pathways consist of an intricate system of afferents, ascending tracts and processing centers in the spinal cord and in the brain that accurately relay bodily encounters with different types of stimuli. The system enables the individual to sense the stimulus, filter it and perceive it at will. Consequently, the individual can often choose the encounter or avoid it if he controls the agent. The motor system is always available to execute his will (i.e., he can find a comfortable bodily position). Viscerosensory mechanisms are different. The individual does not control any of the components involved. The stimuli are not avoidable, and the autonomic nervous system is not commonly mastered.

Misunderstandings concerning the differences between the mechanisms of somatic and visceral pain may promote over-reliance on visceral pain as a harbinger of injury. Osler wrote extensively about the unreliability of chest pain as an indicator of cardiac injury. He noted that "in acute endocarditis, pain is rarely present, and that ulceration of valves or of the wall may proceed to a most extreme degree without any sensory disturbance" (42).

This is certainly an important issue when a patient's perception of pain is used as a clinical endpoint in the guidance of treatment. For example, compared with the body's response to somatic injury, angina is a relatively late manifestation of myocardial ischemia. One fourth of documented myocardial infarctions are "silent". In fact, most infarctions are preceded by silent ischemia, which means that only a minority of ischemic cardiac episodes are experienced as angina. This may relate to the individual patient's overall pain threshold (e.g., related to sensitivity to electrically induced dental pain). It is well known that silent myocardial infarctions are more frequent in diabetics. This may be due to neuropathy blocking or depressing autonomic activation. It has also been documented that people who secrete more endorphins during exercise, such as atheletes, will have more silent ischemia. Naloxone can be used as a pre-treatment to improve the predictive value of exercise-testing in some of these patients (43).

Visceral Hyperalgesia

Because of its neurological mapping and reflex involvement, chronic visceral pain is often expressed as a functional disorder, an important example of which is irritable bowel syndrome. Such disorders often feature extra-organ involvement, such as sexual dysfunction, sleep disruption, and fibromyalgia-like symptoms (44). Often, a prominent affective component is featured, such as anxiety or depression.

Irritable bowel syndrome affects up to 22% of the United States population. Most of these patients report hypersensitive stomachs or mild bowel dysfunction dating back to childhood, though many do not connect this to their diagnosis of IBS. There is probably a genetic predisposition to this syndrome (45). There also appears to be an association with a history of major traumatic events (physical or sexual abuse) or major losses during childhood (46). This may relate to an "embedding" of the pain memory into the central nervous system during a period of intense neural modeling during childhood. Approximately one third of IBS patients develop their symptoms following acute GI infections, though these patients often have other risk factors. This suggests that in susceptible individuals enteric infections and other causes of mucosal inflammation can precipitate ongoing IBS symptoms long after the infection or inflammation is gone (44).

Peripheral Nociceptors

Progressing from the level of peripheral tissues to the peripheral nervous system, there are two types of specialized nociceptors: poorly myelinated A-delta fibers and unmyelinated C-fibers. A-delta fibers are faster transmitters and mediate "first pain", usually having sharp or acute pricking characteristics (see Fig. 1-1). There are two types of A-delta fibers: type I are activated in heat and burn injury, type II are activated by substance P and moderate heat.

C-fibers, which are activated by bradykinin and other mediators, are responsible for the delayed, dull, aching, and burning components of the pain sensation. One group (type I) can secrete neuropeptide neurotransmitters such as substance P and CGRP, and they express the Trk A receptor for nerve growth factor (NGF). The other group (type II) depends on local glial cell-derived growth factors and are sensitized by protons. Most C-fibers are polymodal; that is, they can respond to a broad range of stimuli including thermal, mechanical, and chemical stimulation. One of the most important interfaces between the tissue injury and the nerve impulse is vanilloid receptor-1 (VR-1), which translates the physical injury into a neural impulse. Activating VR-1 opens a calcium channel in the nerve cell. This can be directly activated by capsaicin, heat, protons (H^+ ions), lipids (e.g., cell breakdown products), and substance P. Some C-fibers also have channels that respond directly to cold via CMR-1 receptors, which is thought to be the "cold counterpart" and close molecular cousin to VR-1. These receptors can be also triggered directly by chemicals such as menthol and peppermint, and this activation can cause a "cooling" sensation. Other C-fibers can respond directly to mechanical pressure via an apparatus that is localized in the cell membrane (47).

The two types of C-fibers connect to different areas of the dorsal horn of the spinal cord. C-I fibers synapse with cells in the superficial dorsal horn, and C-II fibers go to the deeper substantia gelatinosa. C-fibers subserving different tissues of the body have their own unique pattern of connection to the spinal cord. C-fibers from the skin terminate in highly topographic fashion in the substantia gelatinosa, whereas nociceptive input from the viscera connect in a more diffuse, less topographic pattern.

In chronic pain states, peripheral nociceptors can undergo a broad range of changes. Individual fibers can become more responsive to a given stimulus—firing at lower thresholds and generating more signals for a given stimulus. High-threshold nociceptors may also reduce their thresholds and thus become recruited into the generation of the pain signal, making it a more complex and intense input than it had been originally. This peripheral sensitization is mediated by several factors including the persistent generation of bradykinin, high concentrations of protons (which are part of the inflammatory milieu), and neurotrophic factors such as NGF released by mast cells and fibroblasts (48).

Nerve Growth Factors

Nerve growth and maintenance are ongoing processes. Peripheral tissues must maintain their complement of nociceptors by secreting nerve growth factors. Nerve growth factors influence the growth, survival, and even the phenotype of peripheral sensory nerves. These factors include nerve growth factor-1 (NGF), which is critical to the development and maintenance of both C-fiber and A-delta type nociceptors. Hypersecretion of NGF may also be responsible for the maintenance of chronic pain states. NGF also mediates the hyperalgesia (e.g., sensitivity to touch) of injured tissue. Therapeutic trials of injections of NGF in the treatment of diabetic neuropathy have resulted in persistent fibromyalgia-like syndromes (49). Because NGF does not cross the blood-brain barrier, this has been attributed to actions on peripheral nerves (50).

In addition to NGF, the family of neurotrophins includes brain-derived neurotrophic factor (BDNF) and neurotrophin-3 (NT-3). Glial-derived neurotrophic factor (GDNF) may have a specific role in maintaining the state of chronic pain. GDNF interacts with type II C-fibers. The different neurotrophins act through a family of specific receptors that activate tyrosine kinase, the Trk receptors. NGF interacts with TrkA, BDNF with TrkB, and NT-3 with TrkC.

Nerves in the Balance: The Ecology of Peripheral Nerve Bundles

Peripheral sensory nerves, both nociceptive and non-nociceptive, exist in a balance within their nerve bundles. This balance is regulated by the secretion of various neurotrophins. Disruption of this balance can lead to abnormal growth of one population. If one population of nerves is injured, another population may become activated. This is invoked as one of the many mechanisms of nerve-damage derived pain (neuropathic pain). In an experimental model that reflects clinical experience, resection of the sciatic nerve causes the destruction of the C-fiber terminals where they synapse in the pain-sensing areas of the superficial dorsal horn of the spinal cord. The loss of these connections causes the endings of large myelinated A fibers to become activated. A-fibers are not nociceptors but rather nerves that carry the sensation of touch. The endings of these large fibers can now invade the superficial dorsal horn region. These large nerves that are activated by touch now carry a signal to an area that interprets the incoming signal as pain. The patient will now experience pain to the non-injurious stimulus of touch. This type of allodynia is commonly seen in patients with chronic low back pain who have undergone surgery and may also be part of the explanation of post-laminectomy syndrome. This syndrome is easy to assess clinically but does not show up on CT, MRI, EMG, or nerve conduction studies. Not only do these cells mediate allodynia, they are relatively resistant to the inhibiting effects of endorphins or opioid medications because A-fibers do not produce opioid receptors. This may be part of the mechanism of the agonizing pain of reflex sympathetic dystrophy and may explain its relative insensitivity to opioid medications (51).

A form of diabetic neuropathy illustrates another mechanism of a persistent pain problem caused by an imbalance in the population of sensory nerves. Loss of tactile A-fibers due to destruction by persistent hyperglycemia can result in mononeuritis multiplex syndrome. In this syndrome, C-fibers remain intact. The oligodendrocytes that form the myelin sheath around the dying A fibers migrate and insulate the pain fibers, which can now transmit their signals with greater efficiency and deliver their signals to the spinal cord unopposed. These patients will experience a loss of tactile function and experience a worsening sensation of painful numbness. Biopsies of the affected areas show drop-out of tactile fibers and abnormal myelination of C-fibers. In experimental models which appear to bear close resemblance to what we see in the clinic, damage to motor or sensory nerves in one dermatome (mimicking that caused by back surgery or rhizotomy) can lead to spontaneous activity among nociceptors in adjacent dermatomes. Schwann cells can then be stimulated to proliferate in peripheral nerve Remak's bundles causing abnormal myelination (and hyper-efficiency) of uninjured peripheral nociceptors (52).

Damage to Pain Nerves as a Cause of Pain

Most of what is taught in medical school about the peripheral nervous system focuses on motor nerves. Because of this, many physicians subscribe to a simple model of the peripheral nervous system—hard-wired, non-changing, with a strict partition between motor and sensory functions. Understanding pain and pain-related disorders requires a reconsideration of the role and actions of the sensory nervous system. The sensory nervous system features constant messages, interactions with motor fibers, and neuroplasticity, a process of constant remodeling and regrowth that is the key to understanding chronic pain. Nerves that carry persistent pain signals will "learn" how to carry these signals more efficiently (hypersensitization), eventually transmitting messages independently of stimuli. These sensitized nerves may eventually recruit other nerves that were not involved in the original response to the initial painful stimulus and provoke their firing. Ultimately the pain may "cross the line" and spread outside its dermatome.

Another "new" concept in pain research is that nerves can heal after injury. The idea that chronic pain can result from injury to nerves is not really new, but it is still not yet widely accepted. The concept of "pain without lesion" (the neuralgias) was first described by Francois Chaussier (1746-1828), a professor at the Ecole de Sante in Paris who is also credited with coining the term *tic douloureux* and with describing the characteristics of neuropathic pain. He associated this type of pain with damage to a nerve trunk or with disruption of branches of nerves. He observed this type of pain in instances where tumors compressed nerves or in wounds severing nerves. He described a type of pain that persisted after healing was complete. He noted that a distinctive sign of neuralgia was that sectioning of the nerve stopped the pain for a certain length of time but that it inevitably returned, often in a more serious form (53).

One would expect that nerve damage would result in lack of function. Certainly if one cuts a motor nerve it results in persistent paralysis. That clinical observation is often interpreted to mean that the motor nerve has died. For hundreds of years, the same was thought to be true for nociceptive fibers. For hundreds of years, physicians treated patients in pain by cutting or damaging pain nerves in the hope that such actions would reduce or eliminate the patient's ability to feel pain. Many surgeries and procedures that are done for pain – from occipital neurectomies for chronic headaches, to many types of back surgeries, to hysterectomies for poorly defined pelvic pain – involve neurodestruction. Some of these procedures do give relief, but often the relief is only temporary and is followed by a worsening of the previous pain.

When peripheral nerves are injured, macrophages are recruited and glial cells are activated to create an environment that supports nerve regeneration. The three major types of glial cells in the CNS are microglia, astrocytes, and oligodendrocytes. Microglia are mediators of CNS inflammation and are a rich source of pro-inflammatory cytokines. Astrocytes surround synapses and can sense synaptic activity; they have glutamate receptors and regulate glucose utilization at the synapse. Oligodendrocytes are myelin-forming cells. Trauma within the CNS can evoke growth of astrocytes and microglia, a process termed *reactive gliosis,* which is stimulated by TNF and IL-1. Microglia themselves can secrete additional IL-1, which is a glial growth factor. Reactive gliosis is a prominent consequence of most neuropathological processes in the CNS and can be associated with the accumulation of immunocompetent cells in the area of pathology and the promotion of continued hyperalgesia.

A key to the understanding of certain persistent pain problems is that the cut surface of a nerve fiber severed distal to its cell body can heal. If it is a motor fiber, it still has lost its connection to its target and the generated signals will not reach the limb and the limb will remain paralyzed. If the nerve is a nociceptor, the healed end can start to generate electrical impulses that will reach the spinal cord and will be interpreted as pain, even though this damaged nerve can now generate signals with an abnormal intensity without any input from the periphery. This is apparently the mechanism of much of the pain associated with advanced cancer, which is usually related to the disruption of nerve fibers by the tumor (54).

Damage to sensory nerves can cause neuropathic pain syndromes that are relatively insensitive to suppression by the anti-nociceptive system. In patients who have had a stroke or spinal cord injury, for example, the nerves that carry touch signals may be destroyed. If enough pain-carrying fibers regenerate, tissues presumed to be anesthetic can generate considerable pain if reinjured or inflamed. This *deafferentation pain* is most common among patients with spinal cord injuries. For example, although a patient with a spinal cord injury may have no normal sensation below the waist, surgery on decubitus ulcers or even a simple bladder infection can still be extremely painful. Without the interference of continuous tactile inputs, some patients with spinal cord injuries can discriminate between different types of pain to the point where they can even identify what type of bacteria is infecting their bladder. This type of pain is also seen in post-operative pain syndromes (e.g., post-thoracotomy pain), where a common finding is pain accompanied by an area of tactile hypoesthesia (55).

Damage to the nociceptors themselves can also give rise to opioid-resistant neuropathic pain. When these nerve fibers are traumatized or severed, opioid receptor proteins manufactured within the nerve cell body cannot be transported down the axon to reach their final destination in the pre-synaptic membrane. That is why surgical procedures designed to destroy or cut pain nerves are generally unsuccessful in providing long-term pain relief. Neurodestructive procedures such as presacral neurectomies for pelvic pain, occipital neurectomies for chronic headaches, and limb amputation for reflex sympathetic dystrophy, which used to be common, have thus fallen out of favor. Partial spinal cord transections and other neuroablative procedures continue to be performed but are reserved primarily for end-stage cancer patients with intractable pain and very limited lifespans (56).

Endogenous Pain Relief

Just as clotting is accompanied by anticoagulation, the complex nociceptive system is balanced by an equally complex anti-nociceptive system. Pain signals arriving from peripheral tissues stimulate the release of endorphins in the periaqueductal gray matter of the brain and enkephalins in the nucleus raphe magnus of the brainstem (Fig. 1-2). Endorphins inhibit the propagation of pain signals by binding to mu-opioid receptors on the pre-synaptic terminals of nociceptors and post-synaptic surfaces of dorsal horn cells. Enkephalins bind to delta-opioid receptors on inhibitory interneurons in the substantia gelatinosa of the dorsal horn, causing release of gamma-aminobutyric acid (GABA) and other mediators that dampen pain signals in the spinal cord. Though endogenous pain control pathways in the brain are widespread, many involve the rostral ventromedial medulla (RVM) (57). Neurons in this area not only mediate endogenous pain-relief but also probably play a role in the action of non-pharmacological pain-relievers, including exercise and placebos. Of note, the relief generated by a placebo can be inhibited by pre-treatment with opioid-antagonists such as naloxone, illustrating the chemical connection between our perceptions and brain chemistry. Dysfunction of this natural pain-relieving mechanism has been invoked to explain certain chronic pain states such as the daily headaches that develop in certain migraineurs. Functional MRI studies of these patients often show iron deposition in the peri-aqueductal gray matter, which is said to be related to fibrosis of endorphin-producing cells (58). Some of the analgesic centers in the brain are not responsive to opioid-agonists. One of these areas can mediate the phenomenon of "stress-induced" analgesia, an activated, "goal oriented" state which can cause profound global analgesia and which is not inhibited by opioid antagonists (59). Pharmacological agonists of this system may include ketamine and phencyclidine, both of which are "dissociative" anesthetics.

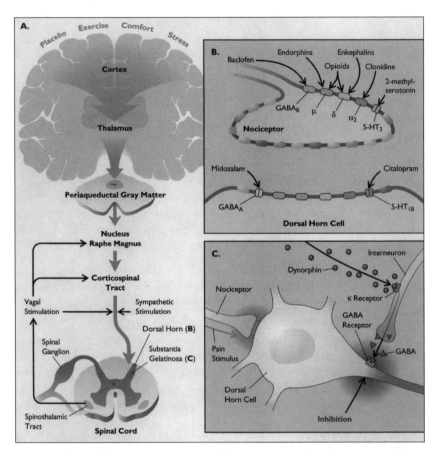

Figure 1-2   Some elements of the antinociceptive system. Panel *A* shows descending antinociceptive pathways that can be triggered by external sensory stimuli to the cerebral cortex (e.g., presenting an individual with a distracting task, offering comforting words, administering a placebo). These tracts generate signals that can travel through the thalamus to neurons in the periaqueductal gray matter, which release enkephalins, or to neurons in descending spinal tracts, which can trigger inhibitory impulses in the corticospinal tract. These inhibitory impulses can be facilitated by vagal stimulation or by the release of norepinephrine by sympathetic nerves. Pain impulses carried by the lateral spinothalamic tract can directly stimulate the periaqueductal gray and nucleus raphe magnus.

Panel *B* shows receptors on the presynaptic surface of the nociceptor and the postsynaptic surface of the dorsal horn cell that can inhibit the transmission of the pain signal. These inhibitory receptors can be stimulated by mediators which include opioids, GABA-A agonists (e.g., midazolam), GABA-B agonists (e.g., baclofen), clonidine, serotonin, or norepinephrine. The most abundant inhibitory receptors are mu-opioid receptors, which can be found on both sides of the synapse. In the resting state, two thirds of these opioid receptors are located on the presynaptic cell membrane and one third are postsynaptic.

Panel *C* shows an inhibitory interneuron in the substantia gelatinosa of the spinal cord which, in response to enkephalin, releases GABA, which inhibits transmission of the pain signal through the dorsal horn cell and dynorphin, which can stimulate inhibitory delta-opioid receptors on nociceptive neurons.

The antinociceptive system has structural components in the spinal cord as well as the brain. For example, spinal interneurons release dynorphin, which activates kappa-opioid receptors and leads to closure of N-type calcium channels in the spinal cord cells that normally relay pain signals to the brain. Following the release of enkephalins, spinal cord cells release other small molecules, including norepinephrine, oxytocin, and relaxin, that can also inhibit the transmission of pain signals (60).

Enkephalin is particularly notable in that it binds to delta-opioid receptors that are selectively exposed on nociceptors that are actively transmitting pain signals. These receptors are usually localized on pre-synaptic vesicles storing neurotransmitters. After the neurotransmitters are released, the receptors are incorporated into the pre-synaptic cell membrane. Active nociceptors thus become more sensitive than inactive nociceptors to both endogenous and exogenous opioids, which can explain how certain opioid analgesics can relieve ongoing pain without impairing the ability to sense pain caused by new injuries.

The natural pain-relieving system may be as important to normal functioning as the pain-signaling system. Because we have the capacity to naturally suppress pain, minor injuries such as a stubbed toe or a cut finger make us dysfunctional for only a few minutes, not for a few days, as might be the case if the pain persisted and intensified until the wound was healed. Just as disorders of the pain-sensing system can give rise to illness and dysfunction, it is very likely that disorders of the pain-relieving system can do the same.

Central Sensitization and the Role of the NMDA Receptor

If pain signals are continuously transmitted to the spinal cord, the central nervous system itself will undergo physiochemical changes resulting in hypersensitivity to pain, increased pain with repeated stimuli ("wind-up"), and resistance to pain-relieving inputs. Ultimately the pain signal can become embedded in the central nervous system like a painful memory, without the need for peripheral input. The analogy to memory is especially fitting because the generation of hypersensitivity in the spinal cord and memory in the brain both share a common chemical pathway involving NMDA (N-methyl-D-aspartate) receptors.

The physical changes that accompany this sensitization process are first seen on the cell membranes of the dorsal horn cells that receive signals from nociceptors. The main chemical mediator used by nociceptors synapsing with the dorsal horn of the spinal cord is glutamate, which can bind to several different types of receptors. AMPA (alpha-amino-3-hydroxy-5-methylisoxazole-4-propionic-acid) receptors are sodium-potassium channels on post-synaptic afferent nerve terminals in the dorsal horn and mediate the transmission of acute pain (Fig. 1-3). Activation of these receptors triggers a transient activating current that generates a signal to the brain via the spinothalamic tract.

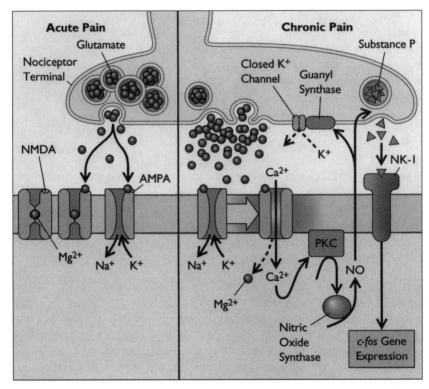

Figure 1-3   Neurochemical differences between acute and chronic pain at the level of the dorsal horn of the spinal cord. Central sensitization and the generation of opioid tolerance are probably related to events that take place throughout the central nervous system. This figure illustrates some of the changes associated with these phenomena at an interface between the peripheral and central nervous systems at the dorsal horn of the spinal cord.

In acute pain, depolarization of a peripheral nociceptor stimulates the release of glutamate into its synapse with an afferent neuron in the dorsal horn of the spinal cord. The membrane of the spinal cord cell contains several different types of receptors for glutamate, including AMPA receptors (whose stimulation opens a sodium-potassium channel) and NMDA receptors (whose stimulation results in calcium influx into the spinal cord cell).

In the resting state, the NMDA-related calcium channel is obstructed by a magnesium ion that prevents calcium influx. Release of glutamate will stimulate AMPA receptors, leading to a depolarizing sodium-potassium flux and transmission of a pain signal to ascending nociceptive tracts in the spinal cord without causing structural changes in the dorsal horn neuron. With repeated pain signals or with very intense stimulation, the resulting ion fluxes can cause changes in the charge of the membrane of the dorsal horn cell resulting in the ejection of magnesium ions from calcium channels, thus "popping the cork" and, in essence, activating NMDA receptors. This leads to neurochemical events associated with the establishment of chronic pain.

Stimulation of NMDA receptors by glutamate and its co-factor glycine gives rise to chemical and structural changes in the membranes of the synapsing cells resulting in sensitization to incoming pain signals and resistance to antinociceptive inputs. One example of the latter is peripheral opioid tolerance. Calcium enters the dorsal horn cell activating

(Cont'd on facing page)

NMDA receptors are a separate class of receptors for glutamate on dorsal horn cells which, when activated, open a channel for the influx of calcium into the spinal cord afferents. In the resting state, this calcium channel is blocked by a magnesium ion. With persistent or intense release of glutamate (e.g., due to very intense or chronic pain), activation of AMPA receptors results in a persistent change in the charge of the cell membrane and the magnesium ion is said to "pop out" of the calcium channel like a cork popping out of a champagne bottle and the NMDA receptor can now be activated (see Fig. 1-3).

In a biochemical sense, this conformational change in the NMDA receptor marks the central transition from acute to chronic pain (61). Calcium ions flowing into the dorsal horn cell activate protein kinase C, which triggers the production of nitric oxide (NO) by nitric oxide-synthase. NO, which is in essence a very short range neurotransmitter, diffuses back across the synaptic cleft and into the nociceptor, stimulating guanyl synthetase-induced closure of potassium channels. Many of these potassium channels are opioid receptors and the nociceptor is thus rendered insensitive (i.e., tolerant or resistant) to opioid-induced suppression of the pain signal by endorphins, enkephalins, and opioid medications (62). This explains the clinical observation that one of the most important mediators of opioid tolerance is unremitting pain, rather than the use of opioid medications. In clinical studies, NMDA-inhibitors such as ketamine or dextromethorphan can reverse opioid tolerance, demonstrating that opioid tolerance is more a biochemical phenomenon than a characterological disorder.

If the pain signal is allowed to persist, NO eventually stimulates the release of substance P from the nociceptors which, by binding to the NK-1 receptors in the dorsal horn membrane, trigger the expression of *c-fos* oncogene, promoting neural remodeling and further hypersensitization. It

---

protein kinase C (PKC) triggering neural nitric oxide synthetase and the production of nitric oxide (NO). NO, a short-range neurotransmitter, crosses back across the synapse stimulating the release of substance P and other growth factors from the nociceptor. These, in turn, bind to NK-1 receptors on the dorsal horn cell triggering, among other changes, enhanced expression of the *c-fos* oncogene, a marker of hypersensitization.

NO also activates guanyl synthetase in the presynaptic nociceptor membrane. This results in the closure of potassium channels associated with opioid receptors and thereby facilitates the transmission of pain signals by antagonizing the effects of endorphin and enkephalin. NMDA activation does not confer tolerance to dynorphin or kappa-opioids, which work by closing calcium channels.

Through sustained stimulation of NK-1 receptors, unremittant chronic pain can eventually stimulate the growth of sensory nerves and remodeling in the spinal cord. This can lead to recruitment of spinal cord nerves subserving other dermatomes which will eventually generate pain signals independent of input from peripheral fibers. This may explain both the perceived increase in the size of a painful area when pain goes undertreated for a prolonged time and one means by which pain can persist despite amputation or resection of the affected peripheral tissue.

is interesting to note that the one chemical abnormality repeatedly documented in controlled studies of patients with fibromyalgia syndrome (a condition that many clinicians continue to consider factitious) is an elevated level of substance P in the spinal fluid (63).

Activation of NMDA receptors has many consequences for nerves in the spinal cord, which can ultimately include cell damage and cell death. NMDA receptors are now being implicated in some of the cell damage that occurs in the brain during strokes, where injured pre-synaptic cells release torrents of glutamate, literally "burning out" and killing post-synaptic cells. One of the most intriguing avenues in stroke research is the therapeutic use of NMDA receptor inhibitors to limit damage in the setting of an acute stroke (64).

Activation of the NK-1 receptor triggers production of *c-fos* oncogene product, a protein that, in many respects, can be regarded as a biochemical footprint of chronic pain. In animal models of chronic pain the *c-fos* oncogene protein can be detected in afferent spinal cord cells that are receiving pain signals. As chronic pain persists, the *c-fos* oncogene protein will become detectable in cells higher up on the spinal cord, appearing outside the dermatome in which the original painful stimulus occurred. This protein will eventually become detectable in the thalamus itself and, at this point, the pain can become virtually untreatable.

c-fos oncogene protein may be a marker for the acquisition of hypersensitivity to pain signals by these different areas of the spinal cord. This would explain how many patients who have persistent pain find that, after months and years of under-treatment, the pain begins to spread to other organs than the one originally involved. For example, patients with long-standing proctitis due to IBS will often develop non-cardiac chest pain if their chronic pain goes untreated. Often, under-treated superficial pain will eventually spread outside its dermatomal boundaries. Unfortunately, when this happens, physicians who are not familiar with the concept of neural plasticity will think that the abnormal area affected by the pain is not "physiologic" and therefore conclude that the patient is either mentally ill or faking.

Stimulation of opioid receptors and other inhibitory receptors on peripheral neurons or at the pre-synaptic terminal in the spinal cord can slow or stop the synaptic release of glutamate and the generation of the pain signal. This may prevent subsequent neural remodeling. This may also explain the unique utility of small doses of intrathecal opioids delivered via an implanted pump in selected pain syndromes. Intrathecal therapy can often provide impressive relief in intractable pain syndromes and works in a complementary fashion with systemically administered opioid medications, which trigger supraspinal antinociceptive pathways. It is interesting to note that opioids do not have much pre-synaptic inhibitory activity on normal peripheral nerves but do inhibit the release of glutamate from inflamed nerves.

Afferent Becomes Efferent: Dorsal Root Reflexes

Although medical schools have taught that neuronal cells transmit signals in one direction exclusively, either towards (afferent) or away (efferent) from the brain, we now know that many neurons can carry signals in both directions. With the prolonged generation of pain signals, a pathological phenomenon called *dorsal root reflex* can become established in which afferent cells in the dorsal horn of the spinal cord release mediators that stimulate nociceptors to fire action potentials antidromically (i.e., backwards) (Fig. 1-4). When this happens, packets of chemicals located at the peripheral terminals of the nociceptors are released. These chemicals include nerve growth factor and substance P, which is not only a neurotransmitter but also a potent inflammatory agent. Pain signals from peripheral nerves are thus heightened, and the cycle of chronic pain continues. Calcitonin-gene related peptide (CGRP) released in the periphery causes vasodilatation, extravasation of proteins, release of bradykinin from vascular endothelial cells, and degranulation of mast cells with release of histamines and serotonin. This causes a long-lasting lowering of nociceptive threshholds. Other peripheral mediators of this type of neurogenic inflammation probably include nitric oxide (NO) and vasoactive intestinal peptide (VIP) (65).

Neurogenic Inflammation

The release of substance P and nerve growth factor into the periphery causes a tissue reaction termed *neurogenic inflammation.* In contrast to the classic inflammatory response to tissue trauma or immune-mediated cell damage, neurogenic inflammation is driven by impulses from the CNS and does not depend on the usual drivers of peripheral inflammation, such as granulocytes or lymphocytes. Substance P causes degranulation of mast cells, and its effects on the vascular endothelium induce the release of bradykinin and production of nitric oxide, a potent vasodilator. Biopsy specimens from neurogenically inflamed tissues (e.g., tendon insertion sites in fibromyalgia, the synovium in certain forms of chronic arthritis, the bladder in interstitial cystitis, the colon in ulcerative colitis) typically show vasodilatation, plasma extravasation, abnormal sprouting of peripheral nerve terminals, and an accumulation of mast cells.

Dorsal root reflexes apparently occur only under circumstances in which there has been prolonged and unsuppressed nociception. This model of central nervous system control over peripheral inflammation explains why many painful conditions do not respond to standard "end-organ oriented" treatments. Some of these syndromes may include certain cases of long-standing rheumatoid arthritis, reflex sympathetic dystrophy, certain cases of chronic headache, severe instances of IBS, and non-cardiac chest pain. Similar findings are commonly seen in inflammatory diseases of the GI tract (e.g., ulcerative colitis, Crohn's disease) and other chronic inflammatory states (e.g., psoriasis, chronic arthritis) (66-70). In some sense, many

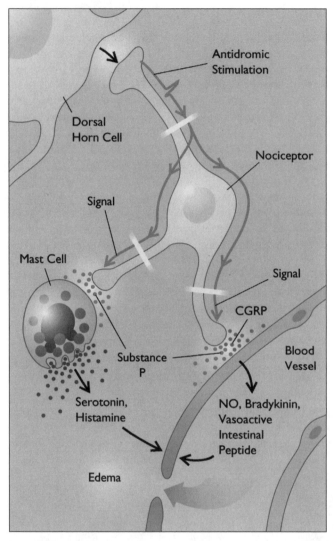

Figure 1-4   Pathophysiology of the dorsal root reflex and the generation of neurogenic inflammation. A dorsal root reflex occurs when afferent neurons in the dorsal horn, after prolonged sensitization, release chemicals (such as nitric oxide) which trigger nociceptors to fire action potentials antidromically (i.e., backwards) into peripheral tissue. This results in the release of inflammatory mediators stored in vesicles in the dendrites of peripheral nociceptors. These mediators include substance P and calcitonin–gene-related peptide (CGRP) whose release triggers vasodilatation, extravasation of proteins, and release of bradykinin from vascular endothelial cells in peripheral tissue. These mediators can also cause degranulation of peripheral tissue. These mediators can also cause degranulation of peripheral mast cells which, in turn, release histamines and serotonin, causing a long-lasting lowering of nociceptive thresholds (i.e., peripheral sensitization). Other peripheral mediators of this process of neurogenic inflammation probably include nitric oxide (NO) and vasoactive intestinal peptide (VIP).

of these diseases could thus be regarded as pain disorders rather than organ disorders. This mechanism explains why we have to treat and suppress certain inflammatory conditions, such as rheumatoid arthritis, within a limited time frame. If we do not, the inflammatory process escapes control by traditional anti-inflammatory medications. This is because these medications are active against immunogenic inflammation, not neurogenic inflammation.

Epidemiology of Chronic Pain

Many factors have long confounded the study of the epidemiology of chronic pain. One is that the study of chronic pain is often partitioned into many syndromes ranging from migraine headaches to fibromyalgia to low back pain. There are at least 600 identifiable pain syndromes (71). Additional confounders include difficulty establishing the point of initial onset, differentiating initial episodes from recurrences, and the lack of reliable methods to enable researchers to distinguish between clinically significant and non-significant pain conditions. Among various populations, the frequency of chronic pain ranges from 7% to 40% (72).

Chronic pain is a major public health problem in the United States. Nearly one third of Americans experience severe chronic pain during their lifetimes. Chronic pain is the most common cause of long-term disability, where it has partially or totally disabled upwards of 30 million people. Over 5 million Americans—more than 4% of the workforce—receive disability pay for disabling chronic pain (73,74). Newly discovered risk factors for the development of chronic pain include trauma, surgery (including breast surgery), thoracotomy, cholecystectomy, back surgery (75), and age.

These new epidemiological insights dovetail well with our increasing understanding of the biology of pain. For example, the ability to sense pain changes as neurophysiological function transforms with age. Advancing age is known to be associated with an increasing prevalence of chronic pain. This ranges from 25% to 65% in the community-dwelling elderly and up to 80% for those in long-term care facilities (76). We now know that there is a biological basis for the common finding that elderly persons often do not show the "classical signs" of acute pain, even in such well-recognized painful syndromes as appendicitis (77) or acute myocardial infarction (78). Indeed, the elderly generally feel less acute pain in response to most acute injuries than younger adults. This is probably due to the deterioration of peripheral C-fibers. Despite this, studies show that the elderly have an increased ability to develop chronic pain. This is likely due to changes in the CNS that translate into an exaggerated capacity for temporal summation, which is the ability of repeated stimuli to cause increasing amounts of pain due to sensitization of nerves in the spinal cord (79). Temporal summation can be measured by administering a fixed painful stimulus repeatedly and asking the subject to assess its intensity. In experimental studies, young subjects will not exhibit temporal summation if the stimuli are spaced more than three seconds apart, but elderly subjects show temporal summation in response to the same stimuli spaced five seconds apart (80). This may be interpreted to mean that a younger person's CNS can recover from the impact of a painful stimulus more rapidly than that of an elderly person.

Furthermore, the elderly patient who is subject to pain will maintain a hyper-excitable state longer, increasing his or her risk of undergoing the neurochemical changes that can lead to chronic pain. Another important age-related change is diminished functioning of descending antinociceptive neural pathways and reduced levels of endogenous opioids such as endorphin and enkephalin (81). This reduction in the natural capacity for pain relief means that elderly patients with chronic pain will have more difficulty coping with it than younger patients. Age-associated changes in neuronal plasticity and deficits in the natural pathways of analgesia put elderly people at increased risk for developing hyperalgesia.

Conclusion

The aim of this chapter has been to show that the perception of injury is mediated by a complex nociceptive system. Nociception is a vital bodily function, without which we cannot survive. Dysfunction of any one of many steps in the nociceptive process can give rise to chronic pain, which can be a destructive and progressive disorder. These dysfunctions can occur in either the peripheral or central nervous system (Table 1-2). By expanding our view of chronic pain, we can frame certain illnesses previously identified with their involved "end organs" as disorders of the nociceptive system much in the same way that we have come to understand that certain cardiovascular and neurological illnesses may really reside in dysfunction of the coagulation system rather than a defect in the heart or the brain.

Table 1-2   Mechanisms of Chronic Pain

Peripheral Nervous System	Central Nervous System
• Sensitization of nociceptors	• Central sensitization
• Activation of silent nociceptors	• Reorganization of synaptic connectivity in the spinal cord
• Collateral sprouting	• Impaired segmental and non-segmental pain inhibition
• Increased activity of damaged axons	
• Abnormal firing of dorsal root ganglion cells	
• Invasion of dorsal root ganglia by sympathetic post-ganglionic fibers	
• Phenotypic switch	

From Nurmikko TJ, Nash TP, Wiles JR. Control of chronic pain. Brit Med J. 1998;317:1438-41; with permission.

A unifying theme for the basis of most chronic pain syndromes is the development of hypersensitivity, a disordering change in the normal relationship between a painful stimulus and response. This implies that the ideal agents for the treatment of chronic pain will be "antihypersensitivity" agents rather than analgesic or antinociceptive drugs (82). Current analgesic therapies, along with the introduction of new therapies aimed at generators of hypersensitivity, such as the recently introduced antagonists to NMDA and NK-1 receptors, should allow us to help most of our patients safely regain control over their chronic pain (83,84).

Our concepts about nociception and chronic pain are continually changing. One constant appears to be the reports of our patients, who have steadfastly remained our most important teachers. This brings to mind the words of Paracelsus, who told us over 400 years ago that "Every physician must be rich in knowledge and not only of that which is written in books. His patients must be his books, they will never mislead him and by them he will never be deceived" (85).

ACKNOWLEDGMENTS

I gratefully acknowledge Dr Vicki Ratner, Ashley and Noel Mayfield, and Maurice Elliott, Chairman Emeritus of Methodist Healthcare, without whose friendship and support this chapter would not have been written and my practice could not have continued.

REFERENCES

1. **Rey R.** The History of Pain. Cambridge, MA: Harvard University Press; 1995.
2. **Ness T.** Historical and clinical perspectives. In: Gebhart GF, ed. Visceral Pain. Seattle: LASP Press; 1995:3-21.
3. **Moisan M.** Narcotic Plants in the Hippocratic Collections. Paris: Belles Lettres; 1978.
4. **Double FJ.** A memorandum on the semiotics and practical considerations concerning pain. Journal generale de medecine (Paris). 1805:359.
5. **Latham RG, ed.** The Works of Thomas Sydenham. London: The Thomas Sydenham Society; 1848.
6. **Pernick M.** A Calculus of Suffering. New York: Columbia University Press; 1985.
7. **Holmes OW.** Medical Essays: 1842-1882. Boston: Houghton Mifflin; 1891.
8. **Runes DD, ed.** Selected Writings of Benjamin Rush. New York: Philosophical Library; 1947.
9. **Landre-Beauvais AJ.** Semiotics and the Features of Illness. Paris: Brosson; 1813:315.
10. **Woof V.** On Being Ill. London: Hogarth Press; 1930:6.
11. **Darmberg C.** Galen: On the Uses of the Parts of the Body of Man. Paris: Ballieres; 1856:539-40.
12. **Boerhaave H.** Aphorisms de chirugie. Paris: Vve Cavalier & Fils; 1753.
13. **McGrath PJ.** Psychosocial and psychiatric aspects of pain in children. In: Dworkin R, Breitbart W, eds. Psychosocial Aspects of Pain. Seattle: IASP Press; 2004.

14. **Apkarian AV.** Functional imaging of pain: new insights regarding the role of the cerebral cortex in human pain perception. Semin Neurosci. 1995;7:279-93.

15. **Levine J, Taiwo Y.** Inflammatory pain. In: Wall PD, Melzack R, eds. Textbook of Pain. London: Churchill Livingstone; 1994.

16. **Rang HP, Perkins MN.** The role of bradykinin receptors in inflammatory pain. In: Borsook D, ed. Molecular Neurobiology of Pain. Seattle: IASP Press; 1997.

17. **Kumazawa T.** Sensitization of polymodal nociceptors. In: Belmonte C, Cervero F, eds. Neurobiology of Nociceptors. Oxford: Oxford University Press; 1996:325-45.

18. **Steranka LR, Manning DC, De Haas CJ.** Bradykinin as a pain mediator. Proc Natl Acad Sci. 1988;85:3245-9.

19. **Levine JD, Lam D, Taiwo Y.** Hyperalgesic properties of of 15-lipooxygenase products of arachadonic acid. Proc Natl Acad Sci. 1986;83:5331-4.

20. **Taiwo Y, Levine J.** Mediation of serotonin hyperalgesia by the cAMP second messenger system. Neuroscence. 1992;48:479-83.

21. **Cunha FQ, Lorenzetti BB, Poole S, Ferreira SH.** Interleukin-8 as a mediator of sympathetic pain. Brit J Pharmacol. 1991;104:765-7.

22. **Mantyh PW, Nelson CD, Sevick MA, et al.** Molecular mechanisms that generate and maintain cancer pain. In: Dostrovsky JO, Carr D, Koltzenberg M, eds. Proceedings of the 10th World Congress on Pain. Seattle: IASP Press; 2003:663-81.

23. **McMahon SB.** NGF as a mediator of inflammatory pain. Philos Trans R Soc Lond Biol Sci. 1996;351:431-40.

24. **Lewis T.** The nocisensor system of nerves and its reactions. Brit Med J. 1937;3:431-5.

25. **McMahon SB, Koltzenburg M.** Novel classes of nociceptors. Trends Neurosci. 1990;3:199-201.

26. **Nilsson J, von Euler AM, Dalsgaard CJ.** Stimulation of connective tissue cell growth by substance P and substance K. Nature. 1985;315:61-3.

27. **Aloe L, Tuveri MA, Carcassi U, Levi-Montacalcini R.** Nerve growth factor in the synovial fluid of patients with chronic arthritis. Arthritis Rheum.1992;35:351-5.

28. **Lowe EM, Anand P, Terenghi G.** Increased nerve growth factor levels in the urinary bladder with idiopathic sensory urgency and interstitial cystitis. Br J Urol. 1997;79:572-7.

29. **McMahon SB, Dmitrieva N, Koltzenberg M.** Visceral pain. Brit J Anesth. 1995; 75:132-44.

30. **Gonzales R, Goldyne ME, Taiwo YO, Levine JD.** Production of hyperalgesic prostaglandins by sympathetic preganglionic neurons. J Neurochem. 1989;53: 1595-8.

31. **McMahon SB, Koltzenberg M.** Silent afferents and visceral pain. In: Fields HL, Liebeskind JC, eds. Progress in Pain Research and Management. Seattle: IASP Press; 1994:11-30.

32. **Stein C, Shafer M, Cabot PJ, Zhang Q, et al.** Opioids and inflammation. In: Borsook D, ed. Molecular Neurobiology of Pain. Seattle: IASP Press; 1997:25-37.

33. **Shafer M, Mousa SA, Zhang Q.** Expression of corticotropin-releasing factor in inflamed tissue is required for peripheral opioid analgesia. Proc Natl Acad Sci. 1996;93:6096-100.

34. **Bonica JJ.** The history of pain concepts and pain therapy. Mt Sinai J Med. 1991;58:191-202.

35. **Cervero F.** Mechanisms of visceral pain: past and present. In: Gebhart GF, ed. Visceral Pain. Seattle: IASP Press; 1995:25-40.

36. **Aidar O, Geohegan WA, Uingewitter LH.** Splanchnic afferent pathways in the central nervous systems. J Neurophysiol. 1952;15:131-8.

37. **Sengupta JN, Gebhart GF.** Mechanoreceptive afferent fibers in the gastrointestinal and lower urinary tract. In: Gebhart GF, ed. Visceral Pain. Seattle: IASP Press; 1995:75-98.

38. **Cevero F.** Sensory innervation of the viscera: peripheral basis of visceral pain. Physiol Rev. 1994;74:95-138.

39. **Sengupta IN, Gebhart GF.** Gastrointestinal afferent fibers and sensation. In: Johnson LR, ed. Physiology of the Gastrointestinal Tract. New York: Raven Press; 1994:483-519.

40. **Malliani A.** The conceptualization of cardiac pain as a nonspecific and un-reliable alarm system. In: Gebhart GF, ed. Visceral Pain. Seattle: IASP Press; 1995: 63-74.

41. **Al-Chaer ED, Feng Y, Willis WD.** Visceral pain: a disturbance in the sensorimotor continuum. Pain Forum. 1998;7:117-25.

42. **Osler W.** Angina pectoris. Lancet. 1910;1:839-44.

43. **Canon RO.** Cardiac pain. In: Gebhart GF, ed. Visceral Pain. Seattle: IASP Press; 1995:373-89.

44. **Nabiloff B, Lembo A, Mayer EA.** Abdominal pain in irritable bowel syndrome. Current Review of Pain. 1999;3:144-52.

45. **Locke GR, Talley NJ, Zinmaster AR.** The irritable bowel syndrome and func-tional dyspepsia: functional disorders. Gastroenterology. 1996;110:A26.

46. **Talley NJ, Boyce PM, Jones M.** Is the association between irritable bowel syn-drome and abuse explained by neuroticism? Gut. 1998;42:47-53.

47. **Koltzenberg M.** The changing sensitivity in the life of the nociceptor. Pain. 1999;6:S93-102.

48. **Mendell LM, Albers KM Davis BM.** Neurotrophins, nociceptors and pain. Microsc Res Tech. 1999;45:252-61.

49. **Apfel SC.** Neurotrophic factors and pain. Clin J Pain. 2000;16:S7-11.

50. **Apfel SC.** Nerve growth factor for the treatment of diabetic neuropathy. Int Rev Neurobiol. 2002;50:393-413.

51. **Baron R.** Peripheral neurotrophic pain: from mechanisms to symptoms. Clin J Pain. 2002;16:S12-20.

52. **Dyck PJ, Giannini C.** Pathologic alterations in the diabetic neuropathies of humans: a review. J Neuropathol Exp Neurol. 1996;55:1181-93.

53. **Mitchell SW.** Lesions of Nerves and Their Consequences. Paris: Masson; 1874:70.

54. **Campbell JN.** Nerve lesions and the generation of pain. Muscle Nerve. 2001;24: 1261-73.

55. **Ji RR, Woolf CJ.** Neuronal plasticity and signal transduction in nociceptive neu-rons: implications for the initiation and maintenance of pathologic pain. Neurobiol Dis. 2001;8:1-10.

56. **Bruehl S, McCubbin JA Harden RN.** Theoretical review: altered pain regulatory systems in chronic pain. Neurosci Biobehav Rev. 1999;23:877-90.

57. **Tavares I, Lima D.** The caudal ventrolateral medulla as an important inhibitory modulator of pain transmission in the spinal cord. J Pain. 2002;3:337-46.

58. **Welch KMA, Nagesh V, Aurora SK, Gelman N.** Periaqueductal gray matter dysfunction in migraine: cause or the burden of illness? Headache. 2001;41:629-37.

59. **Willer JC.** Stress-induced analgesia in humans: endogenous opioids and naloxone-reversible depression of pain reflexes. Science. 1981;212:689-90.

60. **Furst S.** Transmitters involved in antinociception in the spinal cord. Brain Res Bull. 1999;48:129-41.

61. **Bennett GJ.** Update on the neurophysiology of pain transmission and modulation: focus on the NMDA-receptor. J Pain Symptom Manage. 2000;19:S2-6.

62. **Riedel W, Neeck G.** Nociception, pain and antinociception: current concepts. Z Rheumatol. 2001;60:404-15.

63. **Russell IJ.** The promise of substance P inhibitors in fibromyalgia. Rheum Dis Clin North Amer. 2002;28:2-10.

64. **Costigan M, Woolf CJ.** Pain: molecular mechanisms. J Pain. 2000;3:35-44.

65. **Pinter E, Szolcanyi J.** Plasma extravasation in the skin and pelvic organs evoked by antidromic stimulation of the lumbosacral dorsal roots in the rat. Neuroscience. 1995;68:603-14.

66. **McKay DM, Bienenstock J.** The interaction between mast cells and nerves in the gastrointestinal tract. Immunol Today. 1994;15:533-8.

67. **Dvorak AM, McLeod RS, Onderdonk AB.** Human gut mucosal mast cells. Int Arch Allergy Immunol. 1992;98:150-68.

68. **Yonei Y.** Autonomic nervous alterations and mast cell degranulation in the exacerbation of ulcerative colitis. Japan J Gastroenterol. 1987;84:1045-56.

69. **Naukkarinen A, Harvima IT, Aalto ML.** Quantitative analysis of contact sites between mast cells and sensory nerves in cutaneous psoriasis. Arch Dermatol Res. 1991;283:433-7.

70. **Hukkanen M, Gronblad M, Rees R.** Regional distribution of mast cells and peptide-containing nerves in normal and adjuvant arthritic rat synovium. J Rheumatol. 1991;18:177-83.

71. **Mersky H, Bogduk N.** Classification of Chronic Pain: Descriptions of Chronic Pain Syndromes and Definitions of Pain Terms. Seattle: IASP Press; 1994.

72. **Von Korff M.** Epidemiological methods. In: Crombie IK, ed. Epidemiology of Pain. Seattle: IASP Press; 1999.

73. **Sternbach RA.** Survey of pain the United States: the Nuprin pain report. Clin J Pain. 1986;2:49-53.

74. **Hartsell C, Ospina M.** How prevalent is chronic pain? Pain: Clinical Updates. 2003;11:1-4.

75. **Macrae WA, Davies HTO.** Chronic post-surgical pain. In: Crombie IK, ed. Epidemiology of Pain. Seattle: IASP Press; 1999.

76. **Gibson SJ.** Pain and aging: the pain experience over the adult life span. In: Dostrovsky JO, Carr DB, Koltzenberg M, eds. Proceedings of the Tenth World Congress on Pain. Seattle: IASP Press; 2003.

77. **Wroblewski M, Mikulowski P.** Peritonitis in geriatric inpatients. Age Ageing. 1991;20:90-4.

78. **MacDonald JB, Baillie J, Williams BO, Ballantyne D.** Coronary care in the elderly. Age Ageing. 1983;12:17-20.

79. **Gibson SJ, Chang W, Farrell MJ.** Age interacts with frequency in the temporal summation of painful electrical stimuli. In: Abstracts of the Tenth World Congress on Pain. Seattle: IASP Press; 2002:906.

80. **Price DD, Hu JW, Dubner R, Gracely RH.** Peripheral suppression of first pain and central summation of second pain evoked by noxious heat pulses. Pain. 1977;3:57-68.

81. **Washington LL, Gibson SJ, Helme RD.** Age-related differences in the endogenous analgesic response to repeated cold water immersion in human volunteers. Pain. 2000;89:89-96.

82. **Mannion RJ, Woolf CJ.** Pain mechanisms and management: a central perspective. Clin J Pain. 2000;16:S144-56.

83. **Attal N.** Chronic neuropathic pain: mechanisms and treatment. Clin J Pain. 2000;6:S118-30.

84. **Brower V.** New paths to pain relief. Nature Biotechnology. 2000;18:387-91.

85. **Jacobi J, ed.** Paracelsus: Selected Writings. Princeton, NJ: Princeton University Press; 1951:50.

2

■ ■ ■

Reliable Care Through the Activity Paradigm for Back Problems

Stanley J. Bigos, MD

Jane E. McKee, MSN, ARNP

E vidence-based medicine is the current "buzzword" for clinicians who intend to practice data-driven care to improve outcomes (1). Recent developments emphasizing the importance of reliable information may additionally offer the clinician insulation from administrative and legal hassles. Unfortunately, the primary care clinician does not often have the time to use the complicated algorithms commonly associated with reliable care codes or for comprehensive reviews of the literature. In this chapter, we hope to offer both an understanding of recent developments and a simpler, activity-oriented application of data-driven care for patients with back problems.

Applying Reliable Data to Back Problems

The Agency for Health Care Policy and Research (AHCPR) first established evidence-based guidelines in the 1990s. One of the largest endeavors by AHCPR was to develop clinical practice guidelines for back problems. This was felt necessary due to the enormous volume of literature on the subject and the variety of professionals involved in this area.[1]

---

[1]A methodological review of 4600 articles after a literature search of 11,000 abstracts was the basis of AHCPR Guideline 14, Acute Low Back Problems in Adults, published in 1994 (2). A review seven years later recommended few changes to that document other than adding information on prevention and more-tempered comments on the limited effectiveness of back schools, lumbar corsets, and epidural steroid injections (3). The other AHCPR statements have been only strengthened by subsequent reliable studies.

It should be pointed out that the need for reliable information is not limited to workers in health care. The legal profession has had an interest since the 1993 Supreme Court decision *Daubert v. Merrill Dow Pharmaceuticals* altered the Federal Rules of Evidence (FRE) to demand experts have reliable data to substantiate their testimony (4). This was the first change in 70 years to the FRE, which have now been expanded to include medical testimony (5). Thus it seems only a matter of time before the *emphasis* on reliable information becomes a *mandatory requirement* in the medical field as well.

One acknowledged failing of the AHCPR Guide, it must be stated, is the labyrinthine complexity of its algorithms. Lost in their intricacies was the importance of treating reduced activity tolerance rather than just the back pain itself.

The most workable activity paradigm for back pain was published in 1995 by Malmivaara et al, which provided a simpler construct for bringing reliable data to life (6). Malmivaara's activity paradigm has been reiterated in multiple studies in recent years (7-10). McGuirk et al have proven the effectiveness of the activity paradigm and its use in applying reliable data (11).

This chapter illustrates the authors' experience with a user-friendly application of the AHCPR Guide activity paradigm.[2] Use of this paradigm results in reduced disability while avoiding further medical treatments that can lead to chronic problems.

As with the AHCPR Guide, our activity paradigm deals with a patient's reduced activity tolerance whether the back pain is the first acute episode, a recurrent episode, or one that accompanies chronic back problems. While the goals of the paradigm for work-related back problems are obvious, the paradigm has also proven beneficial for non-occupational back problems. More and more information reiterates the importance of exercise to the general health of the everyone, especially the elderly (12,13).

The activity paradigm pivots upon treating activity intolerance rather than just chasing the pain. Three issues are important:

1. If it is determined that *nothing dangerous* is causing the symptoms, this information must be conveyed successfully to the patient.

2. Daily activities should be kept *as normal as possible*. The patient's response should dictate the clinical decisions needed to sort out structural versus nonstructural and nonphysical issues and to differentiate pain problems from back problems.

3. Nonphysical issues (e.g., depression) that may accompany back pain must be addressed. In particular, physicians cannot ignore the devastating impact on many patients that results from being off work. Those who are off work for any reason (lay-off,

---

[2]The authors' utilization of the activity approach within a primary care setting was given the moniker of D4C2 (Data Driven, Dauber Defendable Care Code) due to the influence of data-driven care meeting the defendable criteria of the Daubert Supreme Court decision.

compensation, fired, etc.) have a higher mortality risk rate than for any occupation, even the most dangerous. In fact, so heightened is the risk of death from suicide, cirrhosis, and other stress-related diseases while not working, that being unemployed is equivalent to smoking 10 packs of cigarettes per day (14).

Identifying the Problem

The history and physical examination (H&P) is the initial step in determining if the patient's problem is something that requires urgent attention (Fig. 2-1). Red Flags can be detected through medical history and a review of systems and medications (Table 2-1). The addition of a pain drawing to a Visual Analog Scale can save time and improve the quality of information.

In the absence of serious problems, the H&P helps to determine if the patient has an activity or a pain problem. Those without a limitation, those who refuse activity, or those made invalid by other medical issues should not be confused with patients having a back problem. Basic pain paradigms are more appropriate for the former group.

The patient's responses to queries about Red Flags set the stage for the specific history to either explore further any hints or to continue in a quest for categorizing back problems. The H&P classifies an activity problem as either the result of nerve damage (+) or not the result of nerve damage (–). The classification of neurologically positive or negative provides a prognosis for expected recovery and guides the type of work-up should the patient be slow to recover.

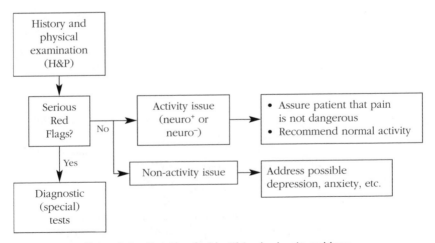

Figure 2-1 Algorithm for identifying back pain problems.

Table 2-1   Red Flags for Potentially Serious Conditions

Possible Fracture	Possible Tumor or Infection	Possible Cauda Equina Syndrome
From Medical History		
• Major trauma (e.g., motor vehicle accident, fall from height) • Minor trauma or even strenuous lifting (in older or potentially osteoporotic patient)	• Age over 50 or less than 20 • History of cancer • Constitutional symptoms (e.g., recent fever or chills, unexplained weight loss) • Risk factors for spinal infection; recent bacterial infection (e.g., urinary tract infection); IV drug abuse; or immune suppression (from steroids, transplant, or HIV) • Pain that is worse when supine; severe nighttime pain	• Saddle anesthesia • Recent onset of bladder dysfunction (e.g., urinary retention, increased frequency, overflow incontinence) • Severe or progressive neurological deficit in lower extremity
From Physical Examination		
		• Unexpected laxity of anal sphincter • Perianal/perineal sensory loss • Major motor weakness: quadriceps (knee extension weakness), ankle/plantar flexors, everters, and dorsiflexers (foot drop)

From Bigos SJ, Chairman. Panel: Bowyer RO, Braen GR, Brown K, Deyo R, Haldeman S, Hart JL, Johnson EW, Keller R, Kido D, Liang MH, Nelson RM, Nordin M., Owen BD, Pope MH, Schwartz RK, Stewart D, Susman J, Triano JJ, Tripp LC, Turk D, Watts C, Weinstein J. Contributors: Battié MC, Bombardier C, Hadler N, Nachemson A, Waddell G, Holland J, Webster J, Schriger D, Shekelle P. Clinical Practice Guideline No. 14, Acute Low Back Problems in Adults, Publication 95-0642. Department of Health and Human Services, Public Health Service, AHCPR, Rockville, MD; 9 December 1994.

Specific History

A pointed history of the present illness provides needed understanding of the quality of symptoms, severity according to limitations, previous similar problems, and the patient's immediate goals. The input will guide the physical examination and subsequent recommendations.

Quality of Symptoms

Guided by a drawing, ask the patient to prioritize from Worst Pain to Least Pain the areas involving pain, weakness, numbness, and stiffness. The physician will want to know if radicular symptoms are intermittent, because electro-diagnostic studies rarely detect surgically significant findings unless symptoms have been constant for 3 or 4 weeks.

Limitations

Limitations provide insight into the severity of the symptoms described. Specifically, the patient should be asked the following questions:

- What activities does your back not let you do? _____
- Date limitation began? _____ Incident? _____
- Specific limitations now:

  Without fearing that you are doing damage, how many:

  1. <u>minutes</u> can you can SIT? _____
  2. <u>minutes</u> can you STAND? _____
  3. <u>minutes</u> or <u>distance</u> you can WALK[3]?
  4. <u>pounds</u> can you LIFT? _____

Answers of less than 20 pounds or 20 minutes are extreme (less than an invalid) and deserve probing. If there is no possibility of damaging the patient, determine if limits are at the point of bringing on or worsening symptoms.

The most important issue is the perceived activity level at which the patient fears further damage. Fear of damage strongly predicates how a patient responds to subsequent activity recommendations. Should a patient decline considering normal activity, responses to the foregoing initial questions about sitting, standing, walking, and lifting allows the clinician a reference for negotiating any limited daily activity. Early in the history patients usually attempt to put their best foot forward. Early face-to-face inquiry tends to provide more reasonable responses. Knowing when limitations began helps the physician determine when the patient qualifies for the slowest 10% to recover (over 4 weeks). Further studies may be warranted depending on the patient's symptoms and life situation.

Previous Similar Problems

Ask the patient about any previous spine or musculoskeletal problems and other reasons for debilitating periods of limited activity. Was surgery required? If so, what kind? When were the latest spinal tests performed?

Goals

The patient's response to the questions "What brings you here today? What do you want me to do for you?" can be a time saver and provide important

---

[3]If walking is limited to less than 300 yards in the elderly, ask "After you have walked as far as possible, can you just stand there and rest to relieve the pain?" (If Yes, consider vascular claudication.) True neuroclaudication requires the individual to sit, bend over, or squat for a few minutes before continuing to walk.

guidance. The manner in which the patient answers this question can be just as important as the answer itself.

Physical Examination

The physical examination obviously provides the physician with important findings. It helps categorize the back problem as neurologically positive or negative and helps determine the expected recovery rate and the type of work-up that may be required should the patient be one of the slowest 10% to recover reasonable activity tolerance.

Only circumferential measurements for atrophy and reflexes are objective examination findings, whether positive or negative. Most of the examination maneuvers are subjective. Subjective data such as sensation and range of motion totally depend upon the patient's interpretation or volition, whereas others can be further qualified with a second maneuver.

The ankle can be flexed up and down and limbs rotated each way to determine whether a pain response to straight leg raising is a true sign of sciatic nerve root tension on the nerve rootlets. Straight leg raising is the most reproducible finding of the physical examination maneuvers. Increased pain with ankle dorsi-flexion and limb internal rotation (but not with ankle plantar flexion) helps differentiate neurological from non-neurological work-up and prognostic considerations.

The following examination should take no longer than 5 minutes. The patient wears shorts or a gown.

Standing

1) Normal walking, then walking on heels (L4-5) and toes (S1-2), followed by a squat and rise (L2-S1); assess general strength (Fig. 2-2). For safety, have the patient hold onto a table or counter before attempting to squat.

   From behind patient:

2) Observe the back during suggested extension, side bending, rotation, and flexion to estimate range relative to that expected for age. There is no need to pull or push to see if the range is full beyond the patient's effort. Seek hints of uncoordinated muscular activity or guarding (commonly termed *dysmetria, spasm,* etc.). A mild nonspecific finding may indicate that something is amiss. Note whether the motion is symmetrical.

Sitting

3) Ankle and knee reflexes (*the only objective finding whether positive or negative*)

4) Circumferential measurements: above and below knee; differences between limbs of more than 1 to 2 cm signify possible atrophy (*objective finding if greater than 2 cm*)

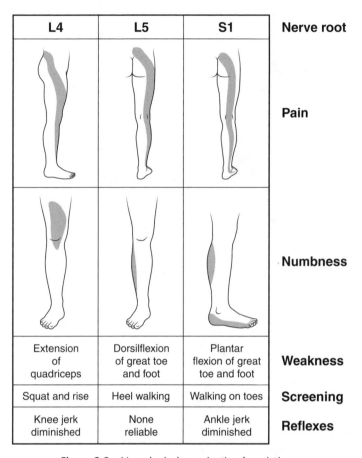

L4	L5	S1	Nerve root
			Pain
			Numbness
Extension of quadriceps	Dorsiflexion of great toe and foot	Plantar flexion of great toe and foot	**Weakness**
Squat and rise	Heel walking	Walking on toes	**Screening**
Knee jerk diminished	None reliable	Ankle jerk diminished	**Reflexes**

Figure 2-2   Neurological examination for sciatica.

5) <u>Lower extremity joints:</u> sitting hip rotation asymmetry (internal rotation loss may signify hip DJD), knee stability (flexed/extended) (Fig. 2-3), foot and ankle motion
6) <u>Muscle strength:</u> a slight loss of strength is most easily detectable in large muscles; observe from strongest to weakest: quadriceps (L2-4), hamstrings (L5-S1), ankle dorsiflexers (L4-5), ankle everters (L5-S1), great toe extensors (L5), toe flexors (S1-2)

Supine

7) <u>Abdomen and pulses:</u> especially important for sero-negative spondy-loathropathies (ankylosing spondylitis, reactive spondylitis, etc.) and in the elderly for aneurysm, or in the presence of a positive Red Flag
8) <u>Straight leg raising (SLR):</u> each lower limb. "Tell me to stop if this bothers you" and "Where is the pain? Back? Same side or opposite side? Hip? Thigh? Knee? Below the knee?" (Fig. 2-4)

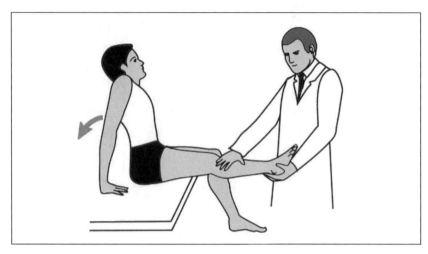

Figure 2-3 Sitting knee extension. Straightening the knee during the knee or foot examination helps qualify nerve root tension. A significantly positive supine straight leg raising should elicit fall-back or complaints of discomfort with sitting knee extension.

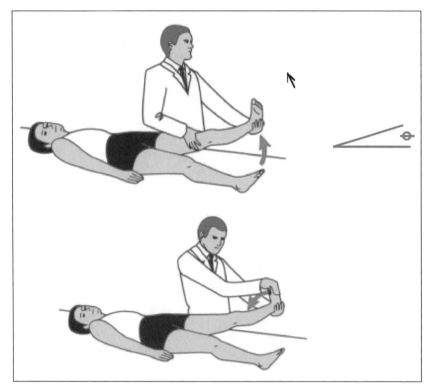

Figure 2-4 Straight leg raising. There is leg pain between 30 and 60 degrees when acute.

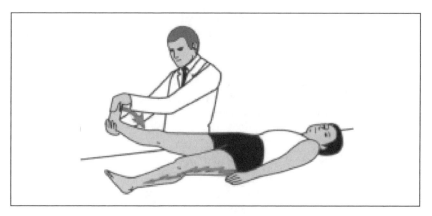

Figure 2-5   Opposite leg raise.

- Check for <u>augmentation</u> of nerve root irritation with straight-leg-raise at the level where pain is first realized with other maneuvers. With the straight leg raised to level of pain is the pain:

  "Worse?" With <u>plantar-flexion</u> of the ankle (*shouldn't be*)

  "Worse?" With <u>dorsi-flexion</u> of the ankle (*a plantar flexion does not stretch the nerve root and should not worsen the pain*)

  "Worse?" With <u>external rotation</u> of the whole limb (*shouldn't worsen the pain*)

  "Worse? With <u>internal rotation</u> of the whole limb (*can be*)

- Perform an opposite (or crossed) leg raise. A reproduction of symptoms in the symptomatic limb when raising the unaffected limb is the strongest predictor of potential anatomic lesion (Fig. 2-5). A raised opposite leg rarely is affected by any augmentation of ankle motion or limb rotation.

- In the presence of <u>neck symptoms</u> evaluate neck motion for guarding, upper extremities for stability of joints and muscle wasting (atrophy), and neurological integrity as assessed in motor (cervical-motor roots appendix), sensory, and reflex examination (always to include Babinski). Anterior neck palpation and at least partial cranial nerve/cerebellar (finger-to-nose coordination, Romberg) testing are also warranted. Always let history warn of a possibility of lung cancer (Pancoast's tumor) and CNS disease in the presence of neck and arm symptoms. Shoulder problems are many times a difficult part of the differential diagnosis with radicular neck symptoms. Without neck or shoulder complaints, it is reasonable to at least check the biceps, triceps, and brachioradialis reflexes and gross grip strength.

Special Studies

Because 90% of patients recover within 4 weeks from any given episode of back pain, special studies should be considered only in the few patients with

Red Flags and in those patients without Red Flags but who have pain duration or unreasonable activity limitation (relative to the patient's needs) of more than 4 weeks. (Work-up is usually sooner for patients whose jobs are in jeopardy.)

The specific diagnostic tests required are determined by the type of symptoms (i.e., neurological or not). Changes on X-rays and other imaging studies are common even at an early age and are poor screening tools.

Initial Care

The goal of initial care is to keep the patient's activity as normal as possible. The purpose is to avoid the unnecessary debilitation of inactivity and the potential socioeconomic complications. Foremost, initial care is based on the problem that is identified by the history and physical examination (Fig. 2-6). Serious problems need urgent referral and are managed according to a different paradigm. Once these serious problems have been adequately attended to, the patient can re-enter the activity paradigm. The point at which the patient enters the activity paradigm depends upon the delay for

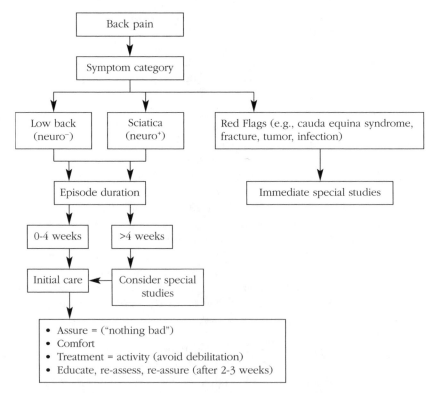

Figure 2-6   Initial care algorithm for patient with back pain.

work-up or treatment in a different paradigm. With prolonged inactivity, conditioning is usually needed to overcome the debilitation. On the other hand, the patient can enter the activity paradigm at initial care if less than a few weeks have lapsed.

Once Red Flags are ruled out, the physician begins with the two most important steps in the activity paradigm: providing assurance and beginning treatment (i.e., activity). First, convey to the patient the good news that nothing serious was detected. This is important to alleviate the patient's fears of physical damage. The second step is to offer help with symptoms and stress the importance of keeping daily activity as normal as possible. Point out that maintaining regular activity will help the patient avoid having to go through the "spring training" of reconditioning that will otherwise be necessary after pain symptoms pass.

Once the patient's fears have been alleviated or removed, the patient is usually willing to return to reasonably normal activity. Should the patient refuse reasonable activity or demand more than one week of limited duty, the physician should, as soon as possible, get another opinion from a colleague or specialist. The consultant is not to take over the care of the patient or recommend limitations or treatment. What is required is confirmation of the diagnosis (as is almost always the case) to convince the patient that there is nothing seriously wrong.

It is important to remember that the AHCPR Guide and the literature upon which it is based are only *guidelines,* not rules. If a patient insists on an X-ray and cannot be convinced that it is not needed, then get *two* views (PA and lateral)! In other words, if an X-ray will provide assurance and spur the patient to resume normal activity, then order it. *The goal of the physician is to do whatever is necessary and reasonable to keep the patient as active as possible.* A reference algorithm should not be allowed to thwart that goal.

Assurance, comfort, and treatment (activity) need be addressed in all patients. If a patient's comfort level allows attendance in physical therapy, then a similar level of activity at work or light duty offers better therapy (in that it keeps the patient functioning at work and therefore involved in his or her usual lifestyle) and avoids the potentially serious complications related to work absence. The following are some of the points that can enhance the patient's understanding of initial care.

Assure and Create Reasonable Expectations

What to say to the patient:

> *We are very good at finding any serious conditions, and at this time we have no hint of anything serious causing your symptoms. Most of them should resolve in the next few weeks. If you are in the slowest 10% to recover, we will consider special studies to look for something serious. The reality is that no one has won the Nobel Prize for explaining the cause of back problems. It's too bad it's such a mystery, because back problems temporarily limit about one third of*

us by age 30, three quarters of us by age 40, and virtually all of us by age 50. Right now, as I've said, we have no hint of anything abnormal going on. That is good news because the outcomes are better in such cases and we can usually avoid a lot of painful reconditioning. Now we need to help you feel more comfortable without prolonging your pain.

Provide Comfort

What to say to the patient:

There are many ways of treating your symptoms but unfortunately no treatment totally wipes out the pain and lets you go about your business as usual. We will recommend the most effective drug combination available, one that allows you to stay as active as possible. Remember that it usually takes twice as long to regain conditioning as it does to lose it, so you have to stay active even though you still have pain. You may have heard of Darvocet, Percocet, Lorcet, or Roxicet. The "-acet" sound is acetaminophen. If a drug is of questionable value when used alone, its manufacturer often adds acetaminophen, aspirin, or ibuprofen to it. That's because they seem to block the pain highway at a different place than the other medication, and thus they work well in combination. We recommend a "Safe-acet" (that is, acetaminophen and another drug). The worst pain episode in cases similar to yours may last for 5 days, but that is rare. So that is the longest you might need serious help with the pain. And we'll try to avoid medication that might cloud your mind or unduly disrupt your normal activities.

If the patient has no hint of kidney or liver dysfunction, or mitigating factor of advanced age, a combination of acetaminophen and NSAIDs is adequate and usually as effective as more dangerous methods (Table 2-2). If the patient says that back manipulation has helped before, remind him or her that it only helps symptoms and does not correct the problem without conditioning. The newer COX-2 inhibitor NSAIDs for patients with peptic ulcer disease and other comorbidities enable many patients to stay active

Table 2-2   Providing the Patient with Back Pain Comfort (Symptom Control Methods)

Treatment		Recommended?
Nonprescription		
1. Acetaminophen, aspirin,* ibuprofen*		Yes
Prescription	**Physical Methods**	
2. NSAIDs*	2. Manipulation (BP only)	Yes
3. Muscle relaxants*	3. Bed rest†	Optional
4. Opioids	4. Temporary modalities†	Optional
5. Sedatives	5. McKenzie method	No
6. Hypnotics	6. Traction	No
7. Steroids	7. Injections	No

* Not to be used together.
† Instructions for home application only.

and to safely avoid mind-altering medications that interfere with activities, sleep, and needed conditioning.

Medication or manipulation (for back pain only) should always be accompanied by encouragement to resume normal activity to avoid disability. If the patient chooses otherwise, negotiate reasonable work activities in accordance with the patient's answers to the history questions related to fear of sitting, standing, walking, and lifting. Prescribe some safe, simple conditioning to aid recovery [e.g., walking, cycling, jogging] along with comfort aides to help the patient minimizes the debilitation of reduced activity.

Treatment

When treating musculoskeletal problems remember the old joke:

"Doctor, after surgery will I be able to play the violin?"

"I would hope so."

"Good! I could never play it before!"

Not surgery, manipulation, injections, medication, or rest will help a patient to play the violin, run a marathon, engage in strenuous activity, or return comfortably to normal activity after being away from it for an extended period. Only conditioning enables a back pain patient to comfortably tolerate unaccustomed activities.

Distinguish between hurt and harm. Conditioning activities need not be more stressful on the back than sitting at bedside before rising in the morning. Some patients require assurance that, although conditioning may not be totally comfortable, nothing will be recommended that is dangerous to the spine and that there is no way to maintain or build activity tolerance without activity. Once activity tolerance is lost, because of either deconditioning or structural change, only hard conditioning, such as spring training or training camp for athletes or boot camp for soldiers, can improve the comfortable activity level.

If the patient avoids some normal activity, a low stress endurance activity can be used to limit the debilitation and reduce the need for "spring training" to get back sufficient endurance to reasonably tolerate regular daily activities. For patients who do not return to work (e.g., those with physically demanding jobs) or those who choose not to return to normal activity, recommend additional daily exercise to limit debilitation (Table 2-3). Such "additional" activity helps stress the importance of staying active.

Education and Reassurance

Education and reassurance should be part of visits for those who do not recover within a few weeks. Reiterate initial assurances and expectations and the importance of normal activity. Reassure the patient that if he or she is not significantly better by the end of 4 weeks special studies will be considered to test for potentially serious conditions.

Table 2-3   Treatment for Reduced Activity Tolerance (Spring Training for the Spine)

If improving but not asymptomatic at 30 days or after appropriate neuro(+) or neuro(–) work-up, begin conditioning to improve comfortable activity tolerance:
- **Phase I**—Endurance Exercises for a few weeks, then add
- **Phase II**—Back Muscle Stamina Exercises as needed for a few weeks, then add
- **Phase III**—General Leg and Abdomen Exercises for a month, and then
  —*Maintenance* – Phase I, 2× per week; Phase II, daily; Phase III, 2-3× per week
  —*Optional* – Nonback stretching (e.g., arms, legs)

Work-Ups and Special Studies

Despite our best diagnostic efforts, 90% of back pain patients will not be diagnosable. The insistence of insurance companies on having a diagnosis has filled our ICD-9 code with many terms (e.g., sprain, strain) that suggest no specific etiology.

We usually seek a work-up for one of two reasons. The first is the presence of Red Flags or chronic general medical problems that can slow recovery. The second reason is slow recovery as determined by the natural history. After 4 continuous weeks of activity limitation, depending on the amount of life interference, a work-up for a potentially correctable lesion may be advisable.

Diagnostic Tests

Some of the most common diagnostic tests for assessing back pain that continues for more than 4 weeks are given below.

Laboratory Studies
Sedimentation rate, blood count, and urine analysis are used as a metabolic general screen if the patient appears ill.

Bone Scan
Bone scan indications include a structural general screen for bony physiological reactions to changes in structural stresses of fracture/dislocation or architecture (e.g., tumor, infection, spondylitis, aging).

Electromyography
Electromyography (EMG) should be considered for constant or near-constant limb symptoms of radiculopathy of 4 or more weeks. (Testing sooner may provide false-negatives because changes take 3 to 4 weeks to be detected.) Consider motor compromise with more than one positive sharp wave or fibrillation potential (if S1 is affected, look for a slowed H-reflex) before considering anatomic verification (if motor testing is 3/5 or weaker, consider anatomic studies). Electromyography is not needed if combined

motor, sensory, and reflex changes indicate obvious L4, L5, or S1 nerve root involvement.

Somato-Sensory Evoked Potentials

Somato-sensory evoked potentials (SEPs) are most helpful in the elderly patient with neuroclaudication from spinal stenosis symptoms, especially in the presence of EMG changes indicating acute motor dysfunction. The SEPs may determine which nerve roots are slow in sensory transmission and can be more sensitive (but less specific) for active compromise than EMG motor changes.

Special Studies and Surgery

At present, surgical correction relates to decompressing nerve roots compromised by disc herniation or the aging of spinal stenosis unless there is acute fracture or dislocation. Many surgical cases do not lead to good results. The results of fusion for reasons other than infection, fracture, tumor, or dislocation are not encouraging (15). Reliable information indicates that good surgical outcomes are only predicted by strong concordant physical and special study findings (16,17). Moreover, although surgical success speeds the recovery, there are no obvious long-term advantages.

Imaging Studies and Physiological Evidence

Imaging studies are important for planning surgery but can be confusing as a sole diagnostic tool (18). Normal aging changes that include disc herniation are present 30% of the time in asymptomatic 30 year olds (2).

Figure 2-7 shows the chances of having a particular finding described as an abnormality on imaging studies in asymptomatic patients. This emphasizes the need for physiological evidence to determine the potential cause of symptoms before seeking concordant imaging pictures. Using imaging alone for diagnosis we only risk finding common age-related changes that may or may not relate to the symptoms. Obtaining physiological evidence of neurological compromise (obvious motor, sensory, and reflex changes or positive sharp waves and fibrillation potentials on EMG) before ordering imaging studies avoids confusion.

Combining physiological testing and anatomic imaging increases the clarity of the diagnostic picture. No level of technical skill can overcome improper identification of the source of the problem. Only concordant strong findings predict a good outcome.

Discography

Neither the results of the AHCPR methodological process nor that used for other reviews like the Cochrane Collaboration found reliable information to support the use of diagnostic discography (19). Four studies by Carragee

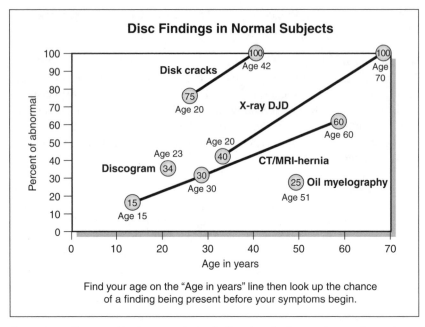

Figure 2-7   Chances of having a particular finding described as an abnormality on imaging studies in asymptomatic patients.

(1999-2000) have been a significant addition to the literature (20-23). The unreliability of high-intensity zone and concordance response for patients was quite condemning, especially with symptoms over 6 months or with abnormal psychological testing. Moreover, discography caused significant symptoms for at least one year in subjects who did not have previous back symptoms. A 2002 presentation to the ISSLS by the same author found discography unable to differentiate a back pain disabled group from a group who whose members were aware that they had back symptoms occasionally but enjoyed unlimited activity (24). Reliable data that meet criteria for either one of the aforementioned reviews do not support intra-discal electro-thermal nucleoplasty (IDET) or a fusion procedure based upon discography.

Diagnosis and Treatment of Common Causes of Back Pain

Sciatica Due to Herniated Disc

Diagnosis
A history of back-related leg symptoms, concordant physiological evidence of nerve root compromise by physical examination or EMG (over 90% at L5

or S1 level), and anatomic findings on MRI or myelography together are indications for surgical consideration.

Treatment

The offending disc and any loose nuclear material within the disc can be excised (discectomy), or a hemi-laminectomy (widening the opening between the lamina) may be performed. However, if the patient can function with less than 3+ EMG findings, recovery commonly occurs within a few months without surgery; there is, however, a recurrence rate of about 60% in the next few years. Surgically decompressing the neural contents can reduce the symptom recurrence rate to about 10%, depending on the balance between subsequent conditioning and the physical daily demands made on the back. Fewer days of work are missed due to back problems for manual workers during the first 4 years following surgery. There seems no difference after 4 years, but surgery is a luxury for speeding recovery when there are very strong findings (25). Generally, the more obvious the findings, the more assured is the recovery following surgical intervention (16,17). The risk of recurrence of herniated disc at the same level is between 2% and 4% (26).

Despite its potential benefits, surgery for a herniated disc does not make the back 18 years young again. Use of the back will still be limited depending on its muscular conditioning relative to what is physically asked of it.

Neuroclaudication from Spinal Stenosis

Diagnosis

Patient history usually reveals a slow gradual decreasing activity tolerance, especially with walking (neuroclaudication) and standing or prolonged extension of the lumbar spine. Symptoms in the back with leg and/or foot symptoms in the patient with spinal stenosis are relieved by flexion of the lumbar spine, which decreases the ligamentous enfolding that can crimp the intra-dural neural contents. Consider screening for diabetes or other general metabolic problems with neuroclaudication before age 60. Most patients have a history of at least intermittent symptoms for months before seeking medical care. Physical examination tends to be unimpressive. Patients are without straight leg raise sciatic tension signs and possibly show signs of symmetrical weakness and atrophy as well as diminished reflexes. EMG changes tend to be minimal due to the gradual nature of the compression. However, EMG can help differentiate new from old changes when acute findings are present (sharps, fibs). SEPs aid EMG in surgical planning as a guide to which nerve root foramina need special attention during surgical decompression. Anatomic studies (either MRI or myelography-CT scan) verify the structural need for central decompressing laminectomy.

Treatment

Foraminal decompression commonly requires partial anterior facetectomy and perhaps partial removal of the inferior pedicle. Surgical decompression is not preventive and should be performed only when the patient feels compromised enough by the walking limitations to undertake the risks. True bowel and bladder compromise can result from stenosis and is an emergency indication for decompression. Those who respond to surgery tend to be the most limited in walking distance (neuroclaudication <300 yards). Segmental fusion may be considered if there is accompanying spondylolisthesis (degenerative slip) with motion.

Spondylolisthesis

Diagnosis

Almost 4% of adults in the United States have slippage of either L4 or L5 vertebra. Most slippage is associated with bony disruption between the facets (spondylolysis) early in life. When one vertebra slips forward more than 25% of the anterior-posterior diameter of the vertebrae below, the nerves at the involved level can become compromised. The limb findings and EMG changes are commonly vaguer than with a herniated disc and may be bilateral or unilateral.

Treatment

Surgical decompression with fusion is usually required to treat spondylolisthesis unless the disc is sufficiently aged, which makes the segment stiffer and more stable. Thus there is a greater chance of further slip with decompression of younger discs in the presence of underdeveloped facet joints. From a clinical outcome standpoint, the younger the patient (e.g., less than 30 years old), the better is the result with fusion.

A tricky diagnostic dilemma can develop when vague back symptoms occur in a patient with spondylolisthesis. Because 25% to 40% of back patients have accompanying leg symptoms, a slip noticed on X-ray can lead to the unverified misdiagnosis of a long-standing slip being the cause of the symptoms. A slip of less than 25%, and even up to 50%, may not cause more back trouble during the working years than no slip at all (27). Later the slip can complicate elderly spinal stenosis but even then most slipped segments stiffen, rarely leaving residual motion that would require fusion to augment decompression.

Arthritis

Arthritis (sero-negative spondyloarthropathy) consists of ankylosing spondylitis, Reiter syndrome, psoriatic spondylitis, and related expressions of spinal symptoms. Except for psoriatic arthritis, these mostly occur in men, with onset at age 20 to 40. They tend to be multi-system diseases that improve with medical observation and a combination of therapies that maximize patient functioning. Once the bones become stiff and brittle, minor trauma can cause fractures with serious consequences. Symptoms include back pain lasting longer than 3 months, worse in the morning (especially stiffness) than evening, improved by mild activity, and taking more than 90 minutes to improve for the duration of the day (28).

Segmental Instability

The concept of increased motion at one segment (other than spondylolisthesis) is based upon relative increased motion that allows measurable stress shielding of the adjacent segments. For example, the hyper-mobile segment takes up all the stress allowing 11 degrees (15 degrees at L5-S1) more motion than adjacent motion segments or more than 5 mm slipping translation (29).

As with fatiguing a wire to break it, until a weak spot develops the spine bends uniformly with the full length sharing the load. When the weak spot develops, the spot, being more lax, takes up more and more of the stress and shields the remaining, stiffer areas from having to bend.

Thus we can evaluate stress shielding with two lateral radiographs centered at the site of possible pathological increase in motion (weak spot or hyper-mobile segment). By superimposing the two films, the translation and angular motion can be correlated and evaluated.

Fusion is indicated for infection, tumor, fracture, or dislocation. As yet the only reasonable elective indication for fusion is for a slip with motion when laminectomy is required to decompress spinal stenosis causing neuroclaudication or similarly involved younger patients with spondylolysis (pars interarticularis) and spondylolisthesis (slip). Most fusions performed today are based upon instability criteria that as yet are not related to a predictable outcome (19).

Motion films provide us with at least some semblance of objective evaluation for instability, though our clinical correlations for aged disc without fracture or dislocation are sketchy at best. The radiologist should be asked if there is more than 5 mm of translation or more than 11 degrees motion at one motion segment compared with the adjacent motion segment.

Fusion must be approached with caution. Fritzell and co-workers (15) found only paltry improvement for a fusion group compared with a non-operative group. There was a rapid convergence toward similar complaints by the two groups, from a 26% difference at 6 months to only a 15% difference on a 100-point visual analog pain scale at 2 years. The non-operative group had the markedly less potential placebo impact of being offered nothing new and no potential cure. The results were unimpressive as the authors had to include the caveat "fusion . . . rarely cures the patient." The "rare cure" caveat must be weighed relative to a reported 17% complication rate with the fusion surgery. Nine percent of the surgery patients had either life-threatening complications or complications that required immediate re-operation In this study, as in other trials, a solid fusion or lack thereof did not influence either a good or a bad result (30-35). Such findings continue to question the whole premise of the procedure.

In summary, a review of the reliable literature leads to the conclusion that, at present, instrumentation fusion for back pain is not justified.

Conditioning

We return to a treatment paradigm with an emphasis on maximizing comfortable activity tolerance whether the problem is due to a period of reduced activity or altered structural or neurological status. Conditioning is necessary for all patients with back pain regardless of its cause and regardless of other treatments that the patient has received or is receiving. Conditioning is needed in patients that have not had surgery as well as in those that have. At this point nothing should stand in the way of conditioning.

Explaining Conditioning

A physician may improve patient understanding of the importance of conditioning by using analogy and examples.

Patient: "When will the pain go away?"

Physician: "Consider a knee injury. It makes no difference whether knee surgery is required or not, recovery only comes after conditioning the thigh muscles to the point of compensating for whatever knee problem remains. With adequate conditioning of the protective muscles, some patients can return to rigorous athletics, not because the knee is normal but because there is adequate muscular compensation to tolerate the required activity. The protective muscles must be conditioned well beyond how they were before the knee problem. Until then, the knee continues to be painful, does not tolerate activity, can be tweaked by any minor mishap, and may even get red and swollen after minor use. It is no different with problems of the spine.

Until our muscles have the endurance to tolerate a desired activity, aches and pains (or worse) will be experienced. Athletes beginning intense preseason training feel stiff and achy, and so do gardeners kneeling and bending in the spring after a prolonged winter's moratorium. Take the latter example. We enjoy gardening, but after we tire or the muscles we are using begin to fatigue, our body is more easily irritated. We may feel achy and sore that night or the next day. It usually takes days of working in the garden before our muscles become conditioned well enough that the pain goes away. If we are older or our muscles are already compensating for a compromised joint, the irritation can cause much more intense symptoms."

Further discussion can help patients realize how a lack of general stamina can prolong symptoms and how training of specific spine muscles provides protection from future problems (36).

Patient: "I want my back to feel as it did when I was in my twenties."

Physician: "Our best science indicates that conditioning involves addressing two weak links that can keep protective muscles from reacting quickly and with enough strength to protect our joints. The most obvious is fatigue of specific muscles. When fatigued, they are weaker and react slower and are unable to do their protective job. If the owner of those muscles becomes tired, the spine muscles also react slower. Fatigue robs us of our coordination and reactions.

There is no treatment, I'm sorry to say, surgical or non-surgical, that makes the back young again after a few weeks of limitation or significant radiculopathy. One third of the population under age 30 doesn't have what we call a "young" back and nobody does over the age of 50. So the key to treatment is improving spine muscle endurance. That is the only way to reduce the frequency and severity of future episodes of back problems."

Phases of Conditioning

The conditioning process starts with a couple of weeks of general conditioning, perhaps 5 days per week for 6 weeks of keeping the pulse rate above 120-130 beats per minute. This is accomplished either by continuously walking or stationary cycling for 30 minutes or by jogging 15-20 minutes. After 2-4 weeks of general conditioning, add specific back muscle conditioning of the erector spinae and gluteal and hamstring muscles. This confers muscular protection at even 4 minutes nightly (Fig. 2-8). Spine muscle conditioning has a proven protective impact that reduces symptoms and back-limiting episodes in people with strenuous jobs (37).

A third phase is not actually treatment of the spine but an attempt to restore what tends to be lost after a period of inactivity due to back pain. This phase is simple but effective reconditioning of arm, legs, and abdominal muscles. Dips, for the arms, can be performed in an armchair. Leg exercises include either squats at the sink or the old ski-conditioning exercise of assuming the sitting position against a wall without a chair. Abdominal muscle conditioning demands only mild exercises. Each of these can be performed in less than 5 minutes and usually can be added after 4 weeks of specific spine muscle conditioning.

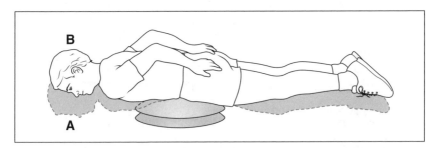

Figure 2-8   Spine muscle conditioning.

Work hardening should be reserved for gradual return to work. Work hardening is a job-oriented treatment plan that is based on an evaluation of the particular job demands of the patient. The basic concept is to encourage the patient to perform as many repetitions of a specific limited task as possible. If unable to tolerate a full circuit, then repetitions need to be built with a portion of the load (three quarters or two thirds of the requirement) until one circuit can be completed. For example, a postal worker who must walk 10 miles per day should start with 7.5 miles, or three quarters of the usual distance; for a store clerk who must lift 15 pounds, encourage repetitive performance at 10 pounds, or two thirds the required amount. Once the person accomplishes more repetitions than are needed, gradually increase the load to the normal level. The speed of progression to the eventual goal can be predicated on many physical and non-physical factors. A work-hardening approach performed in the normal work milieu increases the odds of success and reduces the chances of re-injury.

Approaches to Slow Recovery

Slow recovery (i.e., when at least 10% recovery has not occurred by 6 weeks) is what the activity paradigm attempts to avoid. (Individual recovery of course depends on many factors, but 6 weeks without functional improvement is generally accepted as defining "slow" recovery.) The 10% of patients who are slowest to recover have been proven to take up 90% of resources and similarly affect physician time (37).

Continued disability at 6 weeks is cause for concern that the patient is experiencing slow recovery; however, if steady improvement is occurring, continued activity is still encouraged. When recovery is slow, review the history, physical examination, and special studies to confirm that no Red Flags have emerged. Show concern, however, for slow progress or repeated difficulties in reaching an activity goal. This may be the time to discuss objectively the present threat to the patient's livelihood and future, while perhaps broaching some of the more sensitive issues that can be blocking progress.

Clinicians also are frustrated by a patient's slow recovery or a parade of continuous obstacles to gaining reasonable activity tolerance through conditioning. Sometimes that frustration is communicated directly or indirectly to the patient, making the latter defensive or angry. There are many reasons why a patient may be slow to improve, innumerable combinations of physical, emotional, cognitive, and social factors. Patients benefit more from our honest help than from our character judgments.

Encouraging the Patient to Explore New Career Possibilities

The physician may have to encourage the patient who is unwilling to admit that back pain may force a career re-appraisal or change:

If it is difficult at this time to regain activity tolerance, what are the chances that as you get older it will be easier? What will you do if, for any reason, you can not return to your job because it puts too much stress on you back and causes you too much pain? It may be time to gather some information about your options. You may not need them immediately, but they could be important for planning over the next few years or sometime before retirement age.

Offer suggestions. This can help the patient feel much more in control, knowing that he or she is not tied to a particular outcome—is not, in other words, in a "return to work contest" that is either won or lost. Offer to help the patient start a notebook about potential career opportunities. Suggest that career advisers, schools, employment agencies, and employers are contacted. You can quickly review the patient's notebook on each visit to monitor efforts. This takes little clinician time and requires mostly a reminder. Gathering information and improving the patient's understanding of the issues de-emotionalizes decision-making.

Confronting the Patient Who Refuses to Consider Career Change

Naturally enough, some patients may require coaxing to gather information about possible, if not inevitable, career changes. A complete refusal, however, to even consider preparing for a change in employment or life-style must be confronted by the physician:

It is quite unusual for spine symptoms alone to keep someone from preparing for a new way of making a living. Your future and that of your family are at stake. Usually other issues are involved in these cases. I can recommend a very good counselor who may be able to help you sort out the reasons for your behavior.

This usually initiates a (sometimes contentious) discussion and provides the physician with an opportunity to review common reasons for behavior such as depression and alcohol or drug abuse. Referral to a psychologist or counselor should be offered. If the patient is found to have depression or substance abuse, these problems can then be addressed. Back care can continue for the addicted patient after abstinence or detoxification, but the patient must concurrently participate in Alcoholic Anonymous (AA) or Narcotics Anonymous (NA) meetings *daily* for at least 3 months.

Conclusion

Data-driven care may well become a way of life. This chapter has been an overview of an activity approach to back problems that makes easier use of reliable references such as AHCPR Guide 14 for Back Problems and the Cochrane Collaboration (Table 2-4).

One final comment. The authors had the opportunity in 1999-2000 to participate in an application of this activity paradigm. Back problems were the most frequent issue, but the paradigm had a positive impact on health

Table 2-4   Summary of AHCPR Guide 14, Acute Low Back Problems in Adults

	Recommendation	Optional	Recommendation Against
History and physical examination (34 studies)	• Basic history (B) • History of cancer/infection (B) • Cauda equina syndrome (C) • History of significant trauma (C) • Psychosocial history (C) • Straight leg raising test (B) • Focused neurological examination (B)	• Pain drawing and Visual Analog Scale (D)	
Patient education (14 studies)	• Patient education about back problems (B) • Back school in occupational settings (C)	• Back school in nonoccupational settings (C)	
Medication (23 studies)	• Acetaminophen (C) • NSAIDs (B)	• Muscle relaxants C) • Opioids (short course) (C)	• Opioids used >2 wks (C) • Phenylbutazone (C) • Oral steroids (C) • Colchicine (B) • Antidepressants (C)
Physical treatment methods (42 studies)	• Manipulation during first month of low back pain (B)	• Manipulation for patients with radiculopathy (C) • Manipulation for patients with symptoms >1 month (C) • Self-application of heat/cold to back (D) • Shoe insoles (C) • Corset for prevention in occupational setting (C)	• Manipulation for patients with undiagnosed neurological deficits (D) • Prolonged course of manipulation (D) • Traction (B) • TENS (C) • Biofeedback (C) • Shoe lifts (D) • Corset for treatment (D)

Injections (26 studies)		• Epidural steroid injections for radicular pain to avoid surgery (C)	• Epidural injections for back pain without radiculopathy (D) • Trigger point injections (C) • Ligamentous injections (C) • Facet joint injections (C) • Acupuncture (D)
Bed rest (4 studies)		• Bed rest of 2-4 days for severe radiculopathy (D)	• Bed rest >4 days (B)
Activities and exercise (20 studies)	• Temporary avoidance of activities that increase mechanical stress on spine (D) • Gradual return to normal activities (B) • Low-stress aerobic exercise (C) • Conditioning exercises for trunk muscles after 2 weeks (C) • Exercise quotas (C)		• Back-specific exercise machines (D) • Therapeutic stretching of back muscles (D)
Detection of physiological abnormalities (14 studies)	• Bone scan after 1 month of nonimprovement (C) • Needle EMG and H-reflex tests to clarify 4 weeks of unclear nerve root dysfunction (C) • SEP to plan spinal stenosis surgery (C)		• EMG for clinically obvious radiculopathy (D) • Surface EMG and F-wave tests (C) • Thermography (C)
X-rays of L-S spine (18 studies)	• When Red Flags for fracture present (C) • When Red Flags for cancer or infection present (C)		• Routine use in first month of symptoms in absence of Red Flags (B) • Routine oblique views (B)

(Cont'd)

Table 2-4   Summary of AHCPR Guide 14, Acute Low Back Problems in Adults (Cont'd)

	Recommendation	Optional	Recommendation Against
Imaging (18 studies)	• CT or MRI when strongly suspect cauda equina syndrome, tumor, infection, or fracture (C) • MRI test of choice for patients with previous back surgery (D) • Criteria for imaging tests (B)	• Myelography or CT-myelography for preoperative planning (D)	• Use of imaging test before 1 month in absence of Red Flags (B) • Discography or CT-discography (C)
Surgical considerations (14 studies)	• Consider possible surgical options with persistent and severe sciatica and clinical evidence of nerve root compromise after 1 month of conservative therapy (B) • Standard discectomy and micro-discectomy of similar efficacy in treatment of herniated disc (B) • Chymopapain, after ruling out allergic sensitivity, acceptable but less efficacious than discectomy for herniated disc (C)		• Disc surgery for back pain alone, no Red Flags, and no nerve root compression (D) • Percutaneous discectomy, though less efficacious than chymopapain (C) • Surgery for spinal stenosis within first 3 months of symptoms (D) • Stenosis surgery by imaging tests without cauda equina syndrome or neuroclaudication (D) • Fusion without motion and stenosis fracture, dislocation, tumor, or infection complications (C)
Nonphysical factors	• Social, economic, and nonphysical factors can alter patient response to Sx and Tx (D)		

From Bigos SJ, Chairman. Panel: Bowyer RO, Braen GR, Brown K, Deyo R, Haldeman S, Hart JL, Johnson EW, Keller R, Kido D, Liang MH, Nelson RM, Nordin M, Owen BD, Pope MH, Schwartz RK, Stewart D, Susman J, Triano JJ, Tripp LC, Turk D, Watts C, Weinstein J. Contributors: Battié MC, Bombardier C, Hadler N, Nachemson A, Waddell G, Holland J, Webster J, Schriger D, Shekelle P. Clinical Practice Guideline No. 14, Acute Low Back Problems in Adults, Publication 95-0642. Department of Health and Human Services, Public Health Service, AHCPR, Rockville, MD; 9 December 1994.

throughout. Days missed from work and total costs for care and indemnity for a group using an activity paradigm were *one sixth* the missed days and costs for a group using a pain-oriented guideline (38). The emphasis on activity treats what is truly lost (activity tolerance), while quickly detecting the presence of non-physical (i.e., psychosocial) issues.

An activity approach makes the use of reliable data more logical, even if such data are not the answer to treating all back problems. We have attempted here to provide a simple guide to better results for patients and additional protection for the clinician dealing with back problems.

REFERENCES

1. **Sackett DL, Haynes RB, Guyatt GH, Tigwell P.** Clinical epidemiology: a basic science for clinical medicine. Boston: Little, Brown; 1991:59.

2. **Bigos SJ, Chairman. Panel: Bowyer RO, Braen GR, Brown K, Deyo R, Haldeman S, Hart JL, Johnson EW, Keller R, Kido D, Liang MH, Nelson RM, Nordin M., Owen BD, Pope MH, Schwartz RK, Stewart D, Susman J, Triano JJ, Tripp LC, Turk D, Watts C, Weinstein J. Contributors: Battié MC, Bombardier C, Hadler N, Nachemson A, Waddell G, Holland J, Webster J, Schriger D, Shekelle P.** Clinical Practice Guideline No. 14, Acute Low Back Problems in Adults, Publication 95-0642. Department of Health and Human Services, Public Health Service, AHCPR, Rockville, MD; 9 December 1994.

3. **Shekelle PG, Ortiz E, Rhodes S, et al.** Validity of the AHRQ clinical practice guidelines: how quickly outdated? JAMA. 2001;286:1461-7.

4. Daubert v. Merrill Dow Pharmaceutical, Inc., 509 U.S. 579, 113 S.Ct. 2786, 125 L.Ed.2d 469 (1993).

5. Black v. Food Lion Inc., 171 F.3d 308 (5th Circuit, 1999).

6. **Malmivaara A, Hakkinen U, Aro T, et al.** The treatment of acute low back pain: bed rest, exercises, or ordinary activity? N Engl J Med. 1995;332:351-5.

7. **Burton AK, Waddell G, Tillotson KM, Summerton N.** Information and advice to patients with back pain can have a positive effect: a randomized controlled trial of a novel educational booklet in primary care. Spine. 1999;24:2484-91.

8. **Hagen EM, Eriksen HR, Ursin H.** Does early intervention with a light mobilization program reduce long-term sick leave for low back pain? Spine. 2000;25: 1973-6.

9. **Atcheson SG, Brunner RL, Greenwald EJ, et al.** Paying doctors more: use of musculoskeletal specialists and increased physician pay to decrease workers' compensation costs. J Occup Environ Med. 2001;43:672-9.

10. **Buchbinder R, Jolley D, Wyatt M.** Effect of media campaign on back pain beliefs and its potential influence on management of low back pain in general practice. Spine. 2001;26:2535-42.

11. **McGuirk B, King W, Govind J, et al.** Safety, efficacy, and cost effectiveness of evidence-based guidelines for the management of acute low back pain in primary care. Spine. 2001;26:2615-22.

12. **Indahl A, Haldorsen EH, Holm S, et al.** Five-year follow-up study of a controlled clinical trial using light mobilization and an informative approach to low back pain. Spine. 1998;23:2625-30.

13. **Brown M, Holloszy JO.** Effects of walking, jogging and cycling on strength, flexibility, speed and balance in 60- to 72-year olds. Aging (Milano). 1993;5:427-34.

14. **Ross JF.** Where do real dangers lie? Smithsonian. November 1995:42-53.

15. **Fritzell P, Hägg O, Wessberg P, Nordwall A.** Lumbar fusion versus non-surgical treatment for chronic low back pain: a multi-center randomized controlled trial. Spine. 2001;26:2521-32.

16. **Carragee EJ, Kim DH.** A prospective analysis of magnetic resonance imaging findings in patients with sciatica and lumbar disc herniation: correlation of outcomes with disc fragment and canal morphology. Spine. 1997;22:1650-60.

17. **Schade V, Semmer N, Main CJ, et al.** The impact of clinical, morphological, psychosocial and work-related factors on the outcome of lumbar discectomy. Pain. 1999;80:239-49.

18. **Borenstein DG, O'Mara JW Jr, Boden SD, et al.** The value of magnetic resonance imaging of the lumbar spine to predict low-back pain in asymptomatic subjects: a seven-year follow-up study. J Bone Joint Surg Am. 2001;83:1306-11.

19. The Cochrane Collaboration, 1989-2002.

20. **Carragee EJ, Tanner CM, Yang B, et al.** False-positive findings on lumbar discography: reliability of subjective concordance assessment during provocative disc injection. Spine. 1999;24:2542-7.

21. **Carragee EJ, Tanner CM, Khurana S, et al.** The rates of false-positive lumbar discography in select patients without low back symptoms. Spine. 2000;25:1373-80.

22. **Carragee EJ, Chen Y, Tanner CM, et al.** Can discography cause long-term back symptoms in previously asymptomatic subjects? Spine. 2000;25:1803-8.

23. **Carragee EJ, Paragioudakis SJ, Khurana S.** 2000 Volvo Award winner in clinical studies. Lumbar high-intensity zone and discography in subjects without low back problems. Spine. 2000;25:2987-92.

24. **Carragee EJ, Alamin TF, Grafe M, Miller J.** Provocative discography in volunteer subjects with mild persistent low back pain. ISSLS; Cleveland, June 2002.

25. **Weber H.** Lumbar disc herniation: a controlled, prospective study with ten years of observation. Spine. 1983;8:131-40.

26. **Balderston RA, Gilyard GG, Jones AA, et al.** The treatment of lumbar disc herniation: simple fragment excision versus disc space curettage. J Spinal Disord. 1991; 4:22-5.

27. **van Tulder MW, Assendelft WJ, Koes BW, Bouter LM.** Spinal radiographic findings and nonspecific low back pain: a systematic review of observational studies. Spine. 1997;22:427-34.

28. **Calin A., Fries JF.** Striking prevalence of ankylosing spondylitis in "healthy" W27 positive males and females: a controlled study. N Engl J Med. 1975;293:835.

29. **Bigos SJ, Mills EH, McKee JE, Holland JP.** Spine injury model impairment rating. ABIME. January-March 2001;2(1).

30. **Fischgrund JS, Mackay M, Herkowitz HN, et al.** 1997 Volvo Award winner in clinical studies. Degenerative lumbar spondylolisthesis with spinal stenosis: a prospective, randomized study comparing decompressive laminectomy and arthrodesis with and without spinal instrumentation. Spine. 1997;22:2807-12.

31. **Thomsen K, Christensen FB, Eiskjaer SP, et al.** 1997 Volvo Award winner in clinical studies. The effect of pedicle screw instrumentation on functional outcome and fusion rates in posterolateral lumbar spinal fusion: a prospective, randomized clinical study. Spine. 1997;22:2813-22.

32. **France JC, Yaszemski MJ, Lauerman WC, et al.** A randomized prospective study of posterolateral lumbar fusion: outcomes with and without pedicle screw instrumentation. Spine. 1999;24:553-60.

33. **Grob D, Humke T, Dvorak J.** Degenerative lumbar spinal stenosis: decompression with and without arthrodesis. J Bone Joint Surg Am. 1995;77:1036-41.

34. **McGuire RA, Amundson GM.** The use of primary internal fixation in spondylolisthesis. Spine. 1993;18:1662-72.

35. **Moller H, Hedlund R.** Instrumented and noninstrumented posterolateral fusion in adult spondylolisthesis: a prospective randomized study – part 2. Spine. 2000;25:1716-21.

36. **Gundewall B, Liljeqvist M, Hansson T.** Primary prevention of back symptoms and absence from work: a prospective randomized study among hospital employees. Spine. 1993;18:587-94.

37. **Spengler DM, Bigos SJ, Martin N, et al.** Back injuries in industry: a retrospective study. I—Overview and cost analysis. Spine. 1986;11:241-5.

38. Personal communication from the authors to CMI Division of Wal-Mart Stores, Bentonville, Arkansas; 2000.

3

■ ■ ■

Headache

Joel R. Saper, MD

rimary headache disorders are highly prevalent conditions affecting tens of millions of Americans and hundreds of millions of individuals world-wide (1,2). The life-time prevalence of common headache disorders (i.e., migraine, tension-type headache) can be over 78%, with migraine prevalence greater than 20% in adult females. The economic and quality-of-life burden of migraine alone is substantial, with the most disabled half of migraine sufferers accounting for more than 90% of migraine-related work loss. Barriers to successful care include failure to properly diagnose, underestimation by both the professional and public domains of the morbidity of these conditions, and denied access to appropriate treatment.

Classification of Headaches

Headaches may be classified as *primary* or *secondary* headache syndromes. *Primary headaches* include those in which intrinsic dysfunction of the nervous system, often genetic in origin, predisposes to increased vulnerability to headache attacks. The most common primary headache syndromes include cluster headache, migraine, and tension-type headache. *Secondary headaches* are those in which the headache is secondary to an organic or physiological process, intracranially or extracranially (1).

In 1988 the International Headache Society (IHS) developed a classification of headache disorders and their diagnostic citeria; an update was published in 2004 (3). Table 3-1 is a much shortened version of this extensive classification of primary headaches. Table 3-2 lists some of the more frequently occurring categories of illnesses that produce secondary headaches.

Table 3-1   IHS Classification of Primary Headaches

- Episodic migraine
  —With aura (including basilar [brainstem] migraine)
  —Without aura
- Chronic migraine (new IHS criteria)
- Cluster headache (episodic/chronic)
- Tension-type headache (episodic/chronic)

Table 3-2   Common Secondary Headache Conditions

- Cerebrovascular/cardiovascular ischemia
- Metabolic disorders
- Intracranial mass lesions
- Cerebrospinal fluid (CSF) hypotension/hypertension
- Infectious disorders (systemic, intracranial)
- Endocrine dysfunction
- Cervical (neck) disorders
- Temporomandibular/dental disorders

Secondary Headache

Over 300 entities may produce symptoms of headache, many of which mimic the primary headache disorders. The clinician has the burden of ruling out potentially relevant conditions in patients with recurring or persistent headache. Ruling out secondary headache disorders may in some cases involve ruling out dangerous or life-threatening causes of headache (e.g., brain tumor, cerebral venous thrombosis, subarachnoid hemorrhage). Some signs and symptoms of dangerous headache may include first, worst, or different headache; sudden onset and peak intensity ("thunderclap"); abnormal neurological signs; and fever. Diagnostic testing includes investigation of metabolic, endocrinological, toxic, dental, traumatic, cervical, and infectious disorders, and space-occupying lesions. Disturbances of CSF pressure, ischemic disease, and allergic conditions must be considered. Table 3-3 lists diagnostic tests that should be considered in intractable or variant cases.

Important specific conditions to consider include those of the temporomandibular or dental structures, sphenoid sinuses (image and evaluate for sphenoid sinus disease), carotid and vertebral dissection syndromes, and cerebral venous occlusion. Embolic disease (e.g., carotids, patent foramen ovale [PFO], CSF high or low pressure disorders) must also be considered. A full discussion of the diagnosis and treatment of secondary disorders is beyond the scope of this chapter.

Primary Headache

Migraine Headache
Migraine is a complex neurophysiological disorder characterized by episodic and progressive (chronic migraine) forms of head pain, in association

Table 3-3   Diagnostic Tests for Intractable or Variant Headache

- Physical examination
- Metabolic evaluation
  - —Hematological
  - —ESR/CRP
  - —Endocrinological
  - —Chemistry
  - —Toxicology (drug screens)
- Standard X-rays

- Neuroimaging
  - —CT
  - —MRI/MRA/MRV
  - —Arteriography
- Dental and otological examination
- Lumbar puncture (opening and closing pressures, CSF evaluation)
- Diagnostic blockades
- Cardiac Doppler and ultrasonography (patent foramen ovale, atrial aneurysm)

with numerous neurological and non-neurological (autonomic, psycho-physiological) accompaniments. These can precede, accompany, or follow the headache itself.

Migraine is classified into three major subtypes:

- *Migraine with aura* headaches are characterized by neurological events that occur 30 to 60 minutes before head pain attacks. A migraine aura should last longer than 5 minutes and less than 60 minutes. If an aura is consistently less than 5 minutes in duration, then a *secondary aura* should be suspected (e.g., arteriovenous malformation, epileptic aura). If an aura lasts longer than 60 minutes, it is termed a *prolonged aura* and underlying ischemic/coagulo-pathic/embolic disorders should be ruled out. Only 15% to 20% of migraine attacks are associated with heralding neurological events.

- *Migraine without aura* headaches are attacks of migraine and accompaniments that occur without clear-cut pre-headache neurological symptomatology. This is the most common form of migraine (80-85%).

- *Chronic migraine* is a progressive form of migraine in which intermittent attacks occur at increasing frequency, eventually reaching 15 or more days per month. By definition, chronic migraine occurs on a backdrop of episodic migraine without aura, often accompanied by comorbid neuropsychiatric phenomena. Chronic migraine is frequently associated with medication overuse and "rebound" (discussed later in this chapter). Comorbid conditions associated with migraine, particularly chronic migraine, include depression, anxiety and panic disorders, bipolar disorder, obsessive-compulsive disorder, character disorders, and perhaps fibromyalgia (1-3).

Between 80% and 90% of patients with migraine have a family history. In childhood there is a male-to-female ratio of 1:1, but in adulthood the ratio is 3:1 female-to-male. This is primarily thought to result from the adverse influence on the headache mechanism by estrogen. At very senior ages, the gender ratio again declines to almost 1:1, again confirming that the age extremes (young and senior), during which estrogen is less likely to be influential, reflect reasonable equity.

Each attack generally lasts between 4 and 72 hours and can be accompanied by a wide range of autonomic and cognitive symptoms. Migraine may present with a combination of characteristic signs and symptoms, including a severe, throbbing headache that is unilateral or bilateral, nausea and/or vomiting, sensitivity to light or noise, and worsening of headache with activity. In complex cases, particularly in chronic migraine (see below), a likely association with several neuropsychiatric comorbid disorders occurs.

Predisposed individuals are particularly vulnerable to provocation (triggering) by certain extrinsic and intrinsic events, including hormonal fluctuation, weather changes, certain foods, delayed meals and fasting, extra sleeping time, and stress. Migraine is a brain disorder that generally renders the brain "hypersensitive" and over-responsive to a variety of internal and external stimuli (1,2,4-8). Earlier theories that placed the origin of migraine on constricting and dilating blood vessels are not supported by current research. Inflamed blood vessels, resulting from the effusion of irritating neuropeptides, are important in producing the pain but are only part of the pathogenesis picture, which fundamentally invokes a neural mechanism to the process of migraine. The neurological events during the aura are due to neuronal suppression (cortical spreading depression), not ischemia as once believed. Trigeminal/cervical connections and cervical activation may be important phenomena in the clinical manifestations, pathogenesis, and treatment. The key features of migraine pathogenesis are identified in Table 3-4.

Table 3-4   Key Features of Migraine Pathogenesis

- Trigeminal-mediated perivascular (neurogenic) inflammation resulting in painful vascular and meningeal tissue

- Perivascular release of vasoactive neuropeptides, particularly calcitonin-gene-related-peptide (CGRP)

- Development of allodynia and central sensitization as attacks progress

- Presence of an active "modulator zone" in the dorsal raphe nucleus of the midbrain during migraine attacks

- Activation and threshold reduction of neurons in the descending trigeminal system following C2-C3 cervical stimulation

- Deposition of non-heme iron in the brainstem, roughly correlated to increasingly frequent attacks

- A yet-to-be-defined relationship to nitrous oxide

- Cortical spreading depression (the basis of migraine neurological symptoms)

Tension-Type Headache

Tension-type headache, a controversial disorder, is classified into episodic and chronic forms (3). Episodic tension-type headaches have certain features that overlap with migraine without aura, although there is a general absence of throbbing pain and autonomic accompaniments. Chronic tension-type headaches overlap in clinical features with chronic migraine. Both forms, particularly the episodic, may be present in patients who have otherwise typical migraine headaches. Some authorities believe that these disorders are variant forms of migraine.

Cluster Headache and Its Variants

Cluster headache is one of a group of disorders referred to as the trigeminal autonomic cephalgias (Table 3-5) (9). These disorders are characterized primarily by the presence of short-lasting headaches of variable duration, from seconds (SUNCT syndrome) to 3 hours (cluster headache). Attacks are associated with autonomic features.

Cluster headache is a relatively rare disorder (seen perhaps once or twice a year) that affects more men than women in a ratio of 3:1. Its clinical features include the presence of headache cycles or bouts (clusters) lasting weeks to months and occurring one or more times per year or less. During these periods, short-lasting repetitive headache attacks occur one to eight times daily, lasting from one to three hours (averaging 45 minutes). The attacks are associated with focal orbital or temporal pain, which is always unilateral, of extremely severe intensity, and accompanied by lacrimation, nasal drainage, pupillary changes, and conjunctival injection. Attacks commonly occur during sleeping times or napping and can be provoked by ingestion of alcohol or nitroglycerin. Interestingly, a high likelihood of blue- or hazel-colored eyes; ruddy, rugged, lionized facial features; and a long history of smoking and excessive alcohol intake characterize the majority of men with cluster headache (1). Current concepts of pathophysiology suggest disturbances within the hypothalamus with relevant involvement of autonomic systems (1,2,10) and alterations in melatonin function (11,12). Melatonin "fine tunes" endogenous cerebral rhythms and homeostasis.

Table 3-6 lists the clinical distinctions between cluster headache and migraine.

Table 3-5   Trigeminal Autonomic Cephalgias

- Cluster headache

- Chronic and episodic paroxysmal hemicrania

- SUNCT syndrome (Short-lasting Unilateral Neuralgiaform pain with Conjunctival injection and Tearing)

- Cluster-tic syndrome (association of cluster headache with trigeminal neuralgia symptomatology)

Table 3-6   Clinical Features Distinguishing Cluster Headache from Migraine Headache

Feature	Cluster	Migraine
Location of pain	Always unilateral, periorbital; sometimes occipital referral	Unilateral and bilateral
Age at onset (typical)	20 years or older	10-50 years (can be younger or older)
Gender difference	Majority male	Majority female in adulthood
Time of day	Frequently at night, often same time each day	Any time
Frequency of attacks	1-6 per day	1-10 per month in episodic form
Duration of pain	30-120 min	4-72 hours
Prodromes	None	Often present
Nausea and vomiting	20%	85%
Blurring of vision	Infrequent	Frequent
Lacrimation	Frequent	Infrequent
Nasal congestion/drainage	70%	Uncommon
Ptosis	30%	1-2%
Polyuria	2%	40%
Family history of similar headaches	7%	90%
Miosis	50%	Absent
Behavior during attack	Pacing and agitation	Resting in quiet, dark room

Adapted from Saper JR, Silberstein SD, et al. Handbook of Headache Management, 2nd ed. Baltimore: Lippincott Williams and Wilkins; 1999; with permission.

Cluster headache may occur in an episodic form (bouts or cycles of recurring headaches followed by a period of no headache [remission] lasting weeks to years) or a chronic form (no interim period; headaches occur daily for years without interruption). Treatment differences may exist (2).

Chronic Daily Headache
Chronic daily headache is a frequency-based descriptive term that embodies four overlapping clinical subtypes:

- *Chronic migraine*—with or without medication overuse
- *Chronic tension-type headache*—with or without medication overuse

Table 3-7   Features of Medication Overuse Headache

- Weeks to months of excessive use of abortive agents, with usage exceeding 2-3 days/week
- Insidious increase of headache frequency
- Dependable and predictable headache, corresponding to an irresistible escalating use of offending agents at regular, predictable intervals
- Evidence of psychological and/or physiological dependency
- Failure of alternative acute or preventive medications to control headache attacks
- Reliable onset of headache within hours to days following the last dose of symptomatic treatment

Adapted from Saper JR, Silberstein SD, et al. Handbook of Headache Management, 2nd ed. Baltimore: Lippincott Williams and Wilkins; 1999; with permission.

- *New daily persistent headache*—onset of daily, persistent head pain without the progressive features of chronic migraine but often associated with comorbid and medication overuse features
- *Hemicrania continua*—unilateral, generally persistent hemicranial discomfort with some features of migraine and cluster headache and which in 20% of cases appears to arise as a consequence of head trauma

Medication Overuse Headache

Medication overuse headache ("rebound" headache) is a self-sustaining headache condition characterized by persisting and recurring headache (usually migraine forms) against a background of chronic, regular use of centrally acting analgesics, ergotamine tartrate, or triptans (1,13). The 2004 IHS criteria use the term *medication overuse headache*. The key features of this condition are noted in Table 3-7. Medication overuse headache most likely results from chronic changes to receptors (14). For treatment suggestions, see below.

Treatment of Primary Headache

The key principles in the treatment of headaches and related phenomena are

- Diagnosing the specific primary headache entity and ruling out secondary headache
- Determining attack frequency and severity
- Establishing the presence or absence of comorbid illnesses (e.g., psychiatric, neurological, medical)
- Identifying confounding factors, including external or internal phenomena, such as:
  —Medication use
  —Estrogen replacement

—Hormonal disturbances
—Use of or exposure to toxic substances
—Others
• Identifying previous treatment successes and failures

Pharmacological therapy provides the essential treatment for the majority of patients with primary headache. However, nonpharmacological treatments, such as behavioral modification, exercise, and dietary manipulation, can also be helpful, particularly when combined with pharmacological therapy. In addition, increasing attention has focused on the important contribution that interventional treatments, such as occipital nerve blocks for symptomatic treatment, may provide primary headache patients. Finally, for refractory or complex headache problems, inpatient treatment may be necessary.

Nonpharmacological Treatments

A variety of factors related to health, habits, and education can assist patients with headache. Education on headache triggers and eliminating headache-producing behaviors can be essential. Reduction of medication use and the treatment of rebound (i.e., reduction of the medication that causes "rebound" headache) are fundamental and critical elements in the treatments of patients with chronic headache when medication overuse phenomena exist. Discontinuing smoking, establishing regular eating and sleeping patterns, and regular exercise are reported as very helpful by many patients with headache. Biofeedback and behavioral treatment, together with cognitive behavioral therapy, may be of important value in many cases. Many patients with intractable headaches and some with more treatable headaches appear to have striking linkages between emotional and physiological reactions. There is increasing evidence that limbic-brainstem phenomena may activate headache mechanisms as a result of emotional factors (15,16). Tracy has demonstrated activation of the periaqueductal gray in patients in whom distraction is employed (17). Behavioral therapy and formal psychotherapy may therefore be valuable and even necessary in the treatment of many chronic and recurring headache patients.

Treatment of Medication Overuse Headache

Treatment of medication overuse headache requires that both the physiological and behavioral elements of the disorder be addressed. Continued use of offending medications renders patients refractory to effective treatment. Outpatient and inpatient strategies are available, depending upon the intensity of medication usage and the psychological characteristics of each case. Table 3-8 identifies important principles in the approach to the treatment of medication misuse headache.

Table 3-8   Principles in Treating Medication Overuse Headache

- Discontinuation of offending agent (taper if opioid or barbiturate-containing)
- Aggressive treatment of resulting severe withdrawal headache
- Hydration, including IV fluids and support in severe cases (treat nausea)
- Pharmacological prophylaxis (after medication overuse has terminated)
- Implementation of behavioral therapies
- Use of outpatient or hospitalization techniques for advanced and severe conditions
- Address behavioral elements that are relevant to the medication overuse

Adapted from Saper JR, Silberstein SD, et al. Handbook of Headache Management, 2nd ed. Baltimore: Lippincott Williams and Wilkins; 1999; with permission.

Medication overuse headache in conjunction with behavioral elements that drive the misuse must be distinguished from headaches resulting from toxic substances or other exposure to agents or drugs. The latter have a direct provocative influence, whereas the former is a chronic disorder that emerges as a consequence of receptor disturbances after months of overuse.

It is my view that many cases of medication overuse are prompted, sustained, and otherwise influenced by behavioral dynamics, including obsessive drug-taking, fear of pain, and anxiety. Appropriate treatment of medication overuse headache often requires behavioral intervention, without which successful therapy is not possible.

Pharmacological Treatment of Migraine

The pharmacological treatment of headache involves the use of abortive (acute) and preventive medications (1,2,4,18-24). *Abortive (acute) treatments* are used to terminate evolving or existing attacks. *Preventive treatment* is implemented to reduce the frequency of attacks and prevent overuse of acute medications. Most patients require a combination of these two treatments. *Pre-emptive treatment* is a short-term preventive course of therapy used in anticipation of a predictable event such as a menstrual period or a vacation-related headache. The wide variety of pharmacological agents used in headache management and clinical information regarding their use are listed in Table 3-9. Silberstein (20) summarizes the headache consortium report on evidence-based treatment for primary headaches, a report principally directed at treatment at a primary care level.

Abortive (Acute) Medications

Many agents are used for the acute treatment of migraine. Some agents, such as analgesics, are of general value for pain, whereas others, such as the ergots and triptan medications, are migraine-specific and influence receptor and transmitter systems thought relevant to migraine pathogenesis. Table 3-10 lists the various categories of abortive agents.

Table 3-9   Selected Drugs Used in the Pharmacotherapy of Head, Neck, and Face Pain*

Drug Name	Mg/Dose	Standard Daily Administration	Notes
Symptomatic Drugs			
Analgesics			
**Excedrin	—	Varies	Avoid more than 2 days/wk of use
NSAIDs			
**Naproxen sodium (PO)	275-550	bid-tid	Avoid extended, daily use
Indomethacin (PO)	25-50	bid-tid	As above
Indocin SR (PO)	75	1 q day or bid	As above
Indomethacin (prn)	50	bid-tid	As above
Meclofenamate (PO)	50-200	bid	As above
**Ibuprofen (PO)	600-800	bid-tid	As above
Ketorolac (PO)	10	qid	As above
Ketorolac (IM)	30	tid	Appears particularly valuable when ergot derivatives and narcotics must be avoided and parenteral therapy is necessary. No more than occasional, short-term use is advisable because of renal toxicity, most likely in predisposed patients.
Special Migraine Drugs			
**Isometheptene combinations (Midrin, etc.)	—	2 caps at onset, 1-2 q 30-60 min	Max 5-6 caps/day; 2 days/wk
**Ergotamine tartrate (ET) oral (Cafergot, Wigraine, etc.)	1 mg ET, 100 mg caffeine	2 tabs at onset, 1-2 q 30-60 min	Max 4-6/day; 2 days/wk
**ET suppositories (Cafergot, Wigraine)	2 mg ET, 100 mg caffeine	1/3-1 at onset, may repeat in 60 min	Max 2/day; 2 days/wk
**ET sublingual (Ergomar, Ergostat)	2 mg ET	1 at onset; may repeat after 15 min; 0.25-1 mg SC, IM, IV tid	Max 2/day; 2 days/wk
**Dihydroergotamine (DHE) IM/IV/SC	0.25-1	0.25-1 mg SC, IM, IV tid	Can be used 2-3x/day in conjunction with anti-nauseant, analgesic, etc.; IM more effective than SC

Table 3-9   Selected Drugs Used in the Pharmacotherapy of Head, Neck, and Face Pain* *(Cont'd)*

Drug Name	Mg/Dose	Standard Daily Administration	Notes
Special Migraine Drugs (cont'd)			
**DHE nasal spray	1	1 spray each nostril (2 mg/spray); repeat in 15 min (4 sprays = 2 mg)	Use no more than 2-3×/wk, on separate days
**Sumatriptan (parenteral)	6 SC	May repeat in 1 hr	Cannot be used within 24 hr of ergotamine-related meds or other triptans. Should not be used in presence of cardiovascular and/or cerebrovascular, severe hypertension, Prinzmetal's angina, or peripheral vascular disorders. No more than 2 doses in 24 hr. Limit 2 days/week usage. Do not take within 2 weeks of MAOI discontinuation.
**Sumatriptan (oral)	25-100	Take at headache onset; may repeat at 2 hr; max 100 mg/day	As above
**Sumatriptan (nasal spray)	5 or 20	1 spray in 1 nostril only; may repeat in 2 hr; max 40 mg/24 hr	As above
**Zolmitriptan (oral)	2.5-5	1 at onset; may repeat in 2 hr; max 10 mg/24 hr	As above
**Zolmitriptan (ZMT)	As above	As above	As above
**Naratriptan (oral)	2.5	1 at onset; may repeat in 4 hr; max 5 mg/24 hr	As above
**Rizatriptan (oral and MLT)	5-10	1 at onset; may repeat in 2 hr; max 30 mg/24 hr	As above
**Almotriptan	12.5	1 at onset; may repeat; max 25 mg/24 hr	As above
**Frovatriptan	2.5	1 at onset; may repeat after 6-8 hr; max 7.5 mg/24 hr	As above

(cont'd)

Table 3-9   Selected Drugs Used in the Pharmacotherapy of Head, Neck, and Face Pain* *(Cont'd)*

Drug Name	Mg/Dose	Standard Daily Administration	Notes
Special Migraine Drugs (cont'd)			
**Eletriptan	20-40	1 at onset of HA; may repeat if necessary after 2 hr	As above, because it is metabolized by the cytochrome P-450 hepatic enzyme 3A4, eletriptan should not be used with cimetidine, diltiazam, nicardipine, verapamil, or fluoxetine.
**Valproic acid IV	250-750	1 to 3 dosages/ day IV	See entry under Preventive Drugs section below (page 78)
Antinauseants/Neuroleptics			
Chlorpromazine (PO)	25-100	bid-tid	Limit 3 days/wk, except for persistent nausea; avoid extended use. Monitor for hypotension and cardiac rhythm effects (QT interval).
(Suppository)	25-100	bid-tid	As above
(IM)	25-100	bid-tid	As above
(IV)	2.5-10	bid-tid	As above
Metoclopramide			
(PO–tablet and syrup)	10-20	tid	As above
(parenteral)	10	tid	As above
Promethazine			
(PO)	25-75	tid	As above
(IM)	25-75	tid	As above
Perphenazine			
(PO)	4-8	bid-tid	As above
(IM)	5	bid	As above
Antihistamines			
Hydoxyzine (PO, IM)	25-75	bid-tid or hs	Can be used as a symptomatic or preventive treatment
Cyproheptadine (PO)	2-4	tid-qid	As above
Diphenhydramine (IM, IV)	25-50	1 to 3 dosages per day	Used essentially as acute (abortive) agent
Steroids			
Prednisone (PO)	40-60	In 1 or divided doses	4-10 day program; avoid repeated use

Table 3-9   Selected Drugs Used in the Pharmacotherapy of Head, Neck, and Face Pain* *(Cont'd)*

Drug Name	Mg/Dose	Standard Daily Administration	Notes
Preventive Drugs (avoid sustained use for more than 6 mo w/o trial reduction)			
Tricyclic Antidepressants			
Amitriptyline	10-150	Divided doses or hs	Bedtime dose aids sleep disturbance
Nortriptyline	10-100	As above	As above
Doxepin	10-150	As above	As above
Other Antidepressants			
Fluoxetine	20	20-80 mg/day in divided dose	Actual efficacy for headache uncertain. Administer with care to patients using lipophilic beta-blockers (propranolol, metoprolol, etc.) or switch to hydrophilic beta-blockers such as nadolol. Value for headache of many other antidepressants is under investigation.
Other (SSRIs etc.)			
MAO Inhibitors			
Phenelzine	15-30	15-90 mg/day in divided dose	Dietary and medication restrictions mandatory
Beta-Adrenergic Blockers			
**Propranolol	20-50	tid-qid (standard dose)	Monitor cardiac function, BP, pulse, lipids
Atenolol	50-100	bid	As above
**Timolol	10-20	bid	As above
Metoprolol	50-100	bid	As above
Nadolol	20-120	bid	As above
Calcium Channel Antagonists			
Verapamil	80-160	tid-qid	Monitor cardiac function, BP, pulse, lipids; eliminated by kidneys
Nimodipine	30-60	tid	As above
Diltiazem	30-90	tid	As above

(cont'd)

Table 3-9   Selected Drugs Used in the Pharmacotherapy of Head, Neck, and Face Pain* (Cont'd)

Drug Name	Mg/Dose	Standard Daily Administration	Notes
Ergotamine Derivatives			
**Methysergide	1-2	tid-5×/day	After 6 months of treatment, review cardiac, pulmonary, and retroperitoneal regions for fibrotic changes. Carefully observe contraindications.
Methylergonovine	0.2-0.4	tid-qid	As above
Anticonvulsants			
**Valproic acid	125-500	1-2 g/day in divided doses	Monitor hepatic, metabolic (platelets), and metabolic parameters carefully. Consider dose reduction when used with antidepressants, lithium, verapamil, phenothiazines, benzodiazepines, and other anticonvulsants. Observe warnings carefully; avoid using with barbiturates and perhaps benzodiazepines.
**Valproic acid (ER)	250-1000	500 mg-1 g/day, once per day dosing	As above
**Valproic acid (IV)	250-750	1 to 3 dosages/day IV	As above
Carbamazepine	100-200	300-1200 mg/day in divided doses	Monitor hepatic and metabolic parameters carefully. Consider dose reduction when used with anticonvulsants, lithium, verapamil, and phenothiazines. Observe warnings carefully. *Reduces oral contraceptive efficacy.*
Gabapentin	100-400	1800-3600 mg/day	May cause agitation and other CNS side effects.
Topiramate	25-50	25 mg bid, tapered slowly to 100-200 mg/day	Sedation, cognitive impairment, tingling, abdominal cramps, and risk for renal stones are limiting features. Liver function disturbances, acute myopia, and closed-angle glaucoma (in 1st month) require careful monitoring and immediate discontinuation. Weight loss may occur.

Table 3-9   Selected Drugs Used in the Pharmacotherapy of Head, Neck, and Face Pain* *(Cont'd)*

Drug Name	Mg/Dose	Standard Daily Administration	Notes
Others			
Baclofen	10-20	tid-qid	Increase and decrease dose slowly and allow tolerance to develop; taper when discontinuing
Tizanidine	2-8	2-8 mg tid or prn; max dose 32-36 mg/day	May be used as abortive or preventive agent. Sedation, hypotension, and liver function disturbances must be considered and monitored. Careful use with other alpha-adrenergic agonist agents (e.g., clonidine) and with hepatotoxic agents is recommended. Maximum dose is 36 mg/day.
Lithium	150-300	bid-tid	Reduce dose in conjunction with verapamil, other calcium channel antagonists, and NSAIDs; monitor metabolic parameters
Oxygen inhalation	100% O_2 w/mask	7 L/min for 10-15 min	Must be used at onset of cluster headache; avoid around extreme heat or flame and cigarettes
**Stadol nasal spray (butorphanol)	1 mg/spray; maximum use: 2 dose days/wk		Useful for acute migraine but important side effects. Dependency and addictive potential significant. Avoid in patients with addictive or obsessive drug-taking patterns or history of drug overdose. Avoid in patients with daily or almost daily headache. Withdrawal symptoms can be severe.
Botulinum toxin	Uncertain	Uncertain	Controlled studies have not firmly established efficacy in headache
Melatonin	3-15	Usually hs	Value in cluster headache is tentative but promising; risks in asthma and vasoconstrictive diseases remain to be defined

* Few of the medications listed in this table are either approved specifically for headache or have been shown by controlled studies to be effective for headache. Their inclusion reflects the fact that they have been recommended from various sources as possibly useful for the treatment of some cases of headache. Drugs approved by the FDA for the treatment of migraine, cluster headache, or tension-type headache are designated by (**).

Modified from Saper JR, Silberstein SD, et al. Handbook of Headache Management, 2nd ed. Philadelphia: Lippincott Williams & Wilkins; 1999.

The triptans represent narrow-spectrum, receptor-specific (serotonin [5-HT$_1$]) agonists that stimulate the 5-HT$_1$ receptors to reduce neurogenic inflammation (2,4,18,19). The ergot derivatives are broader spectrum agents, affecting the serotoninergic receptors and the alpha-adrenergic and dopamine receptors (and others). While many patients respond well to the triptans, others appear to require the broader influence of ergot derivatives. Experienced clinicians are adept at administering several of the triptans as well as the ergots. Short-acting, rapidly effective triptans include almotriptan, sumatriptan, rizatriptan, zolmitriptan, and eletriptan; naratriptan and frovatriptan have the longest half-lives. Several delivery formats are available in addition to tablets: injection (sumatriptan), nasal spray (sumatriptan and zolmitriptan), and rapidly dissolving forms (zolmitriptan and rizatriptan).

Patients who have not responded to less potent medications require triptans or ergots for maximum benefit. It is increasingly imperative that the triptans, and probably the ergot derivatives as well, be administered to patients in the early phases of a headache attack in order to bring about maximum benefit and reduce the possibility of recurrence (the return of headache within the same 24-hour period). It is important that clinicians encourage patients to take these medications early, unless patients have a history of medication overuse or would unreasonably anticipate an attack, thus increasing the potential for medication misuse.

Burstein and colleagues (6) have emphasized the importance of early treatment with triptans before central sensitization occurs. Central sensitization is the development of lowered firing threshold in second-order and third-order neurons and perhaps other areas of the brain after 20 to 30 minutes of onset of a migraine headache. Central sensitization brings with it cutaneous allodynia. Burstein and colleagues have shown that once central sensitization and allodynia occur, reversibility of pain is not as likely, and therefore early treatment is more effective. Early treatment, however, may bring with it premature usage and overusage, and the clinician must balance these two important dynamics.

Table 3-10   Abortive Medications Used in the Treatment of Migraine

- Simple and combined analgesics (acetaminophen, Excedrin, NSAIDs, others)

- Mixed analgesics (barbiturate and simple analgesics, aspirin +/- acetaminophen, +/- caffeine); often avoided because of the likelihood of dependency and misuse

- Ergot derivatives, including dihydroergotamine

- Triptan medications, including
  - —Sumatriptan   —Zolmitriptan
  - —Naratriptan   —Frovatriptan
  - —Almotriptan   —Eletriptan
  - —Rizatriptan

Abortive medications are used in conjunction with antinauseants and in combination with each other for maximum efficiency (do *not* combine ergots and triptans). Clinicians must be familiar with important contraindications and safety warnings of each of these medication groups as well as adverse effects and influence on hepatic metabolism, particularly when these drugs are used in combination with others. (For example, in patients with underlying coronary artery disease, triptans may precipitate an anginal episode.)

Finally, for reasons that are not fully understood but perhaps related to the cervical/trigeminal connections, occipital nerve blocks may relieve acute migraine attacks in some individuals. This method has been historically used by anesthesiologists but is increasingly employed by neurologists and others treating headache. Long-term value is rare, but short-term relief is frequently seen.

Preventive Medications

Many agents are available for the prevention of migraine (4,20-22). Prophylaxis should be considered in consultation with the patient. Many experts believe that three attacks per month merits a discussion with the patient. However, one attack every two months that is severe and disabling may likewise warrant consideration of prophylaxis. Thus it is a question of clinical judgment when preventive pharmacotherapy should be introduced. Table 3-11 lists certain clinical guidelines that can be used to make this determination. Abortive medications will continue to be needed in patients receiving prophylactic therapy. After one year of successful prophylaxis, weaning should be considered.

The categories of medications useful in prevention can be found listed in Table 3-12. A wide range of therapies is available, and increasingly useful are those that appear to work on specific neurotransmitter systems.

Table 3-11   Indications for Prophylactic Medications in Patients with Migraine

---

- Disability from migraine headaches (loss of time at work or at home)

- Migraine headaches occurring two or more days per week

- Patient is overusing acute medication (analgesic rebound headache)

- Risk of permanent neurological dysfunction because of the headache condition (hemiplegic migraine, migraine with prolonged aura)

- When acute medications are contraindicated or ineffective

- Patient preference, provided clinical justification exists

Adapted from Saper JR, Silberstein SD, et al. Handbook of Headache Management, 2nd ed. Baltimore: Lippincott Williams and Wilkins; 1999; and Silberstein SD, for the U.S. Headache Consortium. Practice parameter: evidence-based guidelines for migraine headache (an evidence-based review). Report of the Quality Standards Subcommittee of the American Academy of Neurology. Neurol. 2000;55:754-62; with permission.

Table 3-12   Prophylactic Medications for Migraine

- Ttricyclic antidepressants (particularly amitriptyline, nortriptyline, and doxepin)
- Beta-adrenergic blockers (particularly propranolol and nadolol)
- Calcium channel blockers (verapamil)
- Anticonvulsants (valproic acid, gabapentin, topiramate)
- Ergot derivatives (methylergonovine and methysergide)
- Monoamine oxidase inhibitor (for refractory cases)
- Others
  —SSRIs?   —Botulinum toxin?
  —Neuroleptics   —Riboflavin?/coenzyme Q10?
  —Tizanidine

The reader will note that several of these categories do not have influence over vasculature or blood flow, suggesting again that the primary pathogenesis of migraine seems more likely to involve neuronal rather than vascular dynamics.

Tricyclic antidepressants and beta-blockers are well-established, first-line medications for preventive treatment of migraine in those patients who do not have contraindications or restrictions to either medication. Calcium channel blockers are generally not as effective. The anticonvulsants have considerable value and are particularly useful in the presence of neuropsychiatric comorbidities or other conditions, such as seizures or bipolar disorders, that might accompany migraine. Topiramate, at dosages between 75-200 mg/day, has received increasing interest as a result of efficacy data, as well as research, that preliminarily suggest that it may reduce cerebral events related to migraine pathogenesis and progression.

The SSRIs are helpful for neuropsychiatric comorbidities, such as depression and panic and anxiety disorders, but generally do not have a strong anti-migraine influence. Some patients with migraine-related headaches benefit from the antidopaminergic influence of the new neuroleptics (21), although the potential for adverse effects limits their widespread use. Tizanidine, an alpha-adrenergic agonist, has been shown effective in an adjunctive, preventive role (22). Botulinum toxin is increasingly administered for the prevention of migraine. Numerous uncontrolled studies support efficacy, but there is a paucity of controlled data at this time. If botulinum toxin is shown to work for migraine, it is likely to work through a central mechanism, not through a primary muscular influence (23,24).

The treatment of chronic migraine is similar to that of episodic migraine. Treatment is directed at both the daily or almost daily pain and periodic attacks. Because of the likely presence of a progressive course, medication overuse, and neuropsychiatric comorbidities in this population, a more comprehensive approach beyond medications alone (25,26) is required.

This includes cognitive behavioral therapy and other forms of psychotherapy and family therapy. Organic illness must be ruled out with appropriate testing in patients with frequent or daily headache and in those with neurological findings (see below).

Treatment of Cluster Headache

Cluster headache responds and is treated differently than migraine. Because cluster headache attacks generally occur one to eight times daily, the use of abortive medications is limited to the few agents that are safe for such frequent use. Preventive therapy is necessary for cluster headache unless the typical cluster cycle is two weeks in duration or less.

Acute treatments of cluster headache include oxygen inhalation, triptans, ergots, and indomethacin. Also, 100% oxygen, administered via a nonrebreather face mask at 8-10 L/min, can be highly effective and is very safe when used briefly. Parenteral sumatriptan is the most effacious of the triptans for the treatment of cluster headache. Injectable imitrex is most effective due to the rapid onset of the headaches and the delayed gastric emptying experienced with the oral agents. Indomethacin (orally 25-50 mg) is administered at the onset of the attack. As stated earlier, treatment is limited by the need to use medications up to several times a day when effective preventive is not available or has not yet become effective.

Prophylactic treatment of cluster headache is begun at the start of a cluster cycle (which, as mentioned earlier, may last weeks to months) and is tapered to see that the cycle has terminated. Because chronic cluster patterns can continue for years, prophylaxis may be required for many years. Table 3-13 lists the available preventive agents for cluster headache. The most reliable agents for prevention are the steroids, but because of their inherent risks with long-term usage, they are inappropriate except in transitional regimens. Steroids can be used, for example, at the onset of treatment while other preventive agents are being titrated upward; over particularly vulnerable times, such as when traveling; or when other medications are in transition. Table 3-14 shows a recommended prednisone protocol.

Table 3-13   Prophylactic Medications for Cluster Headache

- Verapamil (120-160 mg tid-qid)

- Lithium

- Divalproex/topiramate

- Melatonin 6-15 mg hs

- 7-day prednisone burst (steroids are generally effective for cluster headache prevention, and short-term trials can be dramatically effective, but risks limit utility)

- Ergot derivatives (methylergonovine/methysergide)

Table 3-14   Recommended 7-Day Prednisone Program*

Day	Breakfast (mg)	Lunch (mg)	Dinner (mg)
1	20 (4 pills)	20	20
2	20	20	20
3	20	15 (3 pills)	15
4	15	15	10 (2 pills)
5	10	10	10
6	10	5 (1 pill)	5
7	5	5	—

*5-mg tablets; 60 tablets dispensed; tapered over Days 7-18.

For intractable cases, hospitalization is recommended (see below). In some cases surgical intervention is required, but surgical treatment is limited due to the likelihood of post-surgical painful sequelae. Occipital nerve injection is effective in treating some acute attacks, and subcutaneous occipital stimulation has been recently reported as anecdotally effective (27).

Treatment of Trigeminal Autonomic Cephalgias

Chronic paroxysmal hemicrania (CPH) and episodic paroxysmal hemicrania (EPH), as well as hemicrania continua, are characteristically sensitive to treatment with indomethacin at a dose of 25-50 mg tid (28). SUNCT syndrome may respond to lamotrigine, topiramate, or gabapentin (29).

Interventional Procedures

Because of the relevance of the cervical spine to the descending trigeminal system and headache physiology (trigeminal cervical connection), disturbances at the level of the upper cervical spine, its nerves and joints, have become important targets for the treatment of pharmacologically resistant headaches. Interventional procedures include neuroblockage (nerve, facet, epidural space), radiofrequency and cryolysis procedures, implantations, and stimulation. Premature or excessive use of interventional procedures is unwarranted, but when selective and expertly administered, they clearly have a role in the overall spectrum of diagnosis and treatment for headache conditions. Even more treatments, such as implantable stimulators, are on the horizon.

Table 3-15 summarizes the treatment of primary headaches.

When to Use Opioids

Experience and evidence support the avoidance of sustained opioid administration in the chronic headache population (1,30,31). Use in acute situations

Table 3-15   Therapeutic Categories of Treatment for Primary Headache

- Nonpharmacological treatment
- Pharmacological treatment (acute and preventive)
- Interventional procedures, including
  —Neuroblockade (nerve, facet, epidural space)
  —Radiofrequency and cryolysis procedures
  —Implantations and stimulation
  —Others
- Hospital/rehabilitation programs

when other treatments are contraindicated remains appropriate, but dose and amounts of prescriptions should be limited and monitored carefully to avoid misuse. Sustained opioid administration can be considered in the following limited circumstances:

- When all else fails, following a full range of advanced services, including detoxification
- When standard agents are contraindicated
- In the elderly or during pregnancy

Experience suggests that while some patients with difficult headache problems respond to sustained opioid therapy, there is significant risk for untoward reactions and confounding of the already complex problem. We recommend that sustained opioid therapy for intractable headache not be started on a primary care level but that patients who do not respond to standard treatment be referred to specialists and/or centers where more complex regimens of treatment can be imposed, where rebound can be treated most effectively, and where psychological influences on headache refractoriness can be most effectively addressed. Opioid-induced hyperalgesia reflects the adverse painful effects of chronic opioid administration in some patients and is easily misinterpreted as tolerance, which would ordinarily respond to more medication (32).

Furthermore, nearly 75% of refractory patients placed on daily opioids fail to gain effective control of their headaches (30,31). Approximately one half of those maintained on opioids demonstrated noncompliant drug-related behavior. Despite reports of pain reduction, a major improvement in function was not noted in a significant percentage of patients.

Referral and Hospitalization

It is advisable to refer severe and intractable headache patients to specialists, specialized clinics, and tertiary centers. Hospitalization is also required for many complex patients whose medication misuse or the presence of

---

Table 3-16   Criteria for Hospitalization for Headache

- Severe symptoms that are refractory to outpatient treatment
- Headache accompanied by drug overuse (dependency) or toxicity not treatable as an outpatient
- Intensity of neuropsychiatric and behavioral comorbidity renders outpatient treatment ineffective
- Confounding medical illness
- Treatment urgency in a desperate patient

---

intractable pain and behavioral/neuropsychiatric symptomatology has reached an intensity and complexity that makes outpatient therapy no longer appropriate (33,34). In some patients, confounding medical illness is present, limiting standard treatment administration. Aggressive and thorough diagnostic assessment is mandatory to either rule out organic, toxic, or physiological illness or define unrecognized provocative factors.

Primary care physicians may need to refer patients with complex and intense headache problems to specialists and/or referral centers, which can more effectively address the many issues that arise and have experience in using multiple medication and behavioral regimens simultaneously. Hospitalization for acute and prolonged headache is a complex undertaking, because it must address not only the refractoriness of the symptoms and, in many cases, the oft-present confounding influence of medication overuse headache (rebound) but also the behavioral and psychological factors that often influence these dilemmas. Criteria for hospitalization are summarized in Table 3-16.

For patients who are being treated for medication overuse headache, hospitalization length of stay varies, depending upon the intensity and type of medication that has been overused, the amount of pain and duration of it during the weaning process, the behavioral issues that emerge, and the confounding factors that are often present. Parenteral agents (e.g., dihydroergotamine, diphenhydramine, ketorolac) may be used during hospitalization to control attacks, particularly during rebound withdrawal. Discontinuation of medication and the weaning process bring with them a predictable escalation of headache. Developing a preventive treatment during this time is difficult, because it takes time for medications to work and because generally patients are in a refractory period that may last up to weeks to months after discontinuation of the offending agents.

Conclusion

Primary headaches represent a challenging and important human affliction. There is increasing evidence to support that the primary headaches represent a disease state and the likelihood that pathological markers are present in the brain and may worsen with repetitive attacks. Thus primary headaches may represent a potentially progressive disorder, particularly in the case of migraine. The clinician has the responsibility to make a proper diagnosis as early in the course of the condition as possible and to rule out secondary illnesses that are easily misdiagnosed as a primary headache disorder. The primary care clinician is encouraged to address these conditions with the same seriousness as one would approach any other illness at a primary level and to consider referral of complex or unresponsive patients to more advanced systems of care whenever it becomes apparent that the diagnosis or effective treatment is beyond the services that can be achieved at a primary care level.

REFERENCES

1. **Saper JR, Silberstein SD, et al.** Handbook of Headache Management, 2nd ed. Baltimore: Lippincott Williams and Wilkins; 1999.
2. **Silberstein SD, Lipton RB, Dalessio DJ, eds.** Wolff's Headache and Other Head Pain, 7th ed. New York: Oxford University Press; 2001.
3. **International Headache Society.** The International Classification of Headache Disorders, 2nd ed. Cephalalgia. 2004:24(Suppl 1):9-160.
4. **Goadsby PJ, Lipton RB, Ferrari MD.** Migraine: current understanding and treatment. N Engl J Med. 2002;246:257-70.
5. **Bartsch T, Goadsby PJ.** Stimulation of the greater occipital nerve (GON) enhances responses of dural responsive convergent neurons in the trigeminal cervical complex in the rat. Cephalalgia. 2001;21:401-2.
6. **Burstein RH, Cutrer FM, Yarnitsky D.** The development of cutaneous allodynia during a migraine attack. Brain. 2000;123:1703-9.
7. **Weiller CA, May A, Limmroth V, et al.** Brainstem activation and spontaneous human migraine attacks. Nat Med. 1995;1:658-60.
8. **Welch KM, Nagesh V, Aurora SK, Gelman N.** Periaqueductal gray matter dysfunction in migraine: cause or the burden of illness? Headache. 2001;41:629-37.
9. **Goadsby PJ.** Short-lasting primary headaches: focus on trigeminal autonomic cephalgias and indomethacin-sensitive headaches. Curr Opin Neurol. 1999;12:273-7.
10. **May A, Bahra A, Buchel C, et al.** PET and MRA findings in cluster headache and MRA in experimental pain. Neurol. 2000;55:1328-35.
11. **Leone M, D'Amico D, Moschiano F, et al.** Melatonin vs. placebo in the prophylaxis of cluster headache: a double-blind pilot study with parallel groups. Cephalalgia. 1996;16:494-6.
12. **Peres MF, Rozen TD.** Melatonin in the preventive treatment of chronic cluster headache. Cephalalgia. 2001;21:993-5.
13. **Limmroth V, Katsarav AZ, Fritsche G, et al.** Features in medication overuse headache following overuse of different acute headache drugs. Neurol. 2002;59:1011-4.
14. **Srikiatkhachorn A, Puanguiyom MS, Govitrapon P.** Plasticity of 5-HT^{2a} serotonin receptor in patients with analgesic-induced transformed migraine. Headache. 1998;38:534-9.

15. **Rome HP, Rome JD.** Limbicly augmented pain syndrome (LAPS): kindling, corti-colimbic, sensitization, and the conversions of affective and sensory symptoms in chronic pain disorders. Pain Med. 2000;1:7-23.

16. **Fields HF.** Pain modulation and headache. In: Goadsby PJ, Silberstein SD, eds. Headache. Boston: Butterworth-Heinemann; 1997:38-57.

17. **Tracy I, Ploghaus A, Gati JS, et al.** Imaging attentional modulation of pain in the periaqueductal gray in humans. J Neuroscience. 2002;22:2748-52.

18. **Ferrari MD, Roon KI, Lipton RB, et al.** Oral triptans (serotonin 5-HT$^{1b/1d}$ agonist) in acute migraine treatment: a meta-analysis of 53 trials. Lancet. 2001;358: 1668-75.

19. **Saper JR.** What matters is not the differences between triptans, but the differences between patients. Arch Neurol. 2001;58:1481-2.

20. **Silberstein SD, for the U.S. Headache Consortium.** Practice parameter: evidence-based guidelines for migraine headache (an evidence-based review). Report of the Quality Standards Subcommittee of the American Academy of Neurology. Neurol. 2000;55:754-62.

21. **Silberstein SD, Peres MF, Hopkins MM, et al.** Olanzapine in the treatment of refractory migraine and chronic daily headache. Headache. 2002;42:515-8.

22. **Saper JR, Lake AE 3rd, Cantrell DT, et al.** Chronic daily headache prophylaxis with tizanidine: a double-blind, placebo-controlled, multicenter outcome study. Headache. 2002;42:570-82.

23. **Argoff CE.** A focused review of the use of botulinum toxins for neuropathic pain. Clin J Pain. 2002;18:S177-S181.

24. **Nixdorf DR, Heo G, Major PW.** Randomized control trial of botulism toxin A for chronic myogenous orofacial pain. Pain. 2002;99:465-73.

25. **Saper JR, Lake AE III.** Borderline personality disorder and the chronic headache patient: review and management recommendations. Headache. 2002;42:663-74.

26. **Saper JR.** Chronic daily headache: a clinician's perspective. Headache. 2002;42:538.

27. **Dodick DW.** Suboccipital, subcutaneous stimulation for cluster headache. Personal communication, 2002.

28. **Boes CJ, Dodick DW.** Refining the clinical spectrum of chronic paroxysmal hemicrania: a review of 74 patients. Headache. 2002;42:699-708.

29. **Front CJ, Dodick DW, Bosch EP.** SUNCT responsive to gabapentin. Headache. 2002;42:525-6.

30. **Saper JR, Lake AE III, Hamel RL, et al.** Long-term scheduled opioid treatment for intractable headache: three-year outcome report. Cephalalgia. 2000;20:380.

31. **Saper JR, Lake AE 3rd, Hamel RL, et al.** Daily scheduled opioids for intractable head pain: long-term observations of a treatment program. Neurology. 2004; 62:1687-94.

32. **Mao J.** Opioid-induced abnormal pain sensitivity: implications in clinical opioid therapy. Pain. 2002;100:213-7.

33. **Lake AE III, Saper JR, Madden SF, Kreeger C.** Comprehensive inpatient treatment for intractable migraine: a prospective long-term outcome study. Headache. 1993;33:55-62.

34. **Saper JR, Lake AE III, Madden SF, Kreeger C.** Comprehensive/tertiary care for headache: a 6-month outcome study. Headache. 1999;39:249-63.

4

■ ■ ■

Osteoarthritis and Fibromyalgia

Daniel J. Clauw, MD

O steoarthritis and fibromyalgia are respectively the most common and second-most common rheumatological disorders. Both conditions should typically be diagnosed and managed initially by primary care physicians. However, although most primary care physicians are quite comfortable managing patients with osteoarthritis, most are considerably less comfortable diagnosing and treating fibromyalgia.

There are several reasons why many physicians are uncomfortable with managing fibromyalgia, but most center around the fact that this is a fundamentally different type of pain condition than most other types of chronic pain. In osteoarthritis, pain occurs because of damage and inflammation in the peripheral tissues, in and around the affected joint. Traditional analgesics (e.g., acetaminophen, NSAIDs, opioids) are thus generally effective in treating this type of pain. Moreover, when these therapies do not work, there are others that can address the underlying damage (e.g., arthroplasty) or inflammation (e.g., corticosteroid joint injection).

The pain in fibromyalgia, however, is not due to damage or inflammation of the muscles, joints, and soft tissues. Instead, in fibromyalgia and many other closely related syndromes (e.g., irritable bowel syndrome, temporomandibular joint syndrome, tension headache) the pain is due to an abnormality in how individuals transmit and respond to pain (1,2). A plethora of evidence now exists that the "gain" or "volume" in central pain processing is increased in these conditions, such that normally nonpainful stimuli are painful (allodynia) and normally painful stimuli are more painful (hyperalgesia).

The existence of allodynia and hyperalgesia in these conditions was originally discovered with experimental pain testing (i.e., asking individuals how painful stimuli are) but more recently has been corroborated by objective techniques such as functional imaging. These types of pain have been termed *central* or *non-nociceptive,* because the cause appears to be an abnormal processing of pain signals in the central nervous system, rather than ongoing nociceptive input (e.g., because of damage or inflammation) via sensory nerves. Because of this fundamental difference in pain transmission, the pharmacological therapies that work for fibromyalgia are not "classic" analgesics such as NSAIDs and opioids but neuroactive compounds such as norepinephrine and serotonin that modulate central concentrations of neurotransmitters involved in pain transmission.

Another inherent difference between nociceptive and non-nociceptive pain is that in the latter there is only a modest link between pain and function. For example, in osteoarthritis, studies typically show that when pain worsens, function worsens, and when therapies are given to improve pain, function subsequently improves (3). In fibromyalgia, however, this is less often the case; in many studies, symptoms such as pain are improved but there is no corresponding improvement in function (4). Thus non-pharmacological therapies such as cognitive behavioral therapy and exercise must frequently be combined with symptom-based pharmacological therapy to get meaningful improvements in fibromyalgia.

This chapter discusses and compares these two common chronic pain conditions. Their underlying mechanisms are examined, and the most effective treatments for each are reviewed.

Osteoarthritis

Epidemiology

Osteoarthritis (OA), also termed *degenerative joint disease* (*degenerative disc disease* when it occurs in the spine) is the most common rheumatological disease and the most common form of arthritis. Osteoarthritis is very uncommon in the young; its prevalence increases with age. For example, radiographic evidence of OA of the knee occurs in 27% of those less than age 70 and in 44% of those older than age 80 (5,6). The majority of individuals over age 65 have at least one joint affected by OA.

Etiology

The hallmarks of OA are destruction of cartilage (leading to loss of joint space) and periarticular new bone formation (osteophytes). Until relatively recently, OA had generally been considered a slowly progressive, noninflammatory disease. A more contemporary view is that neither is totally true. In contrast to a slow inexorable progression, many individuals have very stable periods of disease for long periods of time, whereas in others (especially those with obesity, generalized OA, malalignment, or synovitis), there is rapid deterioration of joint space or progression of osteophytic changes (7). There has also been a relatively recent recognition that OA may have a local inflammatory component in some individuals or in some phases of disease. This may be manifest on physical examination (e.g., by finding synovitis or a joint effusion) or with experimental techniques studying synovial fluid (e.g., finding elevated cytokines, metalloproteinases) (8).

Genetics clearly plays a role in OA. Certain subtypes of OA have a strong familial predisposition, such as "nodal" OA of the hands, typically noted in females of European descent. A number of genetic factors have been associated with OA, including genes coding for elements of collagen, synovium, or inflammatory mediators (e.g., IL-1). It is likely that genetic factors influence both the joint distribution of OA as well as the precise underlying cause (9,10).

In contrast to OA of the hands, where there are strong genetic factors in OA affecting other regions of the body, such as the weight-bearing joints of the lower extremities, environmental factors (e.g., obesity, trauma) appear to play a much stronger role in disease expression than genetic factors. Many risk factors for the development of OA have been identified. Perhaps the strongest is age, in that increasing age markedly increases the risk of OA. Obesity is the strongest modifiable risk factor because it is associated with both a higher risk of developing OA and an increased disease progression. The best estimates suggest that the odds ratio for developing OA increases 1.3 times for every ten pounds an individual is overweight (11). Injuries to the joint are also a significant risk for future development of OA, especially if there is concurrent ligament or meniscal damage. Finally, abnormalities of the surrounding tissues (e.g., lower extremity muscle weakness, joint laxity or malalignment) are also a risk factor for progression of OA.

Diagnosis

The diagnosis of OA should be considered in an individual who has pain and/or dysfunction isolated to the joint(s) that are considered to be affected. Osteoarthritis should not be considered as the primary diagnosis if the individual has widespread pain, prominent morning stiffness, or other chronic somatic symptoms.

A careful musculoskeletal history and examination remains the most important diagnostic test for musculoskeletal pain. In contrast to other fields of medicine, where proliferation in technology has largely rendered a physical examination obsolete, in musculoskeletal medicine advanced technology confuses as much as it helps. For example, a high proportion of the healthy, asymptomatic population has a positive antinuclear antibody, positive rheumatoid factor, or abnormal results of imaging studies (50% of individuals over age 60 will have one or more bulging disks on MRI).

The poor specificity and positive predictive value of diagnostic tests are particularly problematic in evaluating an individual for OA. Population-based studies suggest there is a significant disparity between the degree of radiographic OA and the pain and functional limitations that patients with this condition experience. The most dramatic evidence of this is that, in all population databases that have examined OA, between 30% and 60% of individuals with moderate-to-severe radiographic changes of OA are *totally asymptomatic* and approximately 10% of individuals with moderate-to-severe knee pain have normal radiographs (12,13). Some investigators have hypothesized that plain radiography only partly explains pain and other symptoms because this technique does not permit visualization of cartilage defects, bone marrow edema, and other lesions that may be causing pain. Early studies of this hypothesis lent it some support, but more recent studies suggest that although cartilage defects and so on can be detected with more sensitive imaging modalities (e.g., MRI), these modalities lack specificity in that the same abnormalities are likewise seen in a high proportion of the normal population where they do not consistently cause pain (14,15).

This disparity between "peripheral" features and symptoms has also caused investigators to explore the notion that psychological factors may be responsible for this discordance. Studies have suggested that psychological factors such as anxiety and depression account for some of this variance in pain and other symptoms but only to a small degree (16,17).

History

Osteoarthritis should not be considered a likely diagnosis in individuals less than age 40; its incidence begins to rise appreciably after age 50. The patient typically presents with pain involving the affected joint, typically pain that occurs with activity and improves with rest. There will not typically be significant (i.e., >30 minutes) morning stiffness, or redness or warmth of the joint; these are all symptoms of a more robust systemic inflammatory arthritis such as rheumatoid arthritis. A notable exception is a variant of OA of the hands termed *erosive osteoarthritis*. This is especially common in perimenopausal females, and the same joints are involved as in classic OA: the distal interphalangeal (outermost finger) joint, proximal interphalangeal joint (but not the metacarpal joints), and first carpometacarpal joint at the base of the thumb (18). Individuals with erosive OA typically have an early, active inflammatory stage of OA that lasts months-to-years, followed by the classic noninflammatory phase, with osteophytes and loss of joint spcace but no further evidence of inflammation.

Other common locations for OA include the hip (in many cases felt as groin pain), knee, and cervical and lumbar regions. There are certain joints of the body where it is extremely unusual to develop OA, unless there is a history of trauma, such as the elbow and shoulder.

Physical Examination

The most common finding on physical examination is an increase in joint size. The examination should determine if the increase in joint size is due to extra bone (osteophyte) formation (this feels firm to the touch and is not extremely tender) or to soft tissue swelling. Examples of the former are

Heberden's (distal interphalangeal) disease and Bouchard's disease (proximal interphalangeal) noted with "nodal" (hand) OA. The two classic causes of soft tissue swelling are joint effusion and swelling of the joint lining (synovitis). Joint effusions are frequently seen in OA, but signs of synovitis (warmth, redness, soft tissue swelling) are less common. When such features are present, other diagnostic tests (e.g., joint aspiration, sedimentation rate, C-reactive protein) should be performed to help exclude joint infection or systemic inflammatory disease.

An important element of the examination is assessing the patient for tenderness. There is no uniformly agreed upon technique, but it must be determined whether there is any tenderness and, if so, whether it is 1) localized, 2) widespread, or 3) only occurs with "provocative" maneuvers. In OA and other forms of arthritis, the individual will typically only be tender over the joint and will sometimes experience pain if the joint is actively or passively moved. Conditions other than OA have different patterns of tenderness. In regional inflammatory conditions such as bursitis, the individual will typically only be tender over the affected bursae, not the joint. In tendonitis, the tendon may be tender, but more typically the pain can be exacerbated by maneuvers that stretch or use the tendon. In myofascial pain, the individual is tender over an entire region of the body that is typically muscular, whereas in fibromyalgia the tenderness extends throughout the entire body.

The physical examination should also assess for the range of motion, and alignment, of the affected joints. Initially range of motion may only be slightly limited in the planes of initial involvement (e.g., internal rotation is often first noted in hip OA), but in later stages limitations in mobility may be marked.

Diagnostic Testing

Routine blood work is normal in OA. Although there is no evidence of systemic inflammation in OA (thus ESR and C-reactive protein are typically normal), increases in highly sensitive CRP has been shown to be predictive of OA progression (probably by identifying a subset of patients with local inflammatory OA) (19).

Plain radiography is the preferred diagnostic test for confirming the clinical diagnosis of OA. Weight-bearing films of weight-bearing joints are preferable, so that joint width can be more accurately assessed. Radiographs of affected joints will typically show loss of joint space and/or osteophyte formation (20). Other findings on radiographs can include cysts and subchondral sclerosis. Erosions are not typically seen (except in erosive OA) nor is periarticular osteoporosis. However, because of differences in positioning and magnification issues, routine clinical imaging techniques are not nearly sensitive enough to be performed serially to detect disease progression.

Other imaging studies such as MRI may be useful to detect earlier changes of OA (e.g., bone marrow edema) or other accompanying features that suggest an inflammatory component to the disease (e.g., synovitis, joint effusions) (21). MRI also has the advantage of detecting meniscal and ligamentous pathology and radiolucent loose bodies. Again, it is important to emphasize that any of these abnormalities identified in either plain radiography or MRI also commonly occur in many asymptomatic individuals in the population, so the history and physical examination must be consistent with the detected abnormalities in order to establish clinical relevance.

Differential Diagnosis

The precise evaluation of an individual with suspected OA depends largely on the clinical circumstances. For example, if a 70-year-old presents with a five-year history of slowly progressive pain and stiffness localized to his right knee, and the physical examination is normal or reveals only joint tenderness and bony enlargement, then a plain radiograph of the knee showing OA would be adequate to establish the diagnosis. However, a 34-year-old with subacute development of pain and swelling in several joints requires an entirely different approach, especially to rule out infectious or systemic inflammatory disorders. Along these lines, if a chronic effusion is detected, especially in the knee joint where aspiration is simple, the joint should be aspirated to verify a "noninflammatory" fluid (<1000 cell/mm^3) and the lack of crystals consistent with gout or "pseudo-gout" (calcium pyrophosphate deposition disease).

A key issue in considering the differential diagnosis of OA is that the latter frequently co-exists with other musculoskeletal conditions. Two that frequently overlap with OA are bursitis and myofascial pain/fibromyalgia. Co-morbid fibromyalgia is relatively easy to identify because both pain and tenderness have a wider distribution than just the joint. However, the distinction between OA and bursitis is more subtle; both present with localized tenderness because bursae are commonly adjacent to joints. If a careful examination is not performed and bursitis is not identified, and subsequent radiography shows OA of the affected joint, then the individual will be diagnosed with OA and the offending cause of the pain (bursitis) will not be appropriately treated (e.g., by a corticosteroid injection).

In the hip region, trochanteric bursitis frequently simulates symptoms of hip OA. Symptoms include constant or intermittent hip pain, but patients typically also will be unable to sleep on the side at night because of local tenderness over the greater trochanter. Physical examination will detect this tenderness, located in the lateral-most area of the hip region. Anserine bursitis can simulate knee OA and can be detected by identifying tenderness on the medial aspect of the knee 2 to 3 cm below the joint line (where the knee bends).

Treatment

Because OA is a chronic disease, treatments must be given for long periods of time and the cumulative side effects of any therapy must be weighed against the benefits. Because of this, a number of expert guidelines have been published emphasizing a "stepped approach" wherein every patient initially receives therapies that have moderate efficacy and negligible toxicity (e.g., exercise, acetaminophen) and the small number of individuals who fail to respond to these therapies move on to receive more aggressive treatments (22-24).

Non-Pharmacological Therapy

EXERCISE

Aerobic and strengthening exercises have been shown to be of value in improving both pain and function in OA, especially of the knees and hips. Two recent Cochrane reviews of this topic suggest that both types of exercise can be efficacious in OA, with each displaying modest effects (25,26). High and low intensity aerobic exercises seem to be equally useful, and the gains are equal when exercise is performed in a group versus individual format. Strengthening exercises of the quadriceps muscle may be especially helpful for individuals with a history suggesting patellofemoral involvement (e.g., symptoms primarily with getting out of a chair, walking up and down stairs).

The biggest problem with using exercise as a therapeutic modality for OA or other chronic diseases is not that it does not work (it does), but that patients are unlikely to comply long-term with exercise programs (27). Because of this, newer exercise programs that combine cognitive behavioral approaches that increase compliance, motivation, and so on are gaining favor, such as those offered by the Arthritis Foundation.

COGNITIVE BEHAVIORAL THERAPY

Cognitive behavioral therapy (CBT) consists of a program of education and skills training that has been used for many chronic illnesses, especially those characterized by chronic pain. Biofeedback, relaxation, pacing, and cognitive restructuring are examples of CBT. These techniques are designed to allow patients with chronic conditions to gain control over their lives. Even without great reduction in pain, patients learn to accept limitations and move toward meaningful, productive lives. Like exercise, these programs have consistently been shown modestly efficacious for the treatment of OA (28).

COMPLEMENTARY AND ALTERNATIVE THERAPIES

Several complementary and alternative therapies have been shown to be effective in OA The most popular and best supported by evidence is the use of oral glucosamine and/or chondroitin sulfate (discussed below). There is some evidence to support the use of acupuncture in OA, with one meta-analysis suggesting efficacy and others suggesting inconclusive data (29). Other therapies with modest evidence of efficacy include devil's claw, avocado/soybean oils, and SAMe (30).

Pharmacological Therapy

TOPICAL AGENTS

A number of topical compounds have been shown to improve pain associated with OA of the knee, including capsaicin, as well as other irritants or heat-producing substances.

ACETAMINOPHEN (OR PARACETAMOL)

In general, acetaminophen (or paracetamol) is recommended as first-line therapy for OA, especially if an individual has intermittent symptoms and no findings suggesting a local inflammatory element to their disease. Because of the relatively recent recognition that acetaminophen may have more GI toxicity than originally suspected (at doses of >2 g/day) and may be toxic in combination with alcohol and other hepatotoxic drugs, alternatives should be considered in some instances.

NONSTEROIDAL ANTI-INFLAMMATORY DRUGS

Enthusiasm regarding the use of NSAIDs in OA has waxed and waned over the years. Early studies suggested that NSAIDs and acetaminophen were of similar efficacy in OA, but because acetaminophen is better tolerated, until recently treatment guidelines discouraged the initial use of NSAIDs (31,32). Subsequent developments that favored NSAID use over acetaminophen included

1. Studies suggesting that acetaminophen may have more side effects than previously thought
2. Studies showing that many patients with OA had better relief of symptoms with NSAIDs than acetaminophen
3. Development of selective COX-2 specific NSAIDs with decreased toxicity profiles (33,34)

However, the early use of COX-2 selective NSAIDs has been reconsidered given recent data suggesting that COX-2 agents have only modest GI safety advantages over older nonselective NSAIDs and may increase cardiovascular events in some individuals. Furthermore, it has not been conclusively proved that NSAIDS (either COX-2 selective or nonselective) are superior to acetaminophen for OA pain relief.

Choosing a nonselective over a selective COX-2 inhibitor remains controversial, but a few points bear mention:

1. COX-2 inhibitors have never been shown more efficacious than nonselective inhibitors, only to have a better GI toxicity profile.
2. In individuals without risk factors for NSAID-induced gastropathy (e.g., elderly, previous PUD or medication use for PUD), there is no rationale for using a COX-2 over a nonselective COX inhibitor.
3. Individuals with cardiovascular risks that need aspirin for its antiplatelet effects need to take ASA in addition to COX-2 inhibitors

(and perhaps also if they are taking nonselective NSAIDs) to confer the same benefit.

GLUCOSAMINE AND CHONDROITIN SULFATE

Glucosamine and chondroitin sulfate have been shown to be effective in the treatment of pain associated with OA. In general, these drugs take longer to act than acetaminophen or NSAIDs and last longer once they are discontinued. The aggregate data collected on these compounds suggest that their effect lies between the aforementioned classes of compounds (i.e., acetaminophen < glucosamine/chondroitin < NSAIDs) as well as in tolerability (i.e., acetaminophen ≥ glucosamine/chondroitin > NSAIDs). Although early studies suggested a cartilage-sparing effect, subsequent trials have not confirmed this finding, and most feel that these compounds are exerting an analgesic effect in OA.

OTHER ANALGESICS

If the above agents are ineffective, other classes of analgesics can be used to treat OA. Both tramadol and weak opioids, either alone or in combination with acetaminophen, can be useful adjuncts in the treatment of chronic OA pain, especially as "as needed" medications.

Injections

CORTICOSTEROIDS

Injection of corticosteroids into joints affected by OA is an established tool in clinical use. A recent meta-analysis suggests that this treatment is more effective than placebo at one week, but that the effect may not exceed placebo at four weeks (35). Although there are no collaborative data, most physicians will only perform corticosteroid joint injections every 3 to 4 months because of anecdotal reports of acceleration of joint damage with this treatment.

HYALURONIC ACID DERIVATIVES

Several hyaluronic acid derivatives are approved for injection in OA of the knee. These must be given by repeated injections, and recent meta-analyses have suggested that the efficacy of this therapy barely exceeds that of placebo injection (36). Because of the cost and modest incremental benefit of this therapy, it is typically reserved for patients who are not surgical candidates or who are attempting to avoid surgery.

Surgical Therapy

Although there are few data to guide clinicians regarding the optimal timing for surgical therapy in OA, several general guidelines may be helpful. The majority of those who have total arthroplasty for OA of the knee or hip do very well (90% rated good or very good at five years) (37).

Arthroplasty involving other joints is generally somewhat less successful in terms of short- and long-term outcomes but should still be considered. Older individuals (≥80) typically have worse disease at the time of hip or knee arthroplasty, and they note the smallest health gains after surgery. However, younger individuals (or those who are more active) are more likely to need early replacement or revision (i.e., earlier than the expected 10 to 15 year lifespan) of artificial joints. Thus the ideal time to refer for surgery for OA is

1. When the condition is disabling enough that the risk of surgery is justified

2. Not so early that the individual will wear out the prosthesis (and a subsequent replacement) before the end of their life span

3. Not so late that comorbidities will unduly decrease the efficacy of the procedure (e.g., by interfering with rehabilitation) or increase the complications

When to Refer

The primary considerations for referral of the OA patient are to establish the original diagnosis and when surgical or other specialized interventions are being considered. Any number of specialists, including rheumatologists, orthopedists, and others, can assist with the diagnosis of OA in complicated cases. For treatment of established OA, the simplest rule for referral to an orthopedist, physiatrist, or other OA specialist is that the patient is failing to respond adequately to current therapy. Indications for referral to a surgeon have been described in the preceding section.

Future Developments

There are many exciting developments in OA research:

- *Disease-Modifying Drugs*—All of the available pharmacological treatments for OA treat its *symptoms,* but none modify the course of the *underlying disease*. Many classes of drugs are being developed to modify the disease processes. Some of these therapies are aimed at improving the health of subchondral bone, whereas others inhibit enzymes or cytokines that may be causing joint damage. When these drugs are developed, it may be possible to use one class of drug to prevent OA or reverse disease progression and another to treat pain and associated symptoms.

- *Local Biological Therapies*—At present small cartilage defects can be repaired using autologous cells, but the need for two surgeries, and the lack of data regarding long-term efficacy, limit the use of this technique for classic OA. Nonetheless, the proliferation of knowledge in organogenesis and the fact that diseased joints are easily accessible by noninvasive surgeries make OA a perfect candidate for targeted local biological therapies. For example, increases in our understanding of the underlying disease pathophysiology will likely lead to logical targets for local gene therapy for OA (i.e., injected into the affected joint).

- *Biomarkers*—At present there are no biomarkers that can detect the presence or activity of disease, but several substances (e.g., assays for type II collagen synthesis and breakdown) are being studied as potential markers for those at risk for more aggressive OA.

Fibromyalgia

Although the terms we presently use to describe fibromyalgia (FM) are relatively new, the condition is not. For centuries in the medical literature, there have been descriptions of symptom complexes nearly identical to those we now label *fibromyalgia*. Many terms previously used to describe this condition, such as *myofibrositis* or *fibrositis,* were attempts to link the symptom complex to an underlying pathophysiological process. The more generic term we now use to describe this illness reflects the recognition that we know what does *not* cause fibromyalgia, not what *does*. We are fairly certain that there is no *-itis* (i.e., inflammation) of the muscles in FM, and that it is not simply "in the minds" of those afflicted (4).

Nonetheless, the mere existence of FM remains controversial. Some contend that it is a "wastebasket" term to describe patients who otherwise defy explanation, and others suggest that these are primary psychiatric conditions. There are valid arguments refuting many of the current concepts of the definition and pathogenic mechanisms of this illness. However, there is no refuting the existence of large numbers of individuals who suffer from chronic diffuse pain.

Epidemiology

Population-based studies of chronic widespread pain (CWP) have suggested that approximately 10-11% of the population has this symptom at any given time (38,39). Chronic regional pain is found in 20-25% of the population (40). Both chronic widespread and regional pain occur about 1½ times as commonly in women than men.

The 1990 American College of Rheumatology (ACR) criteria for FM require that an individual have both a history of CWP and a finding of 11 of 18 possible tender points on examination (41). Tender points are present in nine paired regions of the body, and if an individual reports pain when these regions are palpated with 4 kg of pressure, this is considered a positive tender point. Using the ACR criteria, the prevalence of FM in industrialized countries has been reported to range from 0.5% to 4% of the population (38,42).

Even though women are only 1½ times as likely to experience CWP as men, they are about ten times as likely to meet criteria for FM. This gender differential for CWP and FM is solely due to the ACR criteria requiring 11 of 18 tender points. Because men are inherently less tender, the finding of ≥11 tender points occurs eleven times more commonly in women than in men (40,42).

The tender-point requirement of the ACR criteria not only causes FM to become almost exclusively a female disorder but also skews FM patients towards displaying high levels of distress. Distress is typically operationalized as some combination of somatic symptoms and symptoms of anxiety/depression. Wolfe said it best when he commented that because of the association between tender points and distress in population-based studies, tender points are a "sedimentation rate for distress" (43). Until recently it had been assumed that because tender points were associated with distress, tenderness (an individual's innate sensitivity to mechanical pressure) was associated with distress (44,45). However, recent studies have suggested that other measures of tenderness are not at all related to measures of distress, just to tender points (46,47). Tender points probably do not accurately assess the tenderness of individuals, because individuals know how much pressure will be applied; individuals who are anxious or "expectant" have a tendency to "bail out" as predictable pressure is applied, because they do not want to experience even brief pain. More sophisticated measures of tenderness that administer stimuli in a random, unpredictable fashion, yield results that are totally independent of psychological status. Thus, eliminating the requirement for 11 of 18 tender points from the FM criteria would lead to a totally different disorder: one affecting far more men, with the group displaying considerably lower levels of distress.

The relationship between FM and distress is not solely due to tender points. CWP alone is somewhat associated with distress (44,48). (This is discussed in detail later in this chapter.) In addition, many individuals with CWP have other somatic symptoms such as fatigue and memory difficulties. This clustering of somatic symptoms in the population gives rise to overlapping syndromes such as fibromyalgia, chronic fatigue syndrome, multiple chemical sensitivity, and somatoform disorders (Fig. 4-1) (49). Population-based studies have been performed using factor analytic techniques to identify the seminal features of these conditions; in such studies the key symptoms that co-aggregate are multifocal pain, fatigue, memory difficulties, and mood disturbances (50). The term *chronic multi-symptom illnesses* (CMI) has been coined by investigators from the Centers for Disease Control and Prevention to describe this symptom complex (51,52).

Population-based studies of individual symptoms (e.g., pain, fatigue) suggest that the greater the number of co-aggregated symptoms, the more

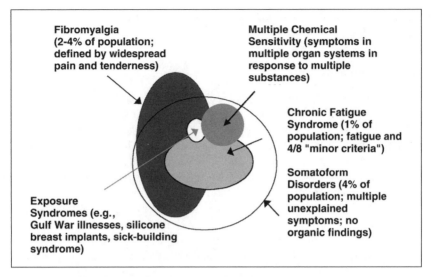

Figure 4-1   Examples of overlapping systemic syndromes characterized by otherwise unexplained chronic pain and fatigue.

unlikely it is that the syndrome will resolve long-term and the more likely that the individual will seek health care (48,53). Other factors that predict the development or persistence of either widespread or regional pain include higher age, a family history of chronic pain, low social support, being an immigrant, being in a lower socioeconomic class, and performing manual labor (54-57).

It is important to note that all of the aforementioned relationships between CWP and other somatic symptoms, as well as distress, also hold true for regional pain syndromes. Chronic low back pain (LBP) has been the best studied in this regard, and it is known that distress can lead to LBP, LBP can lead to distress, and LBP plus other somatic symptoms is less likely to resolve (58). Other relationships have been demonstrated with other regional pain syndromes, with the strongest relationships occurring in other axial (i.e., shoulder, neck) structures (54-56,59).

Pathogenesis and Etiology

Research has indicated a familial component to the development of FM, because family members of FM patients display a higher risk for FM—as well as for common overlapping conditions—than seen in the general population (1,60,61). The same high family history of these related conditions has been noted in most conditions that fall within this spectrum. This co-aggregation of conditions, which include, for example, FM, chronic fatigue syndrome (CFS), irritable bowel syndrome (IBS), and migraine and tension headaches, was originally collectively termed *affective spectrum disorder*

(60) and more recently *central sensitivity syndromes* (62) and *chronic multi-symptom illnesses.*

Environmental Stressors

As with most illnesses that may have a genetic underpinning, environmental factors also may play a prominent role in triggering the development of FM and related conditions. Environmental "stressors" temporally associated with the development of FM or CFS include physical (and particularly skeletal) trauma, certain infections (e.g., hepatitis C, Epstein-Barr virus, parvovirus, Lyme disease), emotional stress, and other regional pain conditions or autoimmune disorders (60,62-64).

An excellent recent example of how illnesses such as FM might be triggered occurred in the Gulf War in 1990 and 1991. The term *Gulf War illnesses* is now commonly used to refer to a constellation of symptoms developed by some 5-15% of the 700,000 U.S. troops deployed to the Persian Gulf in the early 1990s. The symptoms, which include headaches, muscle and joint pain, fatigue, memory disorders, and gastrointestinal (GI) distress (52,65), were seen in troops deployed from the United Kingdom as well (66). The panels of experts who examined potential causes for these symptoms and syndromes found that the sickness could not be traced to any single environmental trigger, and noted the similarities between these individuals and those diagnosed with FM and CFS. The prevailing theory is that during the Gulf War (as well as any other war) individuals were simultaneously exposed to multiple "stressors", and that some of these individuals went on to develop FM or similar syndromes in association with such stressors (67).

Once FM develops, the mechanisms responsible for ongoing symptom expression are likely complex and multifactorial. Because disparate "stressors" can seemingly trigger the development of these conditions, "human stress response" has been closely examined for a causative role. These systems are mediated primarily by the activity of the corticotropin-releasing hormone (CRH) nervous system located in the hypothalamus and locus-ceruleus-norepinephrine/autonomic (sympathetic/LC-NE) nervous system in the brain stem. Recent research suggests that although this system in humans has been highly adaptive, the stress response may be inappropriately triggered by a wide assortment of everyday occurrences that do not pose a real threat to survival, thus initiating the cascade of physiological responses more frequently than can be tolerated (68).

The type of stress and the environment in which it occurs also have an impact on how the stress response is expressed. It has been noted that victims of accidents experience a higher frequency of FM and myofascial pain than those who cause them, which is congruent with animal studies showing that that the strongest physiological responses are triggered by events that are accompanied by a lack of control or support and thus perceived as inescapable or unavoidable (68-70). In humans, daily "hassles" and personally relevant stressors seem to be more capable of causing symptoms than major catastrophic events that do not personally affect the individual (71,72).

These theoretical links between neural stress systems and symptom expression have generally been supported by studies demonstrating alterations of the HPA axis and the sympathetic nervous system (73-80). However, no consistent HPA or autonomic abnormality can be found in the majority of patients with this spectrum of illness. It is plausible that alterations of these stress-response systems identify a population vulnerable to the development of FM. Alternatively, altered neuroendocrine axis activity could cause or occur as a consequence of some FM symptoms. It is likely that these neurobiological alterations are shared with other poorly understood somatic syndromes and psychiatric disorders that frequently co-occur with FM.

Abnormalities in Pain Processing Systems

The most consistently detected objective abnormalities in FM have been involving pain processing systems. Because FM is defined in part by tenderness, considerable work has been performed exploring the potential reason for this phenomenon. One of the earliest findings in this regard was that the tenderness in FM is not confined to tender points but instead extends throughout the entire body (81). Theoretically, such diffuse tenderness could be either primarily due to psychological (e.g., hypervigilance, where individuals are too attentive to their surroundings) or neurobiological (e.g., the plethora of factors that can lead to temporary or permanent amplification of sensory input) factors. Two decades of experimental pain studies in FM have yielded the following conclusions:

1. Fibromyalgia patients cannot *detect* electrical, pressure, or thermal stimuli at lower levels than normals, but the point at which these stimuli *cause* pain or unpleasantness is lower (82).

2. These findings are noted even when stimuli are presented in a random, unpredictable fashion, suggesting that psychological factors such as hypervigilance play a minor role in modulating tenderness (47).

Experimental pain testing has also been used to look for evidence of possible mechanisms of the widespread allodynia and hyperalgesia seen in FM. Such studies have suggested that there may be evidence of a decrease in neural signals that descend from the brainstem, and normally inhibit the upward transmission of pain (70,83). Other studies using different techniques demonstrate that patients with FM exhibit altered temporal summation of pain stimuli administered as a thermal stimulus to skin or as a mechanical stimulus to muscle (84,85). These studies suggest a parallel between the human condition of FM and the "wind-up" phenomenon that leads to hyperalgesia and allodynia that has been extensively studied in animal models (86).

Other data corroborating the veracity of FM patient pain complaints have been collected using paradigms that are not dependent on subjective reports of patients. For example, Lorenz et al demonstrated altered laser-evoked potentials as objective representation of the CNS response to cutaneous stimulation (87). Functional imaging or positron emission tomography, extensively reviewed by Bradley, has been instructive in pain syndromes in general and in FM in particular. Mountz et al were the first to demonstrate reduced thalamic blood flow under resting conditions (a finding noted in other chronic pain states) (88); their findings have been replicated by a different group (89). A recent study by Gracely and colleagues using functional MRI demonstrated that the amount of pressure stimuli required to cause cerebral activation in pain processing regions of the brain (i.e., the primary and secondary somatosensory cortices) was much lower in FM patients than in healthy controls (90). This study has likewise been replicated both with pressure and heat stimuli (91,92).

Biochemical studies performed on samples from FM patients also support the notion that there are central changes in pain processing that may be due to either high levels of pro-nociceptive peptides or low levels of anti-nociceptive peptides. For example, several studies have shown that patients with FM have approximately three-fold higher concentrations of substance P in cerebral spinal fluid (CSF) compared with normal controls (93-96). (Substance P is a neurotransmitter that has pro-inflammatory characteristics in the periphery. It can transmit pain messages in the dorsal horn and becomes active in sustaining pain in chronic pain conditions.) Other chronic pain syndromes, such as OA of the hip and chronic low back pain, are also associated with elevated substance P levels, although CFS (which is not defined on the basis of pain) is not (97). Interestingly, once elevated, Substance P levels do not appear to change dramatically, and also do not become elevated in response to acute painful stimuli. Thus high substance P appears to be a biological marker for the presence of chronic pain.

Other studies have shown that the principal metabolite of norepinephrine, 3-methoxy-4-hydroxyphenethylene (MPHG), is lowered in CSF of FM patients (98). This finding is important for two reasons:

1. A reduction of norepinephrine-mediated pain-inhibitory pathways that descend to the spinal cord may be a potential mechanism for causing the allodynia and hyperalgesia associated with FM.

2. Some of the most effective drug therapies for FM provide augmentation of central adrenergic activity.

Serotonin levels may also be diminished in patients with this spectrum of disorders. Studies by Russell et al (98) and Yunus et al (99) have demonstrated reduced levels of serotonin and its precursor, L-tryptophan, in the blood serum of patients with FM, as well as reduced levels of the principal metabolite 5-HIAA in CSF, all of which suggest that defective serotonin synthesis or metabolism could be a feature of FM, at least in a subset of patients.

Behavioral and Psychological Factors

In addition to neurobiological mechanisms, behavioral and psychological factors play a role in symptom expression in many FM patients. The rate of current psychiatric co-morbidity in patients with FM may be as high as 30-60% in tertiary care settings, and the rate of lifetime psychiatric disorders may be even higher (100,101). Depression and anxiety disorders are the most commonly seen. However, recent data suggest that this high rate of co-morbid mood disorders is partly an artifact of studying these conditions in tertiary care samples. Individuals who meet ACR criteria for FM who are identified in the general population do not have nearly this high a rate of identifiable psychiatric conditions (102,103).

As already noted, population-based studies have demonstrated that distress can lead to pain, and pain to distress. The presence of tender points is associated with higher levels of distress; however, CWP in and of itself may be associated with distress. Individuals with CWP are somewhat more likely to have high levels of distress, and individuals with high levels of distress are more likely to have CWP (104). Recent longitudinal studies have even shown that this may be a bi-directional *causal* relationship rather than just an association, because individuals identified as having only CWP or distress at a particular time are more likely to develop the other symptom if followed longitudinally. However, these associations are modest. There are far more psychologically "normal" individuals who develop CWP than distressed/depressed people who do, and there are far more CWP patients who do not develop distress/depression than who do (104,105). Nevertheless, in instances in which pain leads to distress, a typical pattern is that, as a result of pain and other symptoms of FM, individuals begin to function less well. They may have difficulties with spouses, children, and work inside or outside the home, all of which exacerbate symptoms and lead to maladaptive illness behaviors. These include isolation, cessation of pleasurable activities, and reductions in activity and exercise. In the worst cases, patients become involved with disability and compensation systems, which almost ensures that they will not improve (106).

The complex interaction of biological, behavioral, and psychological mechanisms is not, however, unique to FM. Non-biological factors play a prominent role in symptom expression in all rheumatic diseases. In fact, in conditions such as RA and OA, non-biological factors such as level of formal education, coping strategies, and socioeconomic variables account for more of the variance in pain report and disability than biologic factors such as the joint space width or sedimentation rate (107,108).

Diagnosis

History

Although both pain and tenderness are defining features of FM, the latter is rarely a presenting complaint. The pain of FM frequently waxes and wanes, may be quite migratory, and may be accompanied by dysesthesias or paresthesias following a nondermatomal distribution. In some instances patients will present with "aching all over", whereas in other instances patients experience several areas of chronic regional pain. In this setting, regional musculoskeletal pain typically involves the axial skeleton, or areas of tender points, and may originally be diagnosed as a local problem (e.g., low back pain, lateral epicondylitis). Regional pain involving non-musculoskeletal regions is also common, including a higher-than-expected prevalence of tension and migraine headaches, temporomandibular disorder (TMD or TMJ) syndrome, noncardiac chest pain, irritable bowel syndrome, a number of entities characterized by chronic pelvic pain, and plantar or heel pain.

In addition to pain and tenderness, most individuals with this illness experience a high lifetime and current prevalence of nondefining symptoms (Fig. 4-2). For example, most patients with FM experience fatigue, and at least half of individuals who meet ACR criteria for FM will also meet criteria for chronic fatigue syndrome (CFS). The fatigue is commonly worse after activities, and may be accompanied by memory difficulties. Memory difficulties, especially with attention and short-term memory, may be the most debilitating aspect of their illness (109). Other constitutional symptoms include fluctuations in weight, heat and cold intolerance, and the subjective sensation of weakness.

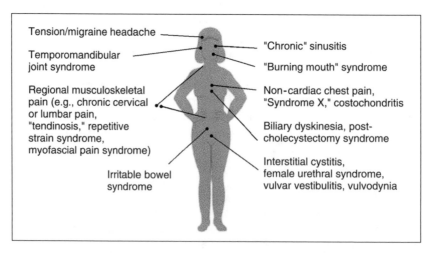

Figure 4-2 Examples of chronic regional pain syndromes where "peripheral" factors (e.g., inflammation, damage to tissues) play a minor or no role in pain.

Patients with FM and related illnesses also display a wide array of "allergic" symptoms, ranging from adverse reactions to drugs and environmental stimuli (as seen in multiple chemical sensitivity), to higher-than-expected incidences of rhinitis, nasal congestion, and lower respiratory symptoms. Although some of these individuals may truly be atopic, many of these symptoms are due to neural (e.g., hypersensitivities, vasomotor rhinitis) mechanisms. Hearing, ocular, and vestibular abnormalities have also been noted, including a high incidence of sicca symptoms, a decreased painful sound threshold, exaggerated nystagmus and ocular dysmotility, and asymptomatic low-frequency sensorineural hearing loss.

Individuals with FM likewise suffer from a number of symptoms of "functional" disorders of visceral organs, including a high incidence of recurrent noncardiac chest pain, heartburn, palpitations, and irritable bowel symptoms. However, prospective studies of randomly selected individuals with FM have detected a high frequency of *objective* evidence of dysfunction of several visceral organs, including echocardiographic evidence of mitral valve prolapse, esophageal dysmotility, and diminished static inspiratory and expiratory pressures on pulmonary function testing. Neurally mediated hypotension, postural orthostatic tachycardia, and syncope also occur more frequently in these individuals. Similar syndromes characterized by visceral pain and/or smooth muscle dysmotility are also seen in the pelvis, including dysmenorrhea, urinary frequency, and urinary urgency, interstitial cystitis, endometriosis, and vulvar vestibulitis or vulvodynia.

Physical Examination
The physical examination in FM is typically normal, except for the finding of tenderness. The tenderness may be virtually anywhere, not just confined to tender points. Although performing a formal tender point count may be useful, it is not essential, because the FM criteria that require 11 or greater (out of a possible 18) tender points were never intended to be used to diagnose individual patients. In fact, most experts in the field estimate that <50% of individuals who have the clinical diagnosis of FM will meet the ACR criteria, largely because many individuals (especially men with FM) do not have at least 11 tender points.

Diagnostic Testing
Considerable clinical judgment is necessary to determine the appropriate diagnostic evaluation for an individual with CWP. For example, three individuals with the same complaints, but who present with six weeks, six months, and six years of symptoms, would require quite different diagnostic work-ups. In general, the individual with the most acute or subacute symptoms generally warrants the most aggressive diagnostic evaluation, whereas an individual with chronic waxing and waning symptoms for many years but a normal physical examination is unlikely to have an unrecognized

autoimmune, hormonal, malignant, or infectious disease, and thus the evaluation can be more limited.

A common problem with diagnostic testing in the chronic pain patient is that of false-positive diagnostic tests. This is true for laboratory testing as well as imaging studies. Antinuclear antibodies are a good example of this problem. As many as 30% of the population may have a 1:40 antinuclear antibody or higher (110), but only 1:2000 individuals has SLE. Therefore less than 1/100 individuals in the population with a positive ANA will have SLE. The same conundrum holds true for rheumatoid factor and many other diagnostic tests. Because FM is several orders of magnitude more common then these autoimmune disorders, ordering such testing in individuals with chronic regional or widespread pain and other common somatic symptoms will lead to much higher rates or false-positive than true-positive tests.

Differential Diagnosis

Disorders that can simulate FM are listed in Table 4-1. The two conditions that arguably most closely simulate FM are hypothyroidism and polymyalgia rheumatica. For this reason, a TSH and ESR are suggested in every person in whom the diagnosis of FM is being entertained. Because FM occurs less frequently in males than females, some have suggested that a further work-up may be in order when a male presents with symptoms consistent with FM. Examples of entities simulating FM that occur more commonly in males are sleep apnea and hepatitis C infection.

Treatment

Fibromyalgia must be managed as a chronic illness. Treatment approaches should include pharmacologic and nonpharmacologic management of symptoms and, importantly, patient education about the nature and course of the illness.

Once this diagnosis (or a similar one) is considered, the practitioner should schedule a prolonged visit, or a series of visits. This "front-loading" of time pays tremendous long-term dividends for both the practitioner and patient. It is necessary for the physician to understand precisely what is

Table 4-1   Conditions That Simulate Fibromyalgia

Common	Less Common
• Hypothyroidism	• Autoimmune disorders (e.g., SLE, RA)
• Polymyalgia rheumatica	• Endocrine disorders (e.g., Addison's disease, Cushing's syndrome, hyperparathyroidism)
• Hepatitis C	
• Sleep apnea	
• Cervical stenosis/Chiari malformation	

bothering the patient, and for the patient to understand the goals of, and rationale for, treatment. In these visits it is important to explore the symptoms the individual is experiencing, the impact they are having on his life, his perception of what is causing the symptoms, and the stressors that may be exacerbating the illness. Once this has been accomplished, the patient should be educated as to the nondestructive nature of this condition, as well as to the fact that meaningful improvement rarely occurs without active participation on his part (i.e., there is no "magic bullet"). The savvy practitioner will soon realize that "labelling" the various disease processes may sometimes be helpful in accomplishing these goals, whereas in other instances such labels are unnecessary and could even be harmful, although there are no data to support this (111,112).

For patients with mild symptoms, such counseling, along with intermittent analgesic therapy, is often enough. For patients whose symptoms are pronounced enough to limit daily function, more aggressive therapy is typically necessary, in many cases using combinations of pharmacological and nonpharmacological approaches. Patients with FM should also be given reputable sources of information from reputable patient advocacy groups (http://www.fmaware.org, www.fmnetnews.com) or academic sites (www.med.umich.edu/painresearch).

Pharmacological Therapy

Several meta-analyses have concluded that the best supported pharmacological therapy for FM is low doses of tricyclic antidepressants (113,114). Tricyclic antidepressants such as amitriptyline and cyclobenzaprine have been effective in treating the pain associated with FM, especially when tolerance-promoting strategies are used (see below) (115,116). This class of compounds has also demonstrated efficacy on co-morbid conditions, including tension and migraine headaches, IBS, and noncardiac chest pain. Tricyclic antidepressants provide the added benefit of improved sleep patterns in patients with disrupted sleep.

Not all tricyclic drugs are of equal efficacy in FM, or in other pain states. Compounds that raise both serotonin and norepinephrine seem to be the most effective. Cyclobenzaprine and amitriptyline are two such tricyclic agents, and have been the best studied in the treatment of FM. No difference has been found in effectiveness between the agents (116). However, the clinical trials performed to date only demonstrate short-term benefits, because neither agent has been shown superior to placebo at six months of study. This could represent tachyphylaxis to these drugs but is more likely due to these studies being under-powered and not designed to administer the optimal dose of the drug.

One prominent issue in the use of tricyclic compounds has been determining the optimal dosage for each individual. Because tolerance to these drugs is problematic, it is recommended to initiate treatment at low doses of 10 mg or less several hours before bedtime, with slow (10 mg every week or two) increases until an optimal dose is achieved (up to 40 mg of cyclobenzaprine or 70 to 80 mg of amitriptyline).

Because of a better side effect profile, newer antidepressants are frequently used in FM. The selective serotonin reuptake inhibitors (SSRIs) have been extensively studied, with conflicting results (117-119). It appears that the SSRIs most selective for increasing serotonin (e.g., citalopram) are the least effective in treating pain. In contrast, less selective SSRIs that have some noradrenergic activity, such as fluoxetine and paroxetine, have been shown to be more effective in pain states, especially at higher doses that may be more noradrenergic. Because of recurring evidence that mixed serotinergic/noradrenergic compounds are the most effective in central pain states, compounds such as venlafaxine are used frequently in FM (e.g., beginning at 37.5 mg once in the morning and slowly escalating), and new compounds such as duloxetine and milnacipran are being tested in these conditions. Patients who do not completely respond to treatment with tricyclic antidepressants may therefore benefit from the addition of a SSRI or mixed noradrenergic/serotinergic reuptake inhibitor (e.g., venlafaxine) during the day.

It is important to note that although pain and depression frequently co-occur, and some classes of antidepressants are effective in treating FM and other central pain states, that the causes of pain and depression are not one and the same. There are ample data in the scientific literature that the sensory and affective aspects of pain are independently processed in the brain. This is not just of theoretical interest: Different pharmacological therapies differently influence the sensory and affective dimensions of pain (120). Within the class of antidepressants, some are relatively efficacious analgesics whereas others are not (121). The effects of antidepressants appear to be largely independent of mood, because *a*) antidepressant effects and analgesic effects typically occur independently of each other in clinical trials; and *b*) doses of antidepressants necessary to produce analgesia are, in many cases, lower than the dosages required to treat MDD (113,122-125).

Pain management may also be achieved in FM patients with the use of tramadol; there also is (again only anecdotal) evidence that high doses of gabapentin can be helpful. No data suggest that opioids are effective in treating non-nociceptive pain conditions such as FM, so these should be used judiciously, but they may be helpful for refractory pain.

Other medications can be used to treat specific residual symptoms. For example, fatigue is a significant problem in this spectrum of illnesses. In a review of the various pharmacological treatments used for fatigue across medical conditions, Guymer et al. concluded that classes of compounds that raise central levels of norepinephrine or dopamine appear to be the most specific for management of fatigue (126). Cognitive dysfunction, a significant problem in some individuals with FM (109), may respond to similar classes of drugs. For insomnia, individuals who do not tolerate tricyclic drugs may benefit from alternatives such as trazadone, zolpidem, or clonazepam. A subset of FM patients with features of autonomic dysfunction, including those who may have neurally mediated hypotension, may benefit from the use of low-dose beta-blockers and/or increased fluid and sodium/potassium intake.

Non-Pharmacological Therapy.

One of the biggest mistakes made in clinical practice in treating FM and similar conditions is the under-utilization of non-pharmacological therapies. Although medications can help improve the *symptoms* of FM such as pain and fatigue, non-pharmacological therapies are more likely to improve the *dysfunction* imposed by these illnesses. When individuals are treated with combinations of symptom-based pharmacological therapy, and also use non-pharmacological therapies to improve function as well as symptoms, a more meaningful improvement is typical.

The two best studied non-pharmacological therapies are cognitive behavioral therapy (CBT) and exercise. Both have been shown efficacious in the treatment of FM, as well as a plethora of other medical conditions (127-133). Both can lead to sustained (e.g., greater than one year) improvements and are very effective when an individual complies with therapy. The challenge for new studies examining these treatments is to improve long-term adherence and compliance, and to move towards using modalities (e.g. the Internet, telemedicine) that will allow a larger number of patients access to these therapies.

Until these studies are performed and can provide formal guidance, there are some general recommendations that have been made with respect to exercise. For example, high-impact exercise may be poorly tolerated in some patients, so only low-impact aerobic activities (e.g., walking, swimming, water aerobics, stationary cycling) should be considered initially. The occurrence of post-exertional worsening of symptoms may be reduced by utilizing low-impact conditioning programs, initiated at a slow pace (sometimes beginning at only 5 min/day) that is gradually increased over time.

Other non-pharmacological therapies, many of which are considered complementary or alternative in western medicine, may have some utility in FM (134,135). As with other diseases, there are few controlled trials to advocate their general use. Trigger-point injections, chiropractic manipulation, acupuncture, and myofascial release therapy are among the more commonly used modalities, which achieve varying levels of success. There is some evidence that the use of alternative therapies give patients a greater sense of control over their illness, and in instances where this is accompanied by an improved clinical state, the decision to use these therapies is between the physician and patient themselves.

When to Refer

Referral should be considered for individuals with FM who do not respond to therapy. For those with significant psychosocial or psychiatric comorbidities, referral to a psychologist, social worker, or psychiatrist who has experience in working with pain patients can be very helpful. Referral to a multidisciplinary pain clinic may also be considered, especially if individuals have elements of both nociceptive pain that might respond to procedures such as nerve blocks and non-nociceptive pain.

Conclusion

Osteoarthritis and fibromyalgia are extremely common conditions that, though both characterized by chronic pain, have markedly different causes and treatments. Osteoarthritis is the prototypical "peripheral" or nociceptive pain syndrome, because the pain is occurring because of loss of cartilage and/or inflammation in the affected joint and the subsequent nociceptive input via peripheral sensory nerves. Other conditions that fall under the same general category of nociceptive pain include systemic inflammatory disorders (e.g., rheumatoid arthritis) and cancer pain. However, certain individuals with these conditions may have elements of non-nociceptive pain, thus accounting for the fact that there is sometimes a mismatch between the degree of joint space damage, the extent of inflammation, the extent of metastatic disease, and the amount of pain an individual is experiencing.

In contrast to osteoarthritis, the pain in fibromyalgia is "central" or nonnociceptive. Table 4-2 summarizes the fundamental differences between these different types of pain in terms of accompanying symptoms as well as effective treatments. In some cases, a peripheral nociceptive abnormality can be identified in an individual, but the distribution of the pain exceeds that noted (e.g., the individual with a single herniated disk who has diffuse back

Table 4-2   Mechanistic Characterization of Chronic Pain

Peripheral (Nociceptive)	Central (Non-Nociceptive)
• Primarily due to inflammation or mechanical damage in periphery	• Primarily due to a central disturbance in pain processing
• NSAID, opioid responsive	• Tricyclic, neuroactive compounds compounds most effective
• Responds to procedures	
• Behavioral factors minor	• Psychological/behavioral factors more prominent
• Examples —Osteoarthritis —Rheumatoid arthritis —Cancer pain	• Examples —Fibromyalgia —Irritable bowel syndrome —Tension and migraine headache —Interstitial cystitis/vulvodynia, non-cardiac chest pain

Table 4-3   Recognizing Central Pain Clinically

- Peripheral factors inadequate to account for symptoms
- Pain outside distribution affected by the suspected peripheral disorder
- Hyperalgesia/allodynia present
- Unresponsiveness to "peripheral therapies"
- Accompanying symptoms (fatigue, cognitive dysfunction, distress)

pain and paresthesias). Table 4-3 gives additional clues that an individual may be experiencing "central" non-nociceptive rather than (or in addition to) peripheral "nociceptive" pain. As noted, the presence of tenderness (allodynia/hyperalgesia) is a mechanistic clue that an individual has a globally heightened state of pain processing. In some cases, the presence of non-nociceptive pain is not suspected until the individual is found to be unresponsive to NSAIDs, opioids, nerve blocks, or other therapies that typically ameliorate nociceptive pain. Finally, non-nociceptive pain is sometimes identifiable by the "company it keeps". Patients with non-nociceptive pain syndromes not only have pain in multiple locations (and it is important to consider headache, frequent sore throat, tender nodes, and visceral pain as "pain"), but also frequently experience fatigue, insomnia, sleep disturbances, memory problems, and so on.

The most important reason to move to this type of classification system is because nociceptive and non-nociceptive pain respond differently to therapeutic interventions. NSAIDs and opioids are more effective for nociceptive than non-nociceptive pain. Individuals with nociceptive pain are also much more likely to benefit from procedures aimed at correcting peripheral abnormalities (e.g., joint replacement, nerve blocks). In contrast, different classes of drugs that primarily work on central nervous system function, such as tricyclic compounds, are more effective for non-nociceptive pain. Although psychological, cognitive, and behavioral factors are more common in non-nociceptive than nociceptive pain conditions, these should be identified and addressed in all chronic pain patients.

A final word. Although this chapter has emphasized identifying and treating non-nociceptive pain in individuals with conditions heretofore suspected of being nociceptive, the converse is also true. For example, although we consider conditions such as fibromyalgia to be primarily non-nociceptive, if these individuals have co-morbid arthritis or other mechanical or inflammatory conditions, these should be identified and treated. This is especially important because we know that continuous peripheral nociceptive input can lead to phenomena such as wind-up and central sensitization. Thus if nociceptive stimuli present in an individual with non-nociceptive pain are not appropriately addressed, the consequences may be doubly unfortunate: The nociceptive pain will go on unabated, and this can worsen the non-nociceptive component of that individual's pain.

REFERENCES

1. **Clauw DJ, Chrousos GP.** Chronic pain and fatigue syndromes: overlapping clinical and neuroendocrine features and potential pathogenic mechanisms. Neuroimmunomodulation. 1997;4:134-53.

2. **Mertz H, Naliboff B, Munakata J, et al.** Altered rectal perception is a biological marker of patients with irritable bowel syndrome. Gastroenterology. 1995;109:40-52.

3. **Bolognese JA, Ehrich EW, Schnitzer TJ.** Precision of composite measures of osteoarthritis efficacy in comparison to that of individual endpoints. J Rheumatol. 2001;28:2700-4.

4. **Rossy LA, Buckelew SP, Dorr N, et al.** A meta-analysis of fibromyalgia treatment interventions. Ann Behav Med. 1999;21:180-91.

5. **Felson DT, Naimark A, Anderson J, et al.** The prevalence of knee osteoarthritis in the elderly. The Framingham Osteoarthritis Study. Arthritis Rheum. 1987;30:914-8.

6. **Lawrence RC, Helmick CG, Arnett FC, et al.** Estimates of the prevalence of arthritis and selected musculoskeletal disorders in the United States [Comments]. Arthritis Rheum. 1998;41:778-99.

7. **Lohmander LS, Felson D.** Can we identify a 'high risk' patient profile to determine who will experience rapid progression of osteoarthritis? Osteoarthritis Cartilage. 2004;12(Suppl A):S49-52.

8. **Steinmeyer J.** Cytokines in osteoarthritis: current status on the pharmacological intervention. Front Biosci. 2004;9:575-80.

9. **Aigner T, Dudhia J.** Genomics of osteoarthritis. Curr Opin Rheumatol. 2003;15:634-40.

10. **Jordan JM, Kraus VB, Hochberg MC.** Genetics of osteoarthritis. Curr Rheumatol Rep. 2004;6:7-13.

11. **Hart DJ, Doyle DV, Spector TD.** Incidence and risk factors for radiographic knee osteoarthritis in middle-aged women. The Chingford Study. Arthritis Rheum. 1999;42:17-24.

12. **Radloff LS, Locke BZ.** The Community Mental Health Assessment Survey and the CES-D Scale. In: Weissman M, Myers JK, Ross CE, eds. Community Surveys of Psychiatric Disorders, 4th ed. New Brunswick, NJ: Rutgers University Press; 1986:177-89.

13. **Unruh A.** Gender variations in clinical pain experience. Pain. 1996;65:123-67.

14. **Felson DT, Chaisson CE, Hill CL, et al.** The association of bone marrow lesions with pain in knee osteoarthritis. Ann Intern Med. 2001;134:541-9.

15. **Hill CL, Gale DR, Chaisson CE, et al.** Periarticular lesions detected on magnetic resonance imaging: prevalence in knees with and without symptoms. Arthritis Rheum. 2003;48:2836-44.

16. **Creamer P, Hochberg MC.** The relationship between psychosocial variables and pain reporting in osteoarthritis of the knee. Arthritis Care Res. 1998;11:60-5.

17. **Creamer P, Lethbridge-Cejku M, Costa P, et al.** The relationship of anxiety and depression with self-reported knee pain in the community: data from the Baltimore Longitudinal Study of Aging. Arthritis Care Res. 1999;12:3-7.

18. **Greenspan A.** Erosive osteoarthritis. Semin Musculoskelet Radiol. 2003;7:155-9.

19. **Sowers M, Jannausch M, Stein E, et al.** C-reactive protein as a biomarker of emergent osteoarthritis. Osteoarthritis Cartilage. 2002;10:595-601.

20. **Gupta KB, Duryea J, Weissman BN.** Radiographic evaluation of osteoarthritis. Radiol Clin North Am. 2004;42:11-41.

21. **Guermazi A, Zaim S, Taouli B, et al.** MR findings in knee osteoarthritis. Eur Radiol. 2003;13:1370-86.

22. **Hochberg MC, Altman RD, Brandt, KD, et al.** Guidelines for the medical management of osteoarthritis. Part I. Osteoarthritis of the hip. Arthritis Rheum. 1995;38:1535-40.

23. **Hochberg MC, Altman RD, Brandt KD, et al.** Guidelines for the medical management of osteoarthritis. Part II. Osteoarthritis of the knee. Arthritis Rheum. 1995;38:1541-6.

24. **Jordan KM, Arden NK, Doherty M, et al.** EULAR Recommendations 2003: an evidence-based approach to the management of knee osteoarthritis. Report of a Task Force of the Standing Committee for International Clinical Studies Including Therapeutic Trials (ESCISIT). Ann Rheum Dis. 2003;62:1145-55.

25. **Sinkov V, Cymet T.** Osteoarthritis: understanding the pathophysiology, genetics, and treatments. J Natl Med Assoc. 2003;95:475-82.

26. **Brosseau L, MacLeay L, Robinson V, et al.** Intensity of exercise for the treatment of osteoarthritis. Cochrane Database Syst Rev. 2003;CD004259.

27. **Campbell R, Evans M, Tucker M, et al.** Why don't patients do their exercises? Understanding non-compliance with physiotherapy in patients with osteoarthritis of the knee. J Epidemiol Community Health. 2001;55:132-8.

28. **Keefe FJ, Caldwell DS.** Cognitive behavioral control of arthritis pain. Med Clin North Am. 1997;81:277-90.

29. **Berman BM, Swyers JP, Ezzo J.** The evidence for acupuncture as a treatment for rheumatologic conditions. Rheum Dis Clin North Am. 2000;26:103-15.

30. **Soeken KL.** Selected CAM therapies for arthritis-related pain: the evidence from systematic reviews. Clin J Pain. 2004;20:13-8.

31. **Bradley JD, Brandt KD, Katz BP, et al.** Comparison of an anti-inflammatory dose of ibuprofen, an analgesic dose of ibuprofen, and acetaminophen in the treatment of patients with osteoarthritis of the knee. N Engl J Med. 1991;325:87-91.

32. **Williams HJ, Ward JR, Egger MJ, et al.** Comparison of naproxen and acetaminophen in a two-year study of treatment of osteoarthritis of the knee. Arthritis Rheum. 1993;36:1196-1206.

33. **Whitcomb DC, Block GD.** Association of acetaminophen hepatotoxicity with fasting and ethanol use. JAMA. 1994;272:1845-50.

34. **Wolfe F, Zhao S, Lane N.** Preference for nonsteroidal antiinflammatory drugs over acetaminophen by rheumatic disease patients: a survey of 1799 patients with osteoarthritis, rheumatoid arthritis, and fibromyalgia. Arthritis Rheum. 2000;43:378-85.

35. **Godwin M, Dawes M.** Intra-articular steroid injections for painful knees: systematic review with meta-analysis. Can Fam Physician. 2004;50:241-8.

36. **Lo GH, LaValley M, McAlindon T, Felson DT.** Intra-articular hyaluronic acid in treatment of knee osteoarthritis: a meta-analysis. JAMA, 2003;290:3115-21.

37. **Kennedy LG, Newman JH, Ackroyd CE, Dieppe PA.** When should we do knee replacements? Knee. 2003;10:161-6.

38. **Wolfe F, Ross K, Anderson J, et al.** The prevalence and characteristics of fibromyalgia in the general population. Arthritis Rheum. 1995;38:19-28.

39. **Croft P, Rigby AS, Boswell R, et al.** The prevalence of chronic widespread pain in the general population. J Rheumatol. 1993;20:710-3.

40. **Wolfe F, Ross K, Anderson J, Russell IJ.** Aspects of fibromyalgia in the general population: sex, pain threshold, and fibromyalgia symptoms. J Rheumatol. 1995;22: 151-6.

41. **Wolfe F, Smythe HA, Yunus MB, et al.** The American College of Rheumatology 1990 Criteria for the Classification of Fibromyalgia. Report of the Multicenter Criteria Committee. Arthritis Rheum. 1990;33:160-72.

42. **White KP, Speechley M, Harth M, Ostbye T.** The London Fibromyalgia Epidemiology Study: the prevalence of fibromyalgia syndrome in London, Ontario. J Rheumatol. 1999;26:1570-6.

43. **Wolfe F.** The relation between tender points and fibromyalgia symptom variables: evidence that fibromyalgia is not a discrete disorder in the clinic. Ann Rheum Dis. 1997;56:268-71.

44. **White KP, Nielson WR, Harth M, et al.** Chronic widespread musculoskeletal pain with or without fibromyalgia: psychological distress in a representative community adult sample. J Rheumatol. 2002;29:588-94.

45. **Croft P, Schollum J, Silman A.** Population study of tender point counts and pain as evidence of fibromyalgia. BMJ. 1994;309:696-9.

46. **Petzke F, Ambrose K, Gracely RH, Clauw DJ.** What do tender points measure? Arthritis Rheum. 1999;42:S342.

47. **Petzke F, Gracely RH, Khine A, Clauw DJ.** Pain sensitivity in patients with fibromyalgia (FM): expectancy effects on pain measurements. Arthritis Rheum. 1999;42:S342.

48. **McBeth J, Macfarlane GJ, Hunt IM, Silman AJ.** Risk factors for persistent chronic widespread pain: a community-based study. Rheumatology (Oxford). 2001;40:95-101.

49. **Nisenbaum R, Reyes M, Mawle AC, Reeves WC.** Factor analysis of unexplained severe fatigue and interrelated symptoms: overlap with criteria for chronic fatigue syndrome. Am J Epidemiol. 1998;148:72-7.

50. **Doebbeling BN, Clarke WR, Watson D, et al.** Is there a Persian Gulf War syndrome? Evidence from a large population-based survey of veterans and nondeployed controls. Am J Med. 2000;108:695-704.

51. **Nisenbaum R, Barrett DH, Reyes M, Reeves WC.** Deployment stressors and a chronic multisymptom illness among Gulf War veterans. J Nerv Ment Dis. 2000; 188:259-66.

52. **Fukuda K, Nisenbaum R, Stewart G, et al.** Chronic multisymptom illness affecting Air Force veterans of the Gulf War. JAMA. 1998;280:981-8.

53. **McBeth J, Macfarlane GJ, Benjamin S, Silman AJ.** Features of somatization predict the onset of chronic widespread pain: results of a large population-based study. Arthritis Rheum. 2001;44:940-6.

54. **Papageorgiou AC, Silman AJ, Macfarlane GJ.** Chronic widespread pain in the population: a seven-year follow-up study. Ann Rheum Dis. 2002;61:1071-4.

55. **Bergman S, Herrstrom P, Hogstrom K, et al.** Chronic musculoskeletal pain, prevalence rates, and sociodemographic associations in a Swedish population study. J Rheumatol. 2001;28:1369-77.

56. **Bergman S, Herrstrom P, Jacobsson LT, Petersson IF.** Chronic widespread pain: a three year followup of pain distribution and risk factors. J Rheumatol. 2002;29:818-25.

57. **White KP, Harth M, Speechley M, Ostbye T.** A general population study of fibromyalgia tender points in noninstitutionalized adults with chronic widespread pain. J Rheumatol. 2000:27:2677-82.

58. **Croft PR, Papageorgiou AC, Ferry S, et al.** Psychologic distress and low back pain: evidence from a prospective study in the general population. Spine. 1995;20: 2731-7.

59. **Nahit ES, Pritchard CM, Cherry NM, et al.** The influence of work related psychosocial factors and psychological distress on regional musculoskeletal pain: a study of newly employed workers. J Rheumatol. 2001;28:1378-84.

60. **Hudson JI, Goldenberg DL, Pope HGJ, et al.** Comorbidity of fibromyalgia with medical and psychiatric disorders. Am J Med. 1993;92:363-7.

61. **Arnold LM, Hudson JI, Hess EV, et al.** Family study of fibromyalgia. Arthritis Rheum. 2004;50:944-52.

62. **Buskila D, Neumann L, Vaisberg G, et al.** Increased rates of fibromyalgia following cervical spine injury: a controlled study of 161 cases of traumatic injury [Comments]. Arthritis Rheum. 1997;40:446-52.

63. **Buskila D, Shnaider A, Neumann L, et al.** Fibromyalgia in hepatitis C virus infection: another infectious disease relationship. Arch Intern Med. 1997;157:2497-2500.

64. **White PD, Thomas JM, Amess J, et al.** The existence of a fatigue syndrome after glandular fever. Psychol Med. 1995;25:907-16.

65. **Bourdette DN, McCauley LA, Barkhuizen A, et al.** Symptom factor analysis, clinical findings, and functional status in a population-based case control study of Gulf War unexplained illness. J Occup Environ Med. 2001;43:1026-40.

66. **Unwin C, Blatchley N, Coker W, et al.** Health of UK servicemen who served in Persian Gulf War. Lancet. 1999;353:169-78.

67. **Clauw DJ.** The health consequences of the first Gulf War. BMJ. 2003;327:1357-8.

68. **Romero LM, Plotsky PM, Sapolsky RM.** Patterns of adrenocorticotropin secretagog release with hypoglycemia, novelty, and restraint after colchicine blockade of axonal transport. Endocrinology. 1993;132:199-204.

69. **Chrousos GP, Gold PW.** The concepts of stress and stress system disorders: overview of physical and behavioral homeostasis. JAMA. 1992;267:1244-52.

70. **Lautenbacher S, Rollman GB.** Possible deficiencies of pain modulation in fibromyalgia. Clin J Pain. 1997;13:189-96.

71. **Raphael KG, Natelson BH, Janal MN, Nayak S.** A community-based survey of fibromyalgia-like pain complaints following the World Trade Center terrorist attacks. Pain. 2002;100:131-9.

72. **Pillow DR, Zautra AJ, Sandler I.** Major life events and minor stressors: identifying mediational links in the stress process. J Pers Soc Psychol. 1996;70:381-94.

73. **Crofford LJ, Pillemer SR, Kalogeras KT.** Hypothalamic-pituitary-adrenal axis perturbations in patients with fibromyalgia. Arthritis Rheum. 1994;37:1583-92.

74. **Crofford LJ.** The hypothalamic-pituitary-adrenal stress axis in fibromyalgia and chronic fatigue syndrome. Z Rheumatol. 1998;57(Suppl 2):67-71.

75. **Demitrack MA, Crofford LJ.** Evidence for and pathophysiologic implications of hypothalamic-pituitary-adrenal axis dysregulation in fibromyalgia and chronic fatigue syndrome. Ann N Y Acad Sci. 1998;840:684-97.

76. **Bennett RM, Cook DM, Clark SR, et al.** Low somatomedin-C in fibromyalgia patients: An analysis of clinical specificity and pituitary/hepatic responses. Arthritis Rheum. 1993;36:S49.

77. **Qiao ZG, Vaeroy H, Morkrid L.** Electrodermal and microcirculatory activity in patients with fibromyalgia during baseline, acoustic stimulation and cold pressor tests. J Rheumatol. 1991;18:1383-9.

78. **Adler GK, Kinsley BT, Hurwitz S, et al.** Reduced hypothalamic-pituitary and sympathoadrenal responses to hypoglycemia in women with fibromyalgia syndrome. Am J Med. 1999;106:534-43.

79. **Petzke F, Clauw DJ.** Sympathetic nervous system function in fibromyalgia. Curr Rheumatol Rep. 2000;2:116-23.

80. **Martinez-Lavin M, Hermosillo AG, Rosas M, Soto ME.** Circadian studies of autonomic nervous balance in patients with fibromyalgia: a heart rate variability analysis. Arthritis Rheum. 1998;41:1966-71.

81. **Granges G, Littlejohn G.** Pressure pain threshold in pain-free subjects, in patients with chronic regional pain syndromes, and in patients with fibromyalgia syndrome. Arthritis Rheum. 1993;36:642-6.

82. **Lautenbacher S, Rollman GB, McCain GA.** Multi-method assessment of experimental and clinical pain in patients with fibromyalgia. Pain. 1994;59:45-53.

83. **Kosek E, Ekholm J.** Modulation of pressure pain thresholds during and following isometric contraction. Pain. 1995;61:481-6.

84. **Price DD, Staud R, Robinson ME, et al.** Enhanced temporal summation of second pain and its central modulation in fibromyalgia patients. Pain. 2002;99:49-59.

85. **Staud R, Vierck CJ, Cannon RL, et al.** Abnormal sensitization and temporal summation of second pain (wind-up) in patients with fibromyalgia syndrome. Pain. 2001;91:165-75.

86. **Price DD.** Psychological and nerual mechanism of the affective dimension of pain. Science. 2000;288:1769-72.

87. **Lorenz J, Grasedyck K, Bromm B.** Middle and long latency somatosensory evoked potentials after painful laser stimulation in patients with fibromyalgia syndrome. Electroencephalogr Clin Neurophysiol. 1996;100:165-8.

88. **Mountz JM, Bradley LA, Modell JG, et al.** Fibromyalgia in women: abnormalities of regional cerebral blood flow in the thalamus and the caudate nucleus are associated with low pain threshold levels. Arthritis Rheum. 1995;38:926-38.

89. **Kwiatek R, Barnden L, Tedman R, et al.** Regional cerebral blood flow in fibromyalgia: single-photon-emission computed tomography evidence of reduction in the pontine tegmentum and thalami. Arthritis Rheum. 2000;43:2823-33.

90. **Petzke F, Clauw DJ, Wolf JM, Gracely RH.** Pressure pain in fibromyalgia and healthy controls: functional MRI of subjective pain experience versus objective stimulus intensity [Abstract]. Arthritis Rheum. 2000;43(9S):2000.

91. **Cook DB, Lange G, Ciccone DS, et al.** Functional imaging of pain in patients with primary fibromyalgia. J Rheumatol. 2004;31:364-78.

92. **Giesecke T, Gracely RH, Grant MA, et al.** Evidence of augmented central pain processing in idiopathic chronic low back pain. Arthritis Rheum. 2004;50:613-23.

93. **Welin M, Bragee B, Nyberg F, Kristiansson M.** Elevated substance P levels are contrasted by a decrease in met-enkephalin-arg-phe levels in CSF from fibromyalgia patients. J Musculoskeletal Pain. 1995;3:4.

94. **Vaeroy H, Helle R, Forre O, et al.** Elevated CSF levels of substance P and high incidence of Raynaud phenomenon in patients with fibromyalgia: new features for diagnosis. Pain. 1988;32:21-6.

95. **Russell IJ, Orr MD, Littman B, et al.** Elevated cerebrospinal fluid levels of substance P in patients with the fibromyalgia syndrome. Arthritis Rheum. 1994;37:1593-1601.

96. **Bradley LA, Alberts KR, Alarcon GS, et al.** Abnormal brain regional cerebral blood flow and cerebrospinal fluid levels of substance P in patients and non-patients with fibromyalgia [Abstract]. Arthritis Rheum. 1996;39(9S):1109.

97. **Evengard B, Nilsson CG, Lindh G, et al.** Chronic fatigue syndrome differs from fibromyalgia: no evidence for elevated substance P levels in cerebrospinal fluid of patients with chronic fatigue syndrome. Pain. 1998;78:153-5.

98. **Russell IJ, Vaeroy H, Javors M, Nyberg F.** Cerebrospinal fluid biogenic amine metabolites in fibromyalgia/fibrositis syndrome and rheumatoid arthritis. Arthritis Rheum. 1992;35:550-6.

99. **Yunus MB, Dailey JW, Aldag JC, et al.** Plasma tryptophan and other amino acids in primary fibromyalgia: a controlled study. J Rheumatol. 1992;19:90-4.

100. **Boissevain MD, McCain GA.** Toward an integrated understanding of fibromyalgia syndrome. I. Medical and pathophysiological aspects. Pain. 1991;45:227-38.

101. **Hudson JI, Hudson MS, Pliner LF, et al.** Fibromyalgia and major affective disorder: a controlled phenomenology and family history study. Am J Psychiatry. 1985;142:441-6.

102. **White KP, Nielson WR, Harth M, et al.** Does the label "fibromyalgia" alter health status, function, and health service utilization? A prospective, within-group comparison in a community cohort of adults with chronic widespread pain. Arthritis Rheum. 2002;47:260-5.

103. **Aaron LA, Bradley LA, Alarcon GS, et al.** Psychiatric diagnoses in patients with fibromyalgia are related to health care-seeking behavior rather than to illness [Comments]. Arthritis Rheum. 1996;39:436-45.

104. **McBeth J, Macfarlane GJ, Silman AJ.** Does chronic pain predict future psychological distress? Pain. 2002;96:239-45.

105. **Benjamin S, Morris S, McBeth J, et al.** The association between chronic widespread pain and mental disorder: a population-based study. Arthritis Rheum. 2000;43:561-7.

106. **Hadler NM.** If you have to prove you are ill, you can't get well: the object lesson of fibromyalgia. Spine. 1996;21:2397-2400.

107. **Hawley DJ, Wolfe F.** Pain, disability, and pain/disability relationships in seven rheumatic disorders: a study of 1522 patients. J Rheumatol. 1991;18:1552-7.

108. **Callahan LF, Smith WJ, Pincus T.** Self-report questionnaires in five rheumatic diseases: comparisons of health status constructs and associations with formal education level. Arthritis Care Res. 1989;2:122-31.

109. **Park DC, Glass JM, Minear M, Crofford LJ.** Cognitive function in fibromyalgia patients. Arthritis Rheum. 2001;44:2125-33.

110. **Tan EM, Feltkamp TE, Smolen JS, et al.** Range of antinuclear antibodies in "healthy" individuals. Arthritis Rheum. 1997;40:1601-11.

111. **Hadler NM.** Fibromyalgia, chronic fatigue, and other iatrogenic diagnostic algorithms. Do some labels escalate illness in vulnerable patients? [Comments]. Postgrad Med. 1997;102:161-6,171.

112. **White KP, Harth M.** Classification, epidemiology, and natural history of fibromyalgia. Curr Pain Headache Rep. 2001;5:320-9.

113. **O'Malley PG, Balden E, Tomkins G, et al.** Treatment of fibromyalgia with antidepressants: a meta-analysis. J Gen Intern Med. 2000;15:659-66.

114. **Arnold LM, Keck PEJ, Welge JA.** Antidepressant treatment of fibromyalgia: a meta-analysis and review. Psychosomatics. 2000;41:104-13.

115. **Godfrey RG.** A guide to the understanding and use of tricyclic antidepressants in the overall management of fibromyalgia and other chronic pain syndromes. Arch Intern Med. 1996;156:1047-52.

116. **Carette S, Bell MJ, Reynolds WJ, et al.** Comparison of amitriptyline, cyclobenzaprine, and placebo in the treatment of fibromyalgia: a randomized, double-blind clinical trial. Arthritis Rheum. 1994;37:32-40.

117. **Goldenberg D, Mayskiy M, Mossey C, et al.** A randomized, double-blind crossover trial of fluoxetine and amitriptyline in the treatment of fibromyalgia. Arthritis Rheum. 1996;39:1852-9.

118. **Wolfe F, Cathey MA, Hawley DJ.** A double-blind placebo controlled trial of fluoxetine in fibromyalgia. Scand J Rheumatol. 1994;23:255-9.

119. **Arnold LM, Hess EV, Hudson JI Jr, et al.** A randomized, placebo-controlled, double-blind, flexible-dose study of fluoxetine in the treatment of women with fibromyalgia. Am J Med. 2002;112:191-7.

120. **Gracely RH, Dubner R, McGrath PA.** Narcotic analgesia: fentanyl reduces the intensity but not the unpleasantness of painful tooth pulp sensations. Science. 1979;203:1261-3.

121. **Fishbain D.** Evidence-based data on pain relief with antidepressants. Ann Med. 2000;32:305-16.

122. **Salerno SM, Browning R, Jackson JL.** The effect of antidepressant treatment on chronic back pain: a meta-analysis. Arch Intern Med. 2002;162:19-24.

123. **Bair MJ, Robinson RL, Katon W, Kroenke K.** Depression and pain comorbidity: a literature review. Arch Intern Med. 2003;163:2433-45.

124. **Carter GT, Sullivan MD.** Antidepressants in pain management. Curr Opin Investig Drugs. 2002;3:454-8.

125. **O'Malley PG, Jackson JL, Santoro J, et al.** Antidepressant therapy for unexplained symptoms and symptom syndromes [Comments]. J Fam Pract. 1999;48:980-90.

126. **Guymer EK, Clauw DJ.** Treatment of fatigue in fibromyalgia. Rheum Dis Clin North Am. 2002;28:367-78.

127. **Williams DA, Cary MA, Glazer LJ, et al.** Randomized controlled trial of CBT to improve functional status in fibromyalgia. American College of Rheumatology, 2000;43:S210.

128. **White KP, Nielson WR.** Cognitive behavioral treatment of fibromyalgia syndrome: a follow-up assessment. J Rheum. 1995;22:717-21.

129. **National Institutes of Health.** Integration of behavioral and relaxation approaches into the treatment of chronic pain and insomnia. NIH Technology Assessment Panel on Integration of Behavioral and Relaxation Approaches into the Treatment of Chronic Pain and Insomnia. JAMA. 1996;276:313-8.

130. **Keefe FJ, Gil KM, Ross SC.** Behavioral approaches in the multidisciplinary management of chronic pain: programs and issues. Clin Psychol Rev. 1986;6:87-113.

131. **Minor MA, Hewett JE, Webel RR, et al.** Efficacy of physical conditioning exercise in patients with rheumatoid arthritis and osteoarthritis. Arthritis Rheum. 1989;32:1396-1405.

132. **Mannerkorpi K, Nyberg B, Ahlmen M, Ekdahl C.** Pool exercise combined with an education program for patients with fibromyalgia syndrome: a prospective, randomized study. J Rheumatol. 2000;27:2473-81.

133. **Janal MN.** Pain sensitivity, exercise and stoicism. J R Soc Med. 1996;89:376-81.

134. **Crofford LJ, Appleton BE.** Complementary and alternative therapies for fibromyalgia. Curr Rheumatol Rep. 2001;3:147-56.

135. **Harris RE, Clauw DJ.** The use of complementary medical therapies in the management of myofascial pain disorders. Curr Pain Headache Rep. 2002;6:370-4.

5

■ ■ ■

Neuropathic Pain

Alec B. O'Connor, MD
Robert H. Dworkin, PhD

N europathic pain has been defined as "spontaneous pain and hypersensitivity to pain in association with damage to or a lesion of the nervous system" (1). It should be distinguished from nociceptive pain and inflammatory pain, which are normal adaptive mechanisms that protect an organism from injury and during healing from injury, respectively. Neuropathic pain further differs from functional pain, which is "hypersensitivity to pain resulting from abnormal central processing of normal input" (1). In neuropathic pain, disease-induced damage to the peripheral or central nervous system leads to pain and abnormal sensations that do not serve to protect the organism from harm.

Correctly identifying pain as neuropathic is important because the management of neuropathic pain differs from the management of other types of pain. Specifically, anticonvulsants, tricyclic antidepressants, and topical lidocaine have proven benefit in neuropathic pain but not in other types of pain, while nonsteroidal antiinflammatory medications do not seem to be as effective in neuropathic pain as in other types of pain (2,3). In addition, recognizing pain as neuropathic may help reveal a previously unknown causative disease.

Because neuropathic pain is relatively common and often chronic, it is frequently encountered in practice by both primary care physicians and specialists. Primary care providers play a central role in the diagnosis and chronic management of patients with neuropathic pain. In addition, prompt diagnosis and treatment of the underlying cause of neuropathic pain may help improve pain control and overall morbidity and mortality for patients. For example, aggressive management of diabetes mellitus and herpes zoster may prevent the development of two of the most common causes of neuropathic pain, painful diabetic neuropathy (PDN) and postherpetic neuralgia (PHN) (4-8).

In this chapter, an overview is presented of neuropathic pain and its characteristic symptoms, then an evidence-based approach to treatment is discussed.

Epidemiology

The exact incidence of neuropathic pain syndromes is unknown. Several years ago, Bennett estimated the incidence of many types of neuropathic pain syndromes including neuropathic low back pain; he concluded that approximately 3.8 million people suffer from neuropathic pain in the United States (9). However, this may be an underestimation. For example, PDN and PHN alone may affect three million and one million patients respectively in the United States (10,11).

The prevalence of neuropathic pain is expected to increase for several reasons. One is that the population as a whole is aging, which will impact the prevalence of neuropathic pain syndromes because a number of them, including PHN, PDN, and central post-stroke pain, are more common in the elderly. Another reason is that patients are surviving longer with HIV-infection, cancer, diabetes, and other diseases which can cause neuropathic pain. Finally, neuropathic pain can result from the increasingly common use of certain medical and surgical interventions to treat cancer and other diseases (e.g., radiation, chemotherapy, mastectomy).

Pathogenesis

Depending on where the lesion or dysfunction occurs within the nervous system, neuropathic pain can be considered primarily peripheral or central in origin. As with other types of pain, a distinction is made between acute and chronic neuropathic pain, the latter typically considered pain that has persisted beyond the normal time of healing or for more than three months (12). Unfortunately, most patients with neuropathic pain are suffering from chronic pain.

Neuropathic pain can be caused by a broad range of different types of disease processes. These include infections, trauma, metabolic abnormalities, chemotherapy, surgery, radiation, neurotoxins, nerve compression, inflammation, and tumor infiltration. Table 5-1 lists the variety of neuropathic pain syndromes. Peripheral and central neuropathic pain syndromes are listed separately, but it is very likely that peripheral and central mechanisms both contribute to the persistence of pain in many of these syndromes.

Despite the large number of neuropathic pain syndromes, most of the research conducted on the mechanisms and treatment of neuropathic pain has studied either PDN or PHN. Knowledge that has been gained from examining these two peripheral neuropathic pain syndromes has generally

Table 5-1   Common Types of Neuropathic Pain

Peripheral Neuropathic Pain

- Alcoholic polyneuropathy
- Chemotherapy-induced polyneuropathy
- Chronic inflammatory demyelinating polyradiculoneuropathy
- Complex regional pain syndrome (formerly called reflex sympathetic dystrophy)
- HIV-associated neuropathy
- Idiopathic sensory neuropathy
- Nerve compression or infiltration by tumor
- Nerve entrapment syndromes (e.g., carpal tunnel syndrome, lumbar radiculopathy)

- Nutritional deficiency-related neuropathies
- Painful diabetic neuropathy (PDN)
- Phantom limb pain
- Post-herpetic neuralgia (PHN)
- Post-radiation plexopathy
- Post-surgical neuralgias (e.g., post-mastectomy pain, post-thoracotomy pain)
- Post-traumatic neuralgias
- Toxic exposure-related neuropathies
- Trigeminal neuralgia (tic douloureux)

Central Neuropathic Pain

- Compressive myelopathy from spinal stenosis
- HIV myelopathy
- Multiple sclerosis pain
- Parkinson's disease pain

- Post-ischemic myelopathy
- Post-radiation myelopathy
- Post-stroke pain
- Spinal cord injury pain
- Syringomyelia

Adapted from Dworkin RH, Backonja M, Rowbotham MC, et al. Advances in neuropathic pain: diagnosis, mechanisms, and treatment recommendations. Arch Neurol. 2003;60:1524-34; with permission.

been assumed to also have application in understanding the mechanisms and treatment of other neuropathic pain syndromes. However, the extent to which different neuropathic pain syndromes share a common collection of pathophysiologic mechanisms and have similar responses to various pharmacological and non-pharmacological treatments is unknown (13).

There is generally agreement that both central and peripheral processes contribute to many chronic neuropathic pain syndromes, and that specific mechanisms may explain the qualitatively different symptoms and signs that patients experience.

For example, Rowbotham and Fields (14-16) have proposed that there are different mechanisms involved in PHN, and that distinct mechanisms result in specific symptoms and signs in different patients; their proposal illustrates how a mechanism-based approach to neuropathic pain may ultimately lead to more focussed treatment. One group of patients experience prominent allodynia (pain produced by a stimulus that does not ordinarily cause pain, such as wind or clothing brushing on skin) but have minimal sensory deficits. In these patients, the intense acute pain of herpes zoster appears to have produced a state of central sensitization which is then maintained by abnormal activity in primary afferent nociceptors (see Chapter 1 for a detailed discussion). These patients respond to treatment with local anesthetics, which may attenuate the abnormal activity in nociceptors. A separate group of patients tends to present with spontaneous pain, little or no allodynia, and marked sensory deficits in the areas of greatest pain. Primary afferent nociceptors do not appear to contribute to pain in these patients, which suggests that their spontaneous pain is caused by a different mechanism, perhaps central hyperactivity resulting from deafferentation. These patients would be expected to have minimal response to treatment with local anesthetics.

The presence of *both* allodynia and sensory deficits in other patients may be explained by a third mechanism—deafferentation accompanied by central reorganization involving sprouting of large myelinated fibers into the substantia gelatinosa where contact is made onto neurons that were formerly innervated only by nociceptors (17). While the evidence supporting the role of central sensitization and other mechanisms in the pathophysiology of neuropathic pain is clearest for PHN, it is very likely that multiple similar mechanisms are involved in other peripheral neuropathic pain syndromes (13).

Diagnosis

The diagnosis of neuropathic pain is based primarily on a characteristic description of pain, but there are no pathognomonic symptoms or signs. The examination often reveals neurological deficits, and imaging may confirm the presence of a causative nervous system lesion. The clinical evaluation of a patient with pain that is possibly neuropathic should focus on determining if the pain is neuropathic and on searching for an underlying explanatory disease process, the treatment of which may have significant implications for the patient.

History

As with all types of pain, a thorough history evaluating the intensity, location, exacerbating and remitting factors, associated symptoms, radiation, and duration of pain will have important diagnostic and treatment implications. However, the quality of neuropathic pain is what usually distinguishes it from other types of pain.

Although various symptoms and signs have been considered characteristic of neuropathic pain, there are few studies that have systematically compared pain quality in patients with neuropathic and non-neuropathic pain syndromes (18). In a research setting, studies have shown that a detailed and accurate history (using the McGill Pain Questionaire) can differentiate neuropathic from non-neuropathic pain (19-25). One study in particular demonstrated that patients with neuropathic pain chose six sensory adjectives significantly more frequently than patients with pain that was not neuropathic (23). These six adjectives were "electric shock," "burning," "tingling," "cold," "pricking," and "itching." Of these adjectives, "electric shock," "burning," and "tingling" were the most commonly used by neuropathic pain patients (53%, 54%, and 48% respectively). These results support the value of these adjectives in identifying patients with neuropathic pain, but the study also demonstrated that some other adjectives typically considered characteristic of neuropathic pain—including "lancinating" and "shooting"—did not differentiate between the patients with neuropathic and non-neuropathic pain.

Patients with neuropathic pain may describe pain that is either stimulus-evoked or spontaneous (stimulus-independent), a distinction that may help indicate the pathophysiologic mechanism of pain, though neuropathic pain from an individual disease may present as either or both. *Spontaneous pain* occurs in the absence of any stimulation, and can be either intermittent or continuous. An individual patient may describe different types of spontaneous pain with different qualities (e.g., "shooting," "burning," or "throbbing"). *Spontaneous continuous pain* is present all or almost all of the time, although patients usually report that it varies in intensity (e.g., PDN is often worse at night). *Spontaneous intermittent pain* is episodic, occurs without stimulation, and usually is of relatively short duration. This type of neuropathic pain is often paroxysmal and described by patients as "electric-like," "stabbing," or "shooting" in quality (e.g., classic tic douloureux).

In contrast to spontaneous pain, some neuropathic pain is stimulus-evoked (also called stimulus-dependent pain). Table 5-2 lists the different types of stimulus-evoked symptoms, including allodynia and hyperalgesia, which is increased pain in response to a normally painful stimulus (e.g., a pinprick). As many as 90% of patients with PHN have allodynia (26). There is a consensus among researchers that the different types of stimulus-evoked symptoms present in individual neuropathic pain patients provide important information about the pathophysiologic mechanisms causing pain. Understanding the mechanisms causing pain in an individual patient would be expected to guide the treatment of that patient to the safest and most effective options, but the clinical application of these distinctions has not yet been fully delineated.

Patients with neuropathic pain may also experience positive and/or negative sensory or motor symptoms. For example, some patients with neuropathic pain will complain of itching, numbness, tingling, or "pins-and-needles" sensations. Other patients may note weakness or spasticity in the affected extremity. In addition, autonomic dysregulation (e.g., causing flushing or sweating) may be present in the distribution of the pain. The

Table 5-2   International Association for the Study of Pain (IASP) Definitions of Pain Terms

Pain Term	Definition
Allodynia	Pain due to a stimulus which does not normally provoke pain
Analgesia	Absence of pain in response to stimulation which would normally be painful
Hyperalgesia	An increased response to a stimulus which is normally painful
Hypoalgesia	Diminished pain in response to a normally painful stimulus
Hyperesthesia	Increased sensitivity to stimulation, excluding the special senses
Hypoesthesia	Decreased sensitivity to stimulation, excluding the special senses
Hyperpathia	A painful syndrome characterized by an abnormally painful reaction to a stimulus, especially a repetitive stimulus, as well as an increased threshold

Adapted from Merskey H, Bogduk N, eds. Classification of Chronic Pain: Descriptions of Chronic Pain Syndromes and Definitions of Pain Terms, 2nd ed. Seattle: IASP Press, 1994; with permission.

presence of abnormal sensory, motor, or autonomic symptoms in the distribution of pain should suggest the possibility of a neuropathic cause.

Physical Examination

A patient presenting with pain that seems to be neuropathic should undergo a detailed neurological exam of the affected area and a general examination focused on the possible causes of a neurological lesion.

Inspection of the skin of the affected area may reveal a rash, scarring, flushing, or sweating. Atrophy, fasciculations, and tremors may also be present. Fallen arches, arthropathy, and pressure ulcers may be seen on the feet of the diabetic with neuropathy.

The sensory examination should assess the different types of sensation. Examination of light-touch sensation using a cotton swab or the examiner's finger may reveal numbness or allodynia. Thermal sensation, using, for example, ice or hot water in a bag or cup, can reveal loss of sensation, allodynia, or hyperalgesia. Hyperalgesia to pinprick or firm pressure may be present. Finally, loss of position or vibration sense (using a tuning fork) may be present in, for example, diabetic neuropathy.

The motor exam should attempt to detect subtle weakness in the distribution of the pain and elsewhere. Abnormalities in reflex testing can be used to identify the presence of subtle motor deficits. In addition, the presence of hypertonia or hypotonia, dystonia, and ataxia may help lead to the diagnosis.

When neuropathic pain without an underlying explanatory illness is suspected, the general exam should search for findings that might suggest an underlying disease, such as cancer or AIDS.

Diagnostic Testing

Unfortunately there is no single test that will diagnose neuropathic pain (or pain in general) in all patients. Testing in cases of suspected neuropathic pain should focus on confirming the presence of a suspected nervous system lesion and on diagnosing the underlying illness causing the pain.

Magnetic resonance imaging can be used to detect abnormalities of the central nervous system and spine that may lead to neuropathic pain. For example, patients with radicular pain may have nerve root compression demonstrable by MRI. Alternatively, lesions in the thalamus or sensory cortex due to, for example, stroke or multiple sclerosis can produce central neuropathic pain.

Nerve conduction velocity tests and electromyography can detect abnormalities of large, myelinated peripheral nerves, but not smaller nerves; this can be useful in diagnosing certain types of neuropathy (e.g., nerve entrapment syndromes). Occasionally biopsy of the skin or nerves of an affected area may be necessary to document the presence of a nervous system lesion and to diagnose the underlying cause of the lesion.

Further diagnostic testing is generally aimed at detecting the disease responsible for causing the pain. For example, testing designed to detect possible cancer in a specific location or to diagnose diabetes or HIV infection (see Table 5-1 for underlying disease processes).

Differential Diagnosis

Differentiating neuropathic pain from non-neuropathic pain can be challenging, because there are no pathognomonic symptoms or signs and often there is not a diagnostic test that confirms the diagnosis. In general, the diagnosis is made by the presence of characteristic pain and neurological symptoms and findings, preferably supported by testing that confirms the presence of a disease that can cause neuropathic pain (see Table 5-1) and/or diagnostic testing that confirms the presence of a nervous system lesion in a location that explains the patient's symptoms.

Any type of pain can be mistaken for neuropathic pain if the history, exam, and diagnostic evaluation are not thorough. As described above, the use of the adjectives "shooting" or "lancinating" to describe pain are not discriminatory. The use of one of the adjectives positively associated with the presence of neuropathic pain (e.g., "electric shock" or "burning") can be suggestive but, as already mentioned, is certainly not pathognomonic.

In some cases, neuropathic pain can coexist with nociceptive pain. For example, in a patient with radicular and low back pain, pain may be partly from mechanical and myofacial causes and partly from nerve root compression.

Psychological illness can also play a significant role in some patients presenting with chronic pain. Patients with somatization disorder or those who are malingering (possibly for drug- or disability-seeking reasons) can describe pain that may be indistinguishable from neuropathic pain.

Treatment

The range of options that have been successfully used to treat neuropathic pain is quite broad, ranging from physical therapy to invasive procedures (e.g., spinal cord stimulation). Primary care physicians should play a central role in the management of both the cause of neuropathic pain and the pain itself. In general, primary care providers will prescribe the first-line pharmacological treatments, but they should refer to a pain specialist if a patient is refractory to first-line treatments or may be a good candidate for an invasive management strategy (e.g., spinal stimulation or intrathecal medications).

Treatment of the Causative Disease

The effective treatment of diseases with the potential to cause neuropathic pain may reduce the likelihood that a patient will develop neuropathic pain. For example, the incidence of diabetic neuropathy has been tightly linked to glucose control (4,5). The aggressive treatment of acute herpes zoster infection with famciclovir, valacyclovir, or acyclovir probably reduces the likelihood of developing PHN (6-8). There is an association between viral load and the severity of HIV neuropathy (27), suggesting that successful antiviral therapy might prevent or treat pain in some patients with HIV neuropathy, though this remains to be proven.

In many cases, established neuropathic pain (both acute and chronic) will be reduced by effective treatment of the underlying causative disease. Nerve entrapment syndromes (e.g., carpal tunnel syndrome, radiculopathy) can improve dramatically with nerve decompression. The acute pain of herpes zoster infection has been shown to improve with the early administration of antiviral therapy (28). In addition, PDN probably improves with intensive glycemic control (5,29,30).

Despite the broad range of etiologies of neuropathic pain, the treatment of the pain is generally approached in a similar way. Certainly when the management of the neuropathic pain caused by a specific disease differs from the general approach, management should be directed at the neuropathic pain of the specific etiology; examples include trigeminal neuralgia, the usual treatment of which includes carbamazepine, phenytoin, and baclofen (31), and complex regional pain syndrome, which has been proven to respond significantly to physical therapy of the affected extremity with additional therapies being applied as needed (32). However, there is currently little evidence that different management strategies are needed for neuropathic pain based on the specific etiology.

Systemic and Topical Pharmacotherapy for Neuropathic Pain

Evidence-based treatment guidelines for the pharmacological management of chronic neuropathic pain have recently been published and will provide the basis for our discussion of treatment (33), although we have made a number of updates because this is a rapidly evolving field. Two important caveats are required before discussing these treatment guidelines. First, the majority of the randomized controlled trials of chronic neuropathic pain have examined only two pain syndromes, PHN and PDN. In addition, the United States Food and Drug Administration has approved medications for the treatment of only three specific neuropathic pain syndromes: PHN (gabapentin, lidocaine patch 5%), PDN (duloxetine), and trigeminal neuralgia (carbamazepine). The applicability of the results of clinical trials in one chronic neuropathic syndrome to other chronic neuropathic syndromes is unknown, but most of the first-line therapies identified in the guidelines have been tested in several types of neuropathic pain with generally similar results.

First-Line Pharmacological Treatments

Although many different medications have been used in the treatment of neuropathic pain (Table 5-3), until recently only tricyclic antidepressants (TCA) had been evaluated in multiple randomized, double-blind, placebo-controlled clinical trials. However, there are now several pharmacological treatments demonstrated to provide statistically significant and clinically meaningful treatment benefits compared with placebo in multiple randomized controlled trials in patients with neuropathic pain (33). These medications were considered first-line because of the weight of consistent evidence supporting their effectiveness.

There are clinical circumstances for each one in the initial treatment of patients with neuropathic pain, although TCAs, tramadol, and opioid analgesics generally require greater caution than gabapentin and the lidocaine patch 5%. In general, decisions regarding which medication to prescribe initially in an individual patient should balance concerns about specific drug side effects, comorbidities (e.g., a patient with co-existing depression may benefit more from an antidepressant than from tramadol), potential risk of opioid abuse or drug overdose, and medication cost or co-payment issues. If an adequate trial of one of these medications fails to provide adequate pain relief, a second medication can be added or the first medication can be changed to a different medicine, depending on how well the first medication was tolerated and whether the first medication produced any benefit.

GABAPENTIN AND PREGABALIN

GABAPENTIN

There are an increasing number of published, double-blind, placebo-controlled, randomized clinical trials of gabapentin in patients with neuropathic pain, including studies of PHN, PDN, mixed neuropathic pain syndromes, phantom limb pain, Guillain-Barré syndrome, and acute and chronic spinal cord injury pain (34-42). Gabapentin at daily dosages up to

Table 5-3   Summary of First-Line Medications for Neuropathic Pain

Medication	Starting Dosage	Titration	Maximum Dosage	Duration of Adequate Trial
α₂-δ ligands				
Gabapentin	100-300 mg qhs or 100-300 mg tid	Increase by 100-300 mg tid every 1-7 days as tolerated	3600 mg daily (1200 mg tid); reduce if low creatinine clearance	3-8 wks for titration plus 1-2 weeks at maximum tolerated dosage
Pregabalin	50 mg tid or 75 mg bid	Increase to 300 mg/d after 3-4 days, then by 150 mg/d every 3-4 days as tolerated	600 mg daily	2-4 wks
Lidocaine patch 5%	Maximum of 3 patches daily for a maximum of 12 hours	None needed	Maximum of 3 patches daily for a maximum of 12 hrs	2 wks
Opioid analgesics (dosages given are for oral morphine)	10-30 mg every four hours as needed*	After 1-2 wks, convert total daily dosage to long-acting opioid analgesic and continue short-acting medication as needed	No maximum with careful titration; consider evaluation by pain specialist at dosages exceeding 120-180 mg daily	4-6 wks
Tramadol	50 mg once or twice daily*	Increase by 50-100 mg daily in divided doses (qid) every 3-7 days as tolerated	400 mg daily (100 mg qid); in patients over 75 years of age, 300 mg daily in divided doses (75 mg qid)	4 wks
Antidepressant analgesics				
Tricyclic antidepressants, especially nortriptyline or desipramine	25 mg qhs*	Increase by 25 mg daily every 3-7 days as tolerated	75-150 mg daily; if blood level of active drug and its metabolite is below 100 ng/mL, continue titration with caution	6-8 wks with at least 1-2 wks at maximum tolerated dosage

Table 5-3   Summary of First-Line Medications for Neuropathic Pain (Cont'd)

Medication	Starting Dosage	Titration	Maximum Dosage	Duration of Adequate Trial
Antidepressant analgesics (cont'd)				
Venlafaxine	37.5 mg bid	Increase by 75 mg/d each week as needed	375 mg/d standard venlafaxine or 225 mg/d extended-release preparation	2-4 wks
Duloxetine	60 mg daily	None needed	60 mg bid	2 wks

* Consider starting with half of the listed dose in geriatric patients or patients especially susceptible to side effects.
Adapted from Dworkin RH, Backonja M, Rowbotham MC, et al. Advances in neuropathic pain: diagnosis, mechanisms, and treatment recommendations. Arch Neurol. 2003;60:1524-34; with permission.

3600 mg significantly reduced pain compared with placebo, and improvements in mood, sleep, and quality of life were also demonstrated in some of the trials. The side effects of gabapentin include dizziness, somnolence, and, less often, mild peripheral edema and gastrointestinal symptoms, all of which require monitoring and potentially dose adjustment, but usually not drug discontinuation. In the elderly, gabapentin may cause or exacerbate cognitive or gait impairment. However, gabapentin is generally very well tolerated, safe, and lacks drug interactions, distinguishing it from most other oral medications used in the treatment of chronic neuropathic pain. Dosing generally starts at 300 mg at bedtime, then 300 mg bid on day two, then 300 mg tid on day three, then gradually increased on a tid dosing schedule by about 300 mg/d until efficacy or the maximum dose of 3600 mg/d is reached; usual effective doses are above 1800 mg/d, though dosage reduction is necessary in patients with renal insufficiency (see Table 5-3).

PREGABALIN

Pregabalin is an α_2-δ ligand closely related to gabapentin that has analgesic, anticonvulsant, and anxiolytic activity. It has recently been found to be effective in treating PHN and PDN in three eight-week long trials, and although side effects appeared to increase in a dose-dependent fashion, pregabalin is generally well tolerated (43-45). FDA approval for treatment of PDN and PHN with pregabalin is anticipated by early 2005, and pregabalin would then become the first agent approved for the treatment of more than one neuropathic pain syndrome. The dosing has varied in the three published trials from 150 to 600 mg/d, and although the 150 mg/d dose was roughly equivalent to the 300 mg/d dose in one trial (44), unpublished data are consistent with a dose-response relationship with greater pain reduction at higher dosages. A starting dosage of either 50 mg tid or 75 mg bid is consistent with the results of the trials, and titration to

300 mg daily can occur several days later. Benefits should be seen within 2 weeks of reaching a target dosage of 300-600 mg daily.

LIDOCAINE PATCH 5%

There are three published, double-blind, vehicle-controlled, randomized clinical trials of lidocaine patch 5% that demonstrated statistically significantly greater pain relief with lidocaine patch 5% compared with vehicle-control patches; two of these studies were conducted in patients with PHN (46,47), and one was conducted in a group of patients with diverse peripheral neuropathic pain syndromes, including PHN (48). Lidocaine patch 5% is a topical preparation, and in patients with normal hepatic function, blood levels are minimal and accumulation does not occur with the 12-hour-on—12-hour-off dosing schedule. Lidocaine patch 5% has excellent safety and tolerability, and the only side effects involve mild skin reactions (e.g., erythema, rash). Systemic absorption from lidocaine patch 5% may occur in patients receiving oral class I antiarrhythmic drugs (e.g., mexiletine) (see Table 5-3).

OPIOID ANALGESICS

Several double-blind, randomized trials of oral opioid analgesics have been published since 1998 in patients with PHN, PDN, phantom limb pain, and a variety of peripheral and central neuropathic pain syndromes (49-55). The results of these studies considered together provide the basis for considering opioid analgesics a first-line treatment for neuropathic pain. The most common side effects of opioid analgesics are constipation, sedation, and nausea. Elderly patients can develop cognitive impairment and gait disturbances, increasing the risk of falls. Because accidental death or suicide can occur with overdose, caution must be used when prescribing opioid analgesics to patients with a history of substance abuse or suicide attempts. Patients treated with opioid analgesics may develop analgesic tolerance (i.e., a reduction in analgesic benefit over time), although a stable dosage can usually be achieved. All patients chronically treated with opioids will develop physical dependence (i.e., withdrawal symptoms develop with abrupt discontinuation or rapid dose reduction), and they must be advised not to abruptly discontinue the medication.

TRAMADOL

There are three published, double-blind, placebo-controlled, randomized clinical trials of tramadol in neuropathic pain, one each in patients with PDN, PHN, and painful polyneuropathy of different etiologies including PDN (56-58). In these trials, tramadol titrated to a maximum dosage of 400 mg daily significantly relieved pain compared with placebo, and beneficial effects of treatment on allodynia and quality of life were also reported. The most common side effects of tramadol include dizziness, nausea, constipation, somnolence, and orthostatic hypotension, which occur more frequently with rapid dose escalation. In elderly patients, tramadol can cause cognitive impairment and gait disturbances, potentially resulting in falls. Tramadol raises the risk of seizures in patients who have a history of seizures or who are also receiving antidepressants, opioids, or other drugs that can reduce the seizure threshold. Serotonin syndrome may occur if tramadol is used concurrently with other serotonergic medications, and dosage adjustment is necessary in patients with renal or hepatic disease. Abuse of tramadol has occurred but is thought to be less common than abuse of opioids (see Table 5-3).

ANTIDEPRESSANTS

TRICYCLIC ANTIDEPRESSANTS (TCAs)

TCAs were the first medications proven effective for neuropathic pain in placebo-controlled trials. Although clinical trials of patients with HIV sensory neuropathy (59,60), cis-platinum neuropathy (61), and spinal cord injury pain (62) found little benefit of amitriptyline over placebo, an accurate summary of the overall efficacy of TCAs in neuropathic pain was provided by Mitchell Max in the title of a review of their efficacy, "Thirteen consecutive well-designed randomized trials show that antidepressants reduce pain in diabetic neuropathy and postherpetic neuralgia" (63). TCAs must be used cautiously in patients with a history of cardiovascular disease, and a screening EKG to check for cardiac conduction abnormalities is recommended before beginning treatment, especially in patients over 40 years of age. In a recent study, nearly 20% of patients treated with a TCA after a myocardial infarction developed adverse cardiac events (64). As with opioid analgesics, TCAs must be used cautiously in patients at risk for suicide or accidental death from overdose. TCAs may block the effects of certain antihypertensive drugs (e.g., clonidine), and they interact with drugs metabolized by P450 2D6. Because all selective serotonin reuptake inhibitors (SSRIs) inhibit P450 2D6, toxic TCA levels may result from coadministration of TCAs and SSRIs. In the elderly, TCAs may cause cognitive impairment and gait disturbances that can result in falls. Additional side effects of TCAs include sedation, anticholinergic effects (including exacerbation of urinary retention), postural hypotension, weight gain, and potentially exacerbation of glaucoma.

Most clinical trials of TCAs in neuropathic pain have examined amitriptyline, but amitriptyline is not recommended in elderly patients because it produces more adverse reactions than nortriptyline and desipramine. In a recent randomized, double-blind trial directly comparing nortriptyline and amitriptyline in patients with PHN, nortriptyline provided equivalent analgesic benefits but was better tolerated than amitriptyline (65). Regardless of which TCA is used, patients should be made to understand that TCAs have an analgesic effect that has been demonstrated to be independent of their antidepressant effect, and that, by prescribing a TCA, the physician is not suggesting depression is causing the pain. In general, starting doses should be relatively low, and the dose should be titrated up slowly until pain is controlled. Antidepressant doses may be required for full effectiveness (see Table 5-3).

VENLAFAXINE

Venlafaxine is a serotonin and norepinephrine reuptake inhibitor that inhibits noradrenergic reuptake at higher dosages. It has been found to be more effective than placebo in trials of patients with postmastectomy pain and PDN (66,67). An additional trial found it superior to placebo and roughly comparable to imipramine in treating painful polyneuropathy (68). A recent study also found it to be effective in preventing post-mastectomy pain syndrome when given perioperatively (69). Side effects may be less than with TCAs, but ECG monitoring should occur in relatively high risk patients because 5% of patients in the PDN trial demonstrated significant ECG changes (67). Both standard and extended release preparations of venlafaxine have been studied. The starting dose of venlafaxine is 75 mg/d, and it can be increased by 75 mg/d each week as needed to a maximum dose of 375 mg/d with standard venlafaxine or to 225 mg/d using the extended-release preparation. The full effect of treatment should be seen in 2-4 weeks.

DULOXETINE

Duloxetine is a new dual reuptake inhibitor of serotonin and norepinephrine. It has been shown to be an effective antidepressant and to significantly improve painful symptoms associated with depression (70). To date it has only been evaluated in PDN, but two trials have demonstrated significant benefits with minimal side effects compared to placebo (71,72). Two additional trials have demonstrated safety over 6 and 12 months (73,74). The latter trial compared duloxetine with "routine care" and found that at one year the duloxetine patients reported better pain conrol, improved quality of life, and reduced adverse events; most of the patients in the "routine care" group were treated with gabapentin, venlafaxine, or amytriptyline. On the strength of these trials duloxetine has recently been approved by the FDA for the treatment of diabetic peripheral neuropathic pain.

Advantages of duloxetine are that it seems to have a favorable side effect profile, it demonstrates efficacy within one week of treatment initiation, and, for certain neuropathic pain patients, it is an effective antidepressant. Unfortunately, it has only been studied in PDN to date. The 60 mg/d dose seems to be almost as effective as the 60 mg bid dose and seems to produce less side effects.

Sequential and Combination Treatment with First-Line Medications
Current understanding of the pathophysiology of neuropathic pain is consistent with the existence of multiple pain mechanisms, which may each

respond differently to medications with different mechanisms of action. Patients who do not respond to one of the first-line medications should usually be treated with one or more of the others. Despite the lack of controlled data, the use of combinations of two or more of these first-line medications can be recommended when patients have a partial response to a single one, and also at the beginning of treatment either to increase the likelihood of a beneficial response or when one of the medications being used requires titration to reach an effective dosage is also being used. Disadvantages of combination therapy include an increased risk of side effects as the number of medications is increased. Of note, the combination of tramadol with SSRIs, which includes the dual reuptake inhibitors venlafaxine and probably duloxetine, should be avoided because of the risk of serotonin syndrome.

Second-Line Medications

When patients do not have a satisfactory response to treatment with one or more of the first-line medications alone or in combination, there are several medications that can be recommended as second-line on the basis of positive results from a single randomized controlled trial or inconsistent results from multiple randomized controlled trials (with one exception). Carbamazepine and lamotrigine can be recommended for patients who have not responded to an adequate trial of gabapentin or pregabalin when treatment with an anticonvulsant is sought (75-78). Lamotrigine is the one second-line pharmacological treatment for which there is evidence of efficacy based on the results of multiple randomized controlled trials in several neuropathic pain syndromes (79-83), but it cannot be considered first-line because of the slow and careful titration required and the risk of severe rash and Stevens-Johnson syndrome associated with its use.

The antidepressants bupropion, citalopram, and paroxetine have shown promise in different neuropathic pain syndromes and could be considered for patients with depression who are intolerant of the first-line antidepressants (84,85).

Nonsteroidal antiinflammatory medications (NSAIDs) have been found to reduce pain severity in sciatica and PDN (86,87), but there is a clinical consensus that NSAIDs and acetaminophen rarely provide clinically meaningful pain relief in patients with neuropathic pain.

Intravenous lidocaine has been shown to be effective in treating PDN (88), but its administration is impracticable and associated with potentially severe systemic adverse effects. Trials with its oral analogue, mexilitine, have shown mixed results (89).

Capsaicin, another topical medication, has produced mixed results in clinical trials and often exacerbates pain when first applied (90).

There is some evidence to support the use of systemic corticosteroids in the management of complex regional pain syndrome (CRPS) (91), but their exact role has not been defined (32).

Other Therapies

NON-INVASIVE THERAPIES

Physical therapy is considered to be the first-line therapy for CRPS (32), having been proven effective in controlled trials (92). Physical therapy may also have a role in the management of other types of neuropathic pain, particularly those compromising limb function or gait.

Transcutaneous electrical nerve stimulation (TENS) has been shown to be effective in treating PDN in unselected as well as refractory patients (93-95). It has also shown promise in radicular and post-thoracotomy pain (96). It is non-invasive, relatively inexpensive, and usually well-tolerated.

Psychoeducational interventions, as part of a multidisciplinary approach, have an established role in the management of chronic nonmalignant musculoskeletal pain (97). It is likely that psychological interventions are beneficial in chronic neuropathic pain, though they have not been studied in this setting.

INVASIVE THERAPIES

In general, patients who are failing first-line pharmacological therapy and who have been identified as possibly benefitting from an invasive therapy, such as a spinal cord stimulation or intrathecal medication, should be referred to a pain management specialist.

Spinal cord stimulation has been studied in CRPS and PHN and found to be effective in reducing pain and improving quality of life in selected, challenging patients (98-101). It has also been studied in patients with other types of neuropathic pain with generally good results (102,103).

Intrathecal opioids or baclofen can be used in patients with debilitating pain or spasticity that cannot be controlled with systemic medications either because of ineffectiveness or intolerable side effects. (Oral opioids often cause side effects before adequate doses can be reached.) Intrathecal opioids require smaller doses because they are delivered to the primary target, the dorsal horn. Intrathecal corticosteroids combined with lidocaine have been used with success in refractory patients with PHN (104), although both intrathecal lidocaine and steroids are associated with a variety of potentially serious adverse reactions, including severe hypotension, neurotoxicity, and adhesive arachnoiditis. Recently a new selective N-type voltage-sensitive calcium channel blocking agent, ziconotide, was found to produce clinically significant pain relief in patients with neuropathic pain from cancer or AIDS that was refractory to high-dose systemic opioids (105).

Sympathetic or somatic/sympathetic regional anesthetic blocks can be performed in certain circumstances, such as in patients with CPRS who are unable to perform physical therapy. However, the need for frequent injections limits their use to short-term therapy (32).

Surgical or chemical sympathectomy has been used in an effort to treat neuropathic pain thought to be sympathetically mediated, but there is little evidence to support this practice (106).

Acupuncture and other alternative therapies are commonly employed by patients with neuropathic pain (107), but there is currently little scientific basis for recommending their use.

Future Developments

Given the difficulty managing some patients with neuropathic pain, prevention of the development of neuropathic pain is a critical area of present research. Different prevention strategies are being explored, including trials immunizing elderly individuals with the varicella vaccine to try to prevent herpes zoster (108) and treating herpes zoster patients pre-emptively with proven PHN treatments—for example, tricyclic antidepressants and opioid analgesics—to try to prevent PHN (109,110). In addition, more effective strategies for providing pre-emptive analgesia may prevent the development of various types of post-surgical neuropathic pain, such as phantom limb and post-mastectomy pain syndromes (69,111,112).

In the future, the pharmacological management of neuropathic pain will likely be aimed at the specific pathophysiologic defects causing pain rather than the disease responsible. One would predict that a mechanism-based treatment would be more precisely targeted and therefore more safe and effective. For example, determining that the pain of a patient with PHN is caused predominantly by central sensitization should allow a provider to choose a treatment proven effective in central sensitization specifically, rather than in neuropathic pain in general.

Although support for the potential of the mechanism-based approach is provided by a considerable body of research, it is not possible at present to identify the specific mechanisms that account for a patient's neuropathic pain symptoms and signs. Moreover, there are few examples of controlled trials in which treatment has been targeted to specific pain mechanisms in neuropathic pain patients. Clinical researchers are examining the extent to which pain mechanisms can be identified from patterns of symptoms, signs, quantitative sensory testing, and response to pharmacological challenges (14,16,113,114), and it is likely that major advances in identifying mechanisms and targeting treatment to them are on the horizon.

Conclusion

Neuropathic pain is a common, debilitating, often chronic disorder. It is important to correctly identify pain as neuropathic because the management of neuropathic pain differs considerably from the management of other types of pain. Furthermore, identifying pain as neuropathic may help uncover a significant underlying causative disease.

Attention to the relevance of neuropathic pain mechanisms to treatment, the possibility of preventing neuropathic pain, and the great interest in the pharmaceutical industry in developing new treatments for neuropathic pain all provide a basis for optimism about our future ability to manage neuropathic pain.

REFERENCES

1. **Woolf CJ.** Pain: moving from symptom control toward mechanism-specific pharmacologic management. Ann Intern Med. 2004;140:441-51.

2. **Backonja M.** Defining neuropathic pain. Anesth Analg. 2003;97:785-90.

3. **Portenoy RK.** Current pharmacotherapy of chronic pain. J Pain Symptom Manage. 2000;19:S16-20.

4. The effect of intensive diabetes therapy on the development and progression of neuropathy. The Diabetes Control and Complications Research Group. Ann Intern Med. 1995;122:561-8.

5. Effect of intensive diabetes treatment on nerve conduction in the Diabetes Control and Complications Trial. Ann Neurol. 1995;38:869-80.

6. **Tyring S, Barbarash RA, Nahlik JE, et al.** Famciclovir for the treatment of acute herpes zoster: effects on acute disease and postherpetic neuralgia. A randomized, double-blind, placebo-controlled trial. Collaborative Famciclovir Herpes Zoster Study Group. Ann Intern Med. 1995;123:89-96.

7. **Jackson JL, Gibbons R, Meyer G, Inouye L.** The effect of treating herpes zoster with oral acyclovir in preventing postherpetic neuralgia. A meta-analysis. Arch Intern Med. 1997;157:909-12.

8. **Tyring SK, Beutner KR, Tucker BA, et al.** Antiviral therapy for herpes zoster: randomized, controlled clinical trial of valacyclovir and famciclovir therapy in immunocompetent patients 50 years and older. Arch Fam Med. 2000;9:863-9.

9. **Bennett GJ.** Neuropathic pain: an overview. In: Borsook D, ed. Molecular neurobiology of pain. Seattle: IASP Press, 1997:109-113.

10. **Schmader KE.** The epidemiology and impact on quality of life of postherpetic neuralgia and painful diabetic neuropathy. Clin J Pain. 2002;18:350-4.

11. **Bowsher D.** The lifetime occurrence of herpes zoster and prevalence of postherpetic neuralgia: a retrospective survey in an elderly population. Eur J Pain 1999;3:335-42.

12. **Merskey H, Bogduk N, eds.** Classification of Chronic Pain: Descriptions of Chronic Pain Syndromes and Definitions of Pain Terms, 2nd ed. Seattle: IASP Press, 1994.

13. **Dworkin RH.** An overview of neuropathic pain: syndromes, symptoms, signs, and several mechanisms. Clin J Pain. 2002;18:343-9.

14. **Rowbotham MC, Petersen KL, Fields HL.** Is postherpetic neuralgia more than one disorder? Pain Forum. 1998;7:231-7.

15. **Fields HL, Rowbotham M, Baron R.** Postherpetic neuralgia: irritable nociceptors and deafferentation. Neurobiol Dis. 1998;5:209-27.

16. **Rowbotham MC, Baron R, Petersen KL, Fields HL.** Spectrum of pain mechanisms contributing to PHN. In: Watson CPN, Gershon AA, eds. Herpes Zoster and Postherpetic Neuralgia, 2nd ed. New York: Elsevier Press, 2001:183-95.

17. **Woolf CJ, Shortland P, Coggeshall RE.** Peripheral nerve injury triggers central sprouting of myelinated afferents. Nature. 1992;355:75-8.

18. **Dworkin RH, Nagasako EM, Galer BS.** Assessment of neuropathic pain. In: Turk DC, Melzack R, eds. Handbook of Pain Assessment, 2nd ed. New York: Guilford Press; 2001:519-48.

19. **Melzack R.** The McGill Pain Questionnaire: major properties and scoring methods. Pain. 1975;1:277-99.

20. **Dubuisson D, Melzack R.** Classification of clinical pain descriptions by multiple group discriminant analysis. Exp Neurol. 1976;51:480-7.

21. **Melzack R, Terrence C, Fromm G, Amsel R.** Trigeminal neuralgia and atypical facial pain: use of the McGill Pain Questionnaire for discrimination and diagnosis. Pain. 1986;27:297-302.

22. **Masson EA, Hunt L, Gem JM, Boulton AJ.** A novel approach to the diagnosis and assessment of symptomatic diabetic neuropathy. Pain. 1989;38:25-8.

23. **Boureau F, Doubrère JF, Luu M.** Study of verbal description in neuropathic pain. Pain. 1990;42:145-52.

24. **Defrin R, Ohry A, Blumen N, Urca G.** Acute pain threshold in subjects with chronic pain following spinal cord injury. Pain. 1999;83:275-82.

25. **Wilkie DJ, Huang HY, Reilly N, Cain KC.** Nociceptive and neuropathic pain in patients with lung cancer: a comparison of pain quality descriptors. J Pain Symptom Manage. 2001;22:899-910.

26. **Bowsher D.** Pathophysiology of postherpetic neuralgia: towards a rational treatment. Neurology. 1995;45:S56-57.

27. **Simpson DM, Haidich AB, Schifitto G, et al, for the ACTG 291 Study Team.** Severity of HIV-associated neuropathy is associated with plasma HIV-1 RNA levels. AIDS. 2002;16:407-12.

28. **Wood MJ, Kay R, Dworkin RH, et al.** Oral acyclovir therapy accelerates pain resolution in patients with herpes zoster: a meta-analysis of placebo controlled trials. Clin Infect Dis. 1996;22:341-7.

29. **Boulton AJ, Drury J, Clarke B, Ward JD.** Continuous subcutaneous insulin infusion in the management of painful diabetic neuropathy. Diabetes Care. 1982;5: 386-90.

30. **White NH, Waltman SR, Krupin T, Santiago JV.** Reversal of neuropathic and gastrointestinal complications related to diabetes mellitus in adolescents with improved metabolic control. J Pediatr. 1981;99:41-5.

31. **Loeser JD.** Cranial neuralgias. In: Loeser JD, Butler SH, Chapman CR, Turk DC, eds. Bonica's Management of Pain, 3rd ed. Philadelphia: Lippincott Williams & Wilkins; 2001:855-66.

32. **Rho RH, Brewer RP, Lamer TJ, Wilson PR.** Complex regional pain syndrome. Mayo Clin Proc. 2002;77:174-80.

33. **Dworkin RH, Backonja M, Rowbotham MC, et al.** Advances in neuropathic pain: diagnosis, mechanisms, and treatment recommendations. Arch Neurol. 2003;60:1524-34.

34. **Rowbotham M, Harden N, Stacey B, et al.** Gabapentin for the treatment of postherpetic neuralgia: a randomized controlled trial. JAMA. 1998;280:1837-42.

35. **Backonja M, Beydoun A, Edwards KR, et al.** Gabapentin for the symptomatic treatment of painful neuropathy in patients with diabetes mellitus. JAMA. 1998;280:1831-6.

36. **Gorson KC, Schott C, Herman R, et al.** Gabapentin in the treatment of painful diabetic neuropathy: a placebo-controlled, double-blind, crossover trial. J Neurol Neurosurg Psychiatry. 1999;66:251-2.

37. **Rice AS, Maton S, for the Postherpetic Neuralgia Study Group.** Gabapentin in postherpetic neuralgia: a randomised, double blind, placebo controlled study. Pain. 2001;94:215-24.

38. **Serpell MG, for the Neuropathic Pain Study Group.** Gabapentin in neuropathic pain syndromes: a randomized, double-blind, placebo-controlled trial. Pain. 2002; 99:557-66.

39. **Bone M, Critchley P, Buggy DJ.** Gabapentin in postamputation phantom limb pain: a randomized, double-blind, placebo-controlled, cross-over study. Reg Anesth Pain Med. 2002;27:481-6.

40. **Pandey CK, Bose N, Garg G, et al.** Gabapentin for the treatment of pain in Guillain-Barré syndrome: a double-blinded, placebo-controlled, crossover study. Anesth Analg. 2002;95:1719-23.

41. **Tai Q, Kirshblum S, Chen B, et al.** Gabapentin in the treatment of neuropathic pain after spinal cord injury: a prospective, randomized double-blind, crossover trial. J Spinal Cord Med. 2002;25:100-5.

42. **Levendoğlu F, Öğün CÖ, Özerbil Ö, et al.** Gabapentin is a first-line drug for the treatment of neuropathic pain in spinal cord injury. Spine. 2003;29:743-51.

43. **Dworkin RH, Corbin AE, Young JP Jr, et al.** Pregabalin for the treatment of postherpetic neuralgia: a randomized, placebo-controlled trial. Neurology. 2003;60:1274-83.

44. **Sabatowski R, Galvez R, Cherry DA, et al.** Pregabalin reduces pain and improvesd sleep and mood disturbances in patients with postherpetic neuralgia: results of a randomised, placebo-controlled clinical trial. Pain. 2004;109:26-35.

45. **Rosenstock J, Tuchman M, LaMoreaux, Sharma U.** Pregabalin for the treatment of painful diabetic peripheral neuropathy: a double-blind, placebo-controlled trial. Pain. 2004;110:628-38.

46. **Rowbotham MC, Davies PS, Verkempinck C, Galer BS.** Lidocaine patch: double-blind controlled study of a new treatment method for post-herpetic neuralgia. Pain. 1996;65:39-44,46.

47. **Galer BS, Rowbotham MC, Perander J, Friedman E.** Topical lidocaine patch relieves postherpetic neuralgia more effectively than a vehicle topical patch: results of an enriched enrollment study. Pain. 1999;80:533-8.

48. **Meier T, Wasner G, Faust M, et al.** Efficacy of lidocaine patch 5% in the treatment of focal peripheral neuropathic pain syndromes: a randomized, double-blind, placebo-controlled study. Pain. 2003;106:151-8.

49. **Watson CPN, Babul N.** Efficacy of oxycodone in neuropathic pain: a randomized trial in postherpetic neuralgia. Neurology. 1998;50:1837-41.

50. **Gimbel JS, Richards P, Portenoy RK.** Controlled-release oxycodone for pain in diabetic neuropathy: a randomized controlled trial. Neurology. 2003;60:927-34.

51. **Huse E, Larbig W, Flor H, Birbaumer N.** The effect of opioids on phantom limb pain and cortical reorganization. Pain. 2001;90:47-55.

52. **Raja SN, Haythornthwaite JA, Pappagallo M, et al.** Opioids versus antidepressants in postherpetic neuralgia: a randomized, placebo-controlled trial. Neurology. 2002;59:1015-21.

53. **Rowbotham MC, Twilling L, Davies PS, et al.** Oral opioid therapy for chronic peripheral and central pain. N Engl J Med. 2003;348:1223-32.

54. **Watson CPN, Moulin D, Watt-Watson J, et al.** Controlled-release oxycodone relieves neuropathic pain: a randomized controlled trial in painful diabetic neuropathy. Pain. 2003;105:71-8.

55. **Morley JS, Bridson J, Nash TP, et al.** Low-dose methadone has an analgesic effect in neuropathic pain: a double-blind randomized controlled crossover trial. Palliative Med. 2003;17:576-87.

56. **Harati Y, Gooch C, Swenson M, et al.** Double-blind randomized trial of tramadol for the treatment of the pain of diabetic neuropathy. Neurology. 1998;50:1842-6.

57. **Sindrup SH, Andersen G, Madsen C, et al.** Tramadol relieves pain and allodynia in polyneuropathy: a randomised, double-blind, controlled trial. Pain. 1999;83:85-90.

58. **Boureau F, Legallicier P, Kabir-Ahmadi M.** Tramadol in post-herpetic neuralgia: a randomized, double-blind, placebo-controlled trial. Pain. 2003;104:323-31.

59. **Kieburtz K, Simpson D, Yiannoutsos C, et al, for the AIDS Clinical Trial Group 242 Protocol Team.** A randomized trial of amitriptyline and mexiletine for painful neuropathy in HIV infection. Neurology. 1998;51:1682-8.

60. **Shlay JC, Chaloner K, Max MB, et al, for the Terry Beirn Community Programs for Clinical Research on AIDS.** Acupuncture and amitriptyline for pain due to HIV-related peripheral neuropathy: a randomized controlled trial. JAMA. 1998;280:1590-5.

61. **Hammack JE, Michalak JC, Loprinzi CL, et al.** Phase III evaluation of nortriptyline for alleviation of symptoms of cis-platinum-induced peripheral neuropathy. Pain. 2002;98:195-203.

62. **Cardenas DD, Warms CA, Turner JA, et al.** Efficacy of amitriptyline for relief of pain in spinal cord injury: results of a randomized controlled trial. Pain. 2002;96:365-73.

63. **Max MB.** Thirteen consecutive well-designed randomized trials show that antidepressants reduce pain in diabetic neuropathy and postherpetic neuralgia. Pain Forum. 1995;4:248-53.

64. **Roose SP, Laghrissi-Thode F, Kennedy JS, et al.** Comparison of paroxetine and nortriptyline in depressed patients with ischemic heart disease. JAMA. 1998;279:287-91.

65. **Watson CPN, Vernich L, Chipman M, Reed K.** Nortriptyline versus amitriptyline in postherpetic neuralgia: a randomized trial. Neurology. 1998;51:1166-71.

66. **Tasmuth T, Hartel B, Kalso E.** Venlafaxine in neuropathic pain following treatment of breast cancer. Eur J Pain. 2002;6:17-24.

67. **Rowbotham MC, Goli V, Kunz NR, Lei D.** Venlafaxine extended release in the treatment of painful diabetic neuropathy: a double-blind, placebo-controlled study. Pain. 2004;100:697-706.

68. **Sindrup SH, Bach FW, Madsen C, et al.** Venlafaxine versus imipramine in painful polyneuropathy: a randomized, controlled trial. Neurology. 2003;60:1284-9.

69. **Reuben SS, Makari-Judson G, Lurie SD.** Evaluation of efficacy of the perioperative administration of venlafaxine XR in the prevention of postmastectomy pain syndrome. J Pain Symptom Manage. 2004;27:133-9.

70. **Fava M, Mallinckrody CH, Detke MJ, et al.** The effect of duloxetine on the painful physical symptoms in depressed patients. Do improvements in these symptoms result in higher remission rates? J Clin Psychiatry. 2004;65:521-30.

71. **Goldstein DJ, Lu Y, Iyengar S, et al.** Duloxetine in the treatment of the pain associated with diabetic neuropathy. Poster presented at the 156th American Psychiatric Association, 17-22 May 2003, San Francisco.

72. **Wernicke JF, Lu Y, D'Souza DN, et al.** Duloxetine at doses of 60 mg and 60 mg bid is effective in the treatment of diabetic neuropathic pain. Poster presented at the American Psychiatric Association, 1-6 May 2004, New York.

73. **Raskin J, Wang F, Clemens JW, D'Souza DN.** Duloxetine for patients with diabetic neuropathic pain: a six-month open label safety study. Poster presented at the 23rd Annual Meeting of the Joint American Pain Society and Canadian Pain Society, 6-9 May 2004, Vancouver.

74. **Wernicke JF, Rosen A, Lu Y, et al.** The safety of duloxetine in the long-term treatment of diabetic neuropathic pain. Poster presented at the American Academy of Pain Medicine, 3-9 March 2004, Orlando.

75. **McQuay HJ, Carroll D, Jadad AR, et al.** Anticonvulsant drugs for management of pain: a systematic review. BMJ. 1995;311:1047-52.

76. **Sindrup SH, Jensen TS.** Efficacy of pharmacological treatments of neuropathic pain: an update and effect related to mechanism of drug action. Pain. 1999;83:389-400.

77. **Collins SL, Moore RA, McQuay HJ, Wiffen P.** Antidepressants and anticonvulsants for diabetic neuropathy and postherpetic neuralgia: a quantitative systematic review. J Pain Symptom Manage. 2000;20:449-58.

78. **Sindrup SH, Jensen TS.** Pharmacologic treatment of pain in polyneuropathy. Neurology. 2000;55:915-20.

79. **Simpson DM, Olney R, McArthur JC, et al, for the Lamotrigine HIV Neuropathy Study Group.** A placebo-controlled trial of lamotrigine for painful HIV-associated neuropathy. Neurology. 2000;54:2115-9.

80. **Simpson DM, McArthur JC, Olney R, et al.** Lamotrigine for HIV-associated painful sensory neuropathies: a placebo-controlled trial. Neurology. 2003;60:1508-14.

81. **Eisenberg E, Luria Y, Braker C, et al.** Lamotrigine reduces painful diabetic neuropathy: a randomized, controlled study. Neurology. 2001;57:505-9.

82. **Vestergaard K, Andersen G, Gottrup H, et al.** Lamotrigine for central poststroke pain: a randomized controlled trial. Neurology. 2001;56:184-90.

83. **Finnerup NB, Sindrup SH, Bach FW, et al.** Lamotrigine in spinal cord injury pain: a randomized controlled trial. Pain. 2002;96:375-83.

84. **McQuay HJ, Tramèr M, Nye BA, et al.** A systematic review of antidepressants in neuropathic pain. Pain. 1996;68:217-27.

85. **Semenchuk MR, Sherman S, Davis B.** Double-blind, randomized trial of bupropion SR for the treatment of neuropathic pain. Neurology. 2001;57:1583-8.

86. **Dreiser RL, Le Parc JM, Velicitat P, Lleu PL.** Oral meloxicam is effective in acute sciatica: two randomised, double-blind trials versus placebo or diclofenac. Inflamm Res. 2001;50(Suppl 1):S17-23.

87. **Cohen KL, Harris S.** Efficacy and safety of nonsteroidal anti-inflammatory drugs in the therapy of diabetic neuropathy. Arch Intern Med. 1987;147:1442-4.

88. **Kastrup J, Petersen P, Dejard A, et al.** Intravenous lidocaine infusion. A new treatment of chronic painful diabetic neuropathy? Pain. 1987;28:69-75.

89. **Mendell JR, Sahenk Z.** Painful sensory neuropathy. N Engl J Med. 2003;348:1243-55.

90. **Mason L, Moore RA, Derry S, et al.** Systematic review of topical capsaicin for the treatment of chronic pain. BMJ. 2004;328:991-5.

91. **Kingery WS.** A critical review of controlled clinical trials for peripheral neuropathic pain and complex regional pain syndromes. Pain. 1997;73:123-39.

92. **Oerlemans HM, Oostendorp RA, de Boo T, et al.** Adjuvant physical therapy versus occupational therapy in patients with reflex sympathetic dystrophy/complex regional pain syndrome type I. Arch Phys Med Rehabil. 2000;81:49-56.

93. **Kumar D, Marshall HJ.** Diabetic peripheral neuropathy: amelioration of pain with transcutaneous electrostimulation. Diabetes Care. 1997;20:1702-5.

94. **Kumar D, Alvaro MS, Julka IS, Marshall HJ.** Diabetic peripheral neuropathy: effectiveness of electrotherapy and amitriptyline for symptomatic relief. Diabetes Care. 1998;21:1322-5.

95. **Alvaro M, Kumar D, Julka IS.** Transcutaneous electrostimulation: emerging treatment for diabetic neuropathic pain. Diabetes Technol Ther. 1999;1:77-80.

96. **Carrol EN, Badura AS.** Focal intense brief transcutaneous electric nerve stimulation for treatment of radicular and postthroacotomy pain. Arch Phys Med Rehabil. 2001;82:262-4.

97. **Allegrante JP.** The role of adjunctive therapy in the management of chronic nonmalignant pain. Am J Med. 1996;101:33S-39S.

98. **Kemler MA, Barendse GAM, van Kleef M, et al.** Spinal cord stimulation in patients with chronic reflex sympathetic dystrophy. N Engl J Med. 2000;343:618-24.

99. **Kemler MA, De Vet HC, Barendse GA, et al.** The effect of spinal cord stimulation in patients with chronic reflex sympathetic dystrophy: two years' follow-up of the randomized controlled trial. Ann Neurol. 2004;55:13-8.

100. **Harke H, Gretenkort P, Ladleif HU, et al.** Spinal cord stimulation in postherpetic neuralgia and in acute hepres zoster pain. Anesth Analg. 2002;94:694-700.

101. **Meglio M, Cioni B, Prezioso A, Talamonti G.** Spinal cord stimulation (SCS) in the treatment of postherpetic pain. Acta Neurochir Suppl. 1989;46:65-6.

102. **Cameron T.** Safety and efficacy of spinal cord stimulation for the treatment of chronic pain: a 20-year literature review. J Neurosurg. 2004;100(3 Suppl):254-67.

103. **Shimoji K, Hokari T, Kano T, et al.** Management of intractable pain with percutaneous epidural spinal cord stimulation: differences in pain-relieving effects among diseases and sites of pain. Anesth Analg. 1993;77:110-6.

104. **Kotani N, Kushikata T, Hashimoto H, et al.** Intrathecal methylprednisolone for intractable postherpetic neuralgia. N Engl J Med. 2000;343:1514-9.

105. **Staats PS, Yearwood T, Charapata SG, et al.** Intrathecal ziconotide in the treatment of refractory pain in patients with cancer or AIDS. JAMA. 2004;291:63-70.

106. **Mailis A, Furlan A.** Sympathectomy for neuropathic pain. Cochrane Database Syst Rev. 2003;2:CD002918.

107. **Brunelli B, Gorson KC.** The use of complementary and alternative medicines by patients with peripheral neuropathy. J Neurol Sci. 2003;218:59-66.

108. **Oxman M.** Immunization to reduce the frequency and severity of herpes zoster and its complications. Neurology. 1995;45(Suppl 8):S41-46.

109. **Bowsher D.** The effects of pre-emptive treatment of postherpetic neuralgia with amitriptyline: a randomized, double-blind, placebo-controlled trial. J Pain Symptom Manage. 1997;13:327-31.

110. **Dworkin RH, Schmader KE.** Treatment and prevention of postherpetic neuralgia. Clin Infect Dis. 2003;36:877-82.

111. **Fassoulaki A, Sarantopoulos C, Melemeni A, Hogan Q.** EMLA reduces acute and chronic pain after breast surgery for cancer. Reg Anesth Pain Med. 2000; 25:350-5.

112. **Fassoulaki A, Patris K, Sarantopoulos C, Hogan Q.** The analgesic effect of gabapentin and mexiletine after breast surgery for cancer. Anesth Analg. 2002;95:985-91.

113. **Woolf CJ, Max MB.** Mechanism-based pain diagnosis. Anesthesiology. 2001; 95:241-9.

114. **Petersen KL, Fields HL, Brennum J, et al.** Capsaicin evoked pain and allodynia in post-herpetic neuralgia. Pain. 2000;88:125-33.

6

■ ■ ■

Pharmacological Treatment
of Pain

Ewan McNicol, MS

Daniel B. Carr, MD

Pain is the most frequent reason patients visit their primary care providers (PCPs) (1). The PCP encounters a spectrum of diverse complaints ranging from migraine to cancer pain. The PCP is expected to treat both acute pain, such as that resulting from minor outpatient procedures, and chronic neuropathic pain. Whether acute or chronic, inadequately treated pain can impair a patient's quality of life. It can slow recovery from injury or surgery, interfere with daily activities, and undermine social interaction.

Although treatment of the patient with chronic pain may require a multidisciplinary approach including consultation with a pain specialist, the PCP may slow or prevent the transition from acute to chronic pain or reverse many of the impairments associated with persistent pain by treating pain aggressively and comprehensively. Considerably more patients with pain are seen by PCPs than by pain specialists (1). Although it is widely acknowledged that pain should be treated aggressively, evidence of under-treatment of pain in primary care persists (2), despite recent leaps in understanding the mechanisms and pharmacology of pain and the announcement of the "decade of pain research" (3). Inadequately treated pain has been documented in pediatric through geriatric populations and in multiple settings (4-9).

Several factors contribute to the gap between research and clinical practice: lack of education in schools of medicine (10); clinician's incorrect attitudes or beliefs about side effects and addiction (11-14); patient concerns about addiction, or beliefs that much pain is not treatable, or feelings that one should not complain about pain (15); regulations that render health care providers less willing to prescribe or dispense opioids because of fear of prosecution (11,16); and institutional economics that have led many institutions not to start, or even do away with, acute pain services (17). Yet, within the last five years two major cases have been brought against physicians in Oregon and California for under-treatment of pain, the latter of which resulted in a $1.5 million settlement for the family of a patient with cancer. The physician in question failed to prescribe adequate medication despite clear documentation that his patient was suffering from severe pain (18). And, apart from these exceptional cases, the Joint Commission for the Accreditation of Healthcare Organizations (JCAHO) now mandates pain assessment and appropriate treatment across all practice settings (19).

Pharmacotherapy is considered the cornerstone of management for acute and chronic pain in all age groups (20). A physician's treatment plan should begin with a thorough pain assessment and pain medication history in order to, if possible, identify the nature (acute versus chronic, nociceptive versus neuropathic) and mechanisms of the patient's pain. The physician should ascertain factors that alleviate or worsen pain; its quality and intensity, radiation, and temporal factors; current drug intake (prescription, over-the-counter, herbal medications, and/or social/recreational); and past treatments (including successes/failures, adverse effects, and allergic reactions). The physician should inquire as to how the patient's pain affects functioning. Health-care practitioners should familiarize themselves with the pharmacodynamics, pharmacokinetics, potential drug-drug or drug-food interactions, and contraindications for any medications prescribed, including those already in use by the patient. Practitioners should also take into account factors such as patient age, concurrent medical conditions, or pregnancy. In the present era of patient-centered care, the patient should be included as an integral and informed part of his or her treatment. Treatment rationales and realistic goals should be agreed upon. Health-care practitioners should also assess individual characteristics that may affect compliance (e.g., patient age, frequency/complexity of regimen, route of administration, insurance co-payments or even noncoverage).

The menu of drug therapies can be broadly divided into opioid analgesics, non-steroidal anti-inflammatory drugs (NSAIDs) (including cyclooxygenase-2 [COX-2] inhibitors), and adjuvant analgesics (drugs whose primary indication is not for pain management). Mild or moderate pain often responds to non-opioid analgesia. Severe pain may require an opioid with or without an NSAID. Neuropathic pain may not respond adequately to either regimen, however, and the addition of or substitution with an adjuvant analgesic may be required.

Etiology and Treatment Selection

Pain is traditionally categorized according to its etiology and temporal course. *Acute pain* is elicited primarily by injury, infection, or trauma, and includes the pain evoked by surgery. Activation of nociceptors at the site of tissue damage leads to a response in both the central and autonomic nervous systems. A-delta and C fibers are involved in nociceptive transmission from periphery to the spinal cord; these pathways are rich in opioid receptors and hence nociceptive pain is typically opioid-responsive. Pain resolves as the injury heals but can be prevented or minimized by aggressive pain management.

Chronic pain may be a consequence of chronic disease (e.g., arthritis, fibromyalgia, AIDS), one-time damage to the peripheral and central nervous system (e.g., herpes zoster, stroke), or a sequel to inadequately treated acute pain. It is not the duration of pain that differentiates chronic from acute pain; rather, it is the inability of the body to restore itself to previous homeostatic levels (21). In many cases, the original tissue damage has healed, but central and/or peripheral sensitization and self-sustaining activity within nociceptive circuits ("wind-up") lead to persistent pain in the absence of continuing insult (see Chapter 1 for a detailed discussion). Chronic pain generally requires chronic therapy, because treatments do not alter the underlying pathological process.

In some diseases, such as cancer, patients may experience both acute and chronic pain. Patients may have long-standing pain due to chemotherapy-induced neuropathy along with acute pain due to procedures such as bone marrow aspiration. Although different strategies may be required to treat pain of distinct mechanisms or etiology, many medications may be useful across a range of pain types. This chapter surveys the drug treatment of pain, subject to the broad constraint that much of the evidentiary basis for pain treatment compares unfavorably with corresponding literature for other high-impact public health problems (22,23).

Pharmacotherapy

General Principles: The WHO "Ladder"

The World Health Organization (WHO) developed a series of guidelines in 1986 to address deficiencies in the treatment of cancer pain (24). A central component of these guidelines is the analgesic three-step "ladder" (Fig. 6-1). The guidelines suggest that

> [I]f pain occurs, there should be prompt oral administration of drugs in the following order: nonopioids (aspirin and paracetamol); then, as necessary, mild opioids (codeine); then strong opioids such as morphine, until the patient is free of pain. To calm fears and anxiety, additional drugs – "adjuvants" – should be used. To maintain freedom from pain, drugs should be given "by the clock", that is every 3-6 hours, rather than 'on demand'. This three-step approach of administering the right drug in the right dose at the right time is inexpensive and 80-90% effective. Surgical intervention on appropriate nerves may provide further pain relief if drugs are not wholly effective.

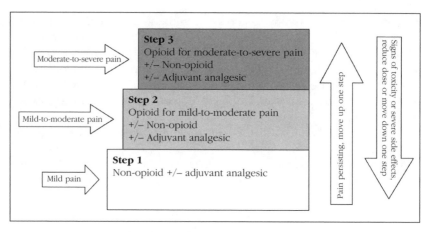

Figure 6-1   The WHO analgesic ladder.

The WHO ladder and accompanying guidelines have been disseminated worldwide. In addition it has been used in pain models other than for cancer and remains a cornerstone of many pain management guidelines. To date, however, no randomized controlled trials (RCTs) have been conducted to validate WHO claims regarding the effectiveness of the ladder, either in treating cancer pain or in other pain models (25). A 1995 prospective case series involving more than 2000 patients reported adequate analgesia in 88% of cases, but it did not compare outcomes with those achieved before introduction of the ladder (26). A recent systematic review of the use of NSAIDs in cancer pain concluded that for the first step of the ladder (the management of mild pain) the results strongly suggest that NSAID alone is superior to placebo and adequate for this purpose, at least in the short-term. However, the review did not find sufficient evidence to substantiate the second step of the ladder (the treatment of mild-to-moderate pain) in which WHO recommends the addition of a "weak" opioid to the patient's regimen. It may be advisable for a patient to increase to "maximum acceptable" the dose of the NSAID (or adjuvant drug) before the addition of, or replacement with, an opioid (27).

There are inherent difficulties in developing RCTs comparing the WHO ladder with other treatment regimens, which may explain the scarcity of literature reporting such trials (25). In the meantime, it appears that the ladder will remain a central component of the physician's pain management strategy. Other WHO recommendations, such as the administration of medications by mouth, and the importance of administering medications "around the clock" are generally accepted as good practice

Advantages of the oral route of drug administration include dependability, ease of access for patients, convenience, rapid onset, and relatively low cost. Oral administration of drugs can manage most cancer pain, pain of other serious illnesses (e.g., HIV/AIDS, sickle disease), and post-operative pain. Physiological limitations, however, such as dysphagia from mucositis after bone marrow transplant, nausea from chemotherapy, malabsorption from gastrointestinal (GI) dysfunction such as fistula, or the dumping syndrome in HIV/AIDS or post-operative ileus, or the need to swallow an impractical number of tablets may require other routes of administration. Intramuscular injections should be avoided because of the discomfort they produce, and the variability of responses depending upon tissue perfusion at the site and/or the technique used to administer the drug. Intramuscular doses may actually end up being deposited in the superficial adipose tissue (especially in women) and not in muscle.

Nonopioid Analgesics

Nonopioid analgesics include NSAIDs (including the subset of selective COX-2 inhibitors) and acetaminophen. Currently more than 20 NSAIDs are available (Table 6-1).

Indications for Use

NSAIDs are recognized as an important tool in treating both acute and chronic pain. They are indicated for pain of inflammation but may also be used in non-inflammatory conditions (20). Both NSAIDS and acetaminophen may be used alone for mild-to-moderate pain or combined with opioids (in combination preparations or separately) for moderate-to-severe pain.

Efficacy

Although many classes of NSAIDs are available and several NSAIDs exist within each class, it is unclear which class or agent is most efficacious, and if there are clinical differences between these agents that justify their cost differences. Additionally, it is uncertain which opioid and NSAID combinations are the most efficacious for pain or even what may be the additional benefit of combining an NSAID with an opioid in treating cancer pain (27,28). NSAIDs have a ceiling for analgesia but not for side effects; administration of doses above the recommended range may increase risk of toxicity without an accompanying increase in analgesic efficacy (29). If a particular NSAID does not provide adequate analgesia for an individual patient, despite maximizing the prescribed dose, another NSAID may be successful, even one from the same class.

Advantages/Benefits

Advantages of NSAID and acetaminophen therapies include wide availability, familiarity to patients and families, effectiveness for pain of diverse etiologies, ease of administration, lack of physical or psychological dependence, additive analgesia when combined with opioids, and in many cases their relatively low cost. Disadvantages include a ceiling for analgesic effect versus dose (hence the need for addition of an opioid to treat moderate-to-severe

Table 6-1   Dosing Information: NSAIDs and Acetaminophen

Agent	Usual Analgesic Adult Dosing (mg)*	Dosing Interval (hours)	Maximum Dose (mg)	Comments
Acetaminophen	325-650	4-6	4000	Available as rectal, liquid, and sustained-release formulations. Possible fatal hepatotoxicity in overdosage. No peripheral antiinflammatory or antiplatelet properties.
Salicylates				
Aspirin	325-650**	4-6	4000**	Available as rectal, liquid, and sustained-release formulations. Do not use in children <12 years old with suspected viral infection because of potential development of Reye's syndrome.
Choline magnesium trisalicylate	500-1500	8-12	4500	Minimal platelet effect; use with caution in renal failure and GI disease.
Diflunisal	500-1000 initial, then 250-500	8-12	1500	Less GI toxicity than aspirin.
Propionic Acids				
Fenoprofen	200*	4-6	3200	Slightly more GI side effects than ibuprofen.
Flurbiprofen	100	6-12	300	Slightly more GI side effects than ibuprofen.
Ibuprofen	200-400**	4-6	1200**	Lowest incidence of GI side effects. Weaker antiinflammatory properties.
Ketoprofen	25-50**	6-8	300	Higher incidence of side effects than ibuprofen.
Naproxen	500 initial, then 250**	6-8	1250**	Slightly higher incidence of side effects than ibuprofen.
Naproxen Sodium	550 initial, then 275**	6-8	1375**	Slightly higher incidence of side effects than ibuprofen.
Oxazoprin	600	24	1200	—
Acetic Acids				
Diclofenac	50**	8	150**	Similar action and side effects to naproxen.
Etodolac	200-400	8-12	1200	Similar side effects to ibuprofen. Similar action to naproxen.

(cont'd)

Table 6-1   Dosing Information: NSAIDs and Acetaminophen (Cont'd)

Agent	Usual Analgesic Adult Dosing (mg)*	Dosing Interval (hours)	Maximum Dose (mg)	Comments
Acetic Acids (cont'd)				
Indomethacin	25-50	8-12	200	High incidence of side effects including GI, dizziness, and headaches.
Ketorolac	IV: 30-60 initial, then 15-30 Oral: 10	IV: 6 Oral: 4-6	IV: 120 Oral: 40 (or 120 combined IV and oral)	Patients under 50 kg, or above age 65, should receive the lower dose of ketorolac (30 mg followed by 15 mg). Limit treatment to 5 days. May precipitate renal failure.
Sulindac	150-200	12	400	Similar in tolerance to naproxen. Safest NSAID for use in mild renal impairment.
Tolmetin	400	8	2000	—
Enolic Acids				
Meloxicam	7.5-15	24	15	—
Piroxicam	10-40	24	40	Higher doses associated with increase in GI adverse effects.
Anthranilic Acids				
Mefenamic acid	500 initial, then 250	4	1500	Use limited to 7 days. Minor anti-inflammatory effects. Indicated for short-term relief of mild-to-moderate pain.
Nabumetone	1000	12-24	2000	Minimal effect on platelet aggregation.

* Oral unless specified.
** Anti-inflammatory doses may be higher.
Dosage information from Wickersham RM, Novak KK, eds. Drug Facts and Comparisons. St. Louis: Wolters Kluwer; 2002.

pain), risk of side effects, including GI bleeding and renal toxicity, and the availability of few parenteral formulations (30).

Mechanism of Action

The primary mechanism of action of NSAIDs is by inhibition of the enzyme cyclooxygenase (COX), thereby preventing the subsequent formation of prostaglandins responsible for inflammation. In addition to this peripheral effect, NSAIDs act centrally at the brain or spinal cord as well as on other inflammatory mediators. Acetaminophen has no anti-inflammatory properties. Its mechanism of action is not well defined but may be due to inhibition of an isoform of COX, COX-3, that is found only in the central nervous system (20). Both NSAIDs and acetaminophen also have antipyretic properties.

Toxicities and Adverse Effects
Perhaps reflecting the unlimited access to, and vast quantities consumed of, these drugs, NSAIDs account for more reports of toxicity than any other type of agent (31). They are responsible for multiple side effects, primarily as a consequence of inhibition of the production of prostaglandins not involved in the inflammatory process. Risk factors for toxicity include dose, duration of therapy, patient age, and renal impairment.

GASTROINTESTINAL EFFECTS
Prostaglandins maintain the protective layer of the gastric mucosa. Reduction of prostaglandin production by NSAIDs impairs this protective barrier. Ulceration and bleeding can occur, even without symptoms. A 1996 meta-analysis concluded that, overall, ibuprofen was associated with the lowest relative risk of GI complications, followed by diclofenac. Azapropazone, tolmetin, ketoprofen, and piroxicam ranked highest for risk (32). The concurrent use of proton pump inhibitors, such as pantoprazole and omeprazole, or the prostaglandin analog misoprostol may reduce the risk of both gastric and duodenal ulcers. The benefit of proton pump inhibitors is thought to be greater than that of histamine-2 receptor antagonists (ranitidine, famotidine, etc.) in this setting (20). In addition, NSAIDs can cause local irritation of the gastric mucosa. Symptoms include heartburn and upper abdominal pain (33). Prevention of local effects can be achieved by taking the NSAID with food or by administering an enteric-coated formulation. Acetaminophen does not damage the gastric mucosa.

HEMATOLOGICAL EFFECTS
Most NSAIDs interfere with platelet aggregation. Choline magnesium trisalicylate, nabumetone, and salsalate have reduced or no effect on aggregation. Aspirin causes irreversible inhibition of platelet aggregability; up to seven days are required for the synthesis of normally adherent platelets after discontinuation of aspirin therapy (33). All other non-selective NSAIDs reversibly inhibit aggregation; therefore inhibition lasts only as long as sufficient systemic quantities of the drug remain. Acetaminophen has no antiplatelet effects.

RENAL EFFECTS
All NSAIDs can cause renal impairment by preventing synthesis of renal vasodilator prostaglandins and by other mechanisms (20). Patients are at particular risk post-operatively because they may be volume depleted. Injected ketorolac is most commonly implicated; consequently such therapy is restricted to five days.

CENTRAL NERVOUS SYSTEM EFFECTS

Mild effects including dizziness, headache, reduced attention span, and loss of short-term memory have all been reported with NSAIDs, possibly as a consequence of central prostaglandin inhibition (20,33).

HEPATIC EFFECTS

Acetaminophen can cause fatal hepatic necrosis with acute overdose. Hepatic injury can also occur at therapeutic doses when patients regularly consume alcohol, are fasting, or have pre-existing hepatic dysfunction. NSAIDs may also occasionally produce liver damage (20).

Contraindications

NSAIDs are contraindicated in patients with a history of hypersensitivity to aspirin or to other NSAIDs and in patients with active peptic ulceration. They should be used with caution in the elderly or pregnant, in breast-feeding mothers, and in patients with coagulation problems, history of GI ulceration, or history of hepatic, renal or cardiac insufficiency. Aspirin should be avoided in patients under the age of 12 due to the potential for Reye's syndrome.

Drug Interactions

NSAIDs interact with multiple classes of drugs. Only the most common or most serious are listed here.

1. *Anticoagulants*—Anticoagulants include warfarin, heparin, and low-molecular weight heparins. Interactions of these agents with NSAIDs are associated with increased risk of hemorrhage.

2. *ACE Inhibitors*—Co-administration may cause reduced antihypotensive effects, increased risk of renal impairment, and hyperkalemia.

3. *Methotrexate*—Interaction with NSAIDs may cause reduced excretion and possible toxicity.

4. *Antidiabetics*—Co-administration enhances the effects of sulphonylureas.

Drug interactions with acetaminophen are less common but prolonged use may enhance the effects of warfarin.

Dosage

The recommended dose range for individual NSAIDs is listed in Table 6-1. It is suggested that the use of lower risk NSAIDs in low dosage should substantially reduce the morbidity and mortality due to serious GI toxicity (32). If pain relief is not achieved at the maximum recommended dose, then the particular drug should be replaced with an NSAID from the same or another class (20).

COX-2 Inhibitors (Coxibs)

Their Roles in the Body

With the discovery and isolation of separate isoforms of cyclooxygenase, it was recognized that at least two forms of COX are expressed in tissues. COX-1 is thought to play a protective role. It is found under normal physiological conditions in the GI tract (maintaining gastric mucosa), vascular system (preserving platelet function), kidneys (preserving renal blood flow in the presence of volume depletion), and most other tissues. COX-2 is expressed constitutively only in the CNS and kidneys. In other organs it is thought to be induced only when the body is exposed to insult through trauma, surgery, or inflammation.

Although recent evidence suggests that the above theory is oversimplified, the clinical availability of newer NSAIDs selective for the COX-2 isoenzyme (COX-2 inhibitors, or coxibs) may nevertheless offer reduced organ toxicity, in particular reduction in both GI adverse effects and bleeding time (34). However, COX-2 inhibitors (a misnomer, in that all such agents currently available inhibit COX-1 to some extent) do not reduce the incidence of renal side effects observed with non-selective NSAIDs and may, in fact, increase the incidence of cardiac events (34,35). Reduction of thrombotic events with low-dose aspirin therapy is based on selective irreversible inhibition of COX-1-mediated platelet thromboxane production. The selective inhibition of prostacyclin formation by COX-2 selective NSAIDs prevents inhibition of thrombosis by prostacyclin, resulting in unopposed action of platelet thromboxane. A 2001 meta-analysis suggested that there may indeed be a potential for increase in cardiovascular event rates with the presently available COX-2 inhibitors (36), although a later reappraisal failed to confirm this concern (37).

In late 2004, rofecoxib (Vioxx) was withdrawn by its manufacturer when a large retrospective study linked high-dose therapy (>25 mg/day) to a threefold increase in acute cardiac events when compared with other NSAIDs (35), and when early data from a randomized, double-blind, multicenter clinical trial, APPROVe (Adenomatous Polyp Prevention on Vioxx), demonstrated an increased risk of confirmed cardiovascular events in patients taking rofecoxib versus placebo after 18 months of use (38). Despite the fact that the former study did not demonstrate a similar risk for celecoxib, the possibility that increased risk of cardiovascular events may be a class effect of coxibs has been suggested (39). Post-release experience with this new class of NSAIDs is still accumulating.

Their Place in Therapy

The coxibs are generally significantly more expensive than non-selective NSAIDs. Justification for use is based on demonstrating that their benefits, in comparison to non-selective NSAIDs, outweigh this additional cost. The 2002 American Pain Society (APS) guidelines for the management of pain in osteoarthritis (OA), rheumatoid arthritis (RA), and juvenile chronic arthritis (40) state that the question of "whether NSAIDs (either COX-2 selective or nonselective) are superior to acetaminophen for OA pain relief" remains unresolved. With respect to RA, they state that "the COX-2 selective NSAIDs should be used as additional [to disease modifying drugs] analgesic and anti-inflammatory agents if needed, unless the patient is at an increased risk for significant hypertension or renal disease or does not respond to COX-2 selective NSAIDs. In either of these cases, the non-selective NSAIDs should be considered; however, the effects on hypertension or the kidneys may be the same." British National Health guidelines contradict APS recommendations for the use of COX-2 in RA therapy, advising that they should only be used in RA (or OA) patients who may be at "high-risk" for developing GI adverse effects (41). Similarly, a 2003 cost-effectiveness analysis concluded that the risk reduction seen with coxibs, in comparison to nonselective NSAIDs, does not offset their increased costs in the management of average-risk patients with chronic arthritis. This analysis concluded that coxibs may provide an acceptable incremental cost-effectiveness ratio in the sub-group of patients with a history of bleeding ulcers (42).

The 2003 APS guidelines for analgesic use in the treatment of acute and cancer pain suggest that coxibs may provide clinical advantages for short-term or intermittent use in patients with bleeding disorders or at high risk of peptic ulcer disease (20). It follows then, that the place of COX-2 inhibitors in pain management has not yet been fully defined. The safety profile of these agents in the perioperative or acute setting may offset their higher cost. Risk reduction of coxibs in chronic therapy may be insufficient to justify their use except in a, as yet unspecified, subset of patients at "high risk" for adverse GI events. Further evidence of the safety profile of the coxibs will be required before recommending their routine administration.

The two COX-2 selective agents currently available in the United States are celecoxib and valdecoxib (Table 6-2). Generally, they appear to be equally efficacious. However, patients may respond differently to different agents. Celecoxib and valdecoxib are mostly metabolized by the cytochrome

Table 6-2   Dosing Information: COX-2 Inhibitors

Agent	Usual Analgesic Adult Dosing (mg)*	Comments
Celecoxib	400 mg initial, followed by an additional 200 mg if needed on day 1; maintenance dose: 200 mg twice daily as needed	Contraindicated in patients with sulfonamide allergy
Valdecoxib	20 mg twice daily as needed	Contraindicated in patients with sulfonamide allergy

* Dose may be lower for chronic use in rheumatoid arthritis or osteoarthritis.
Dosage information from Wickersham RM, Novak KK, eds. Drug Facts and Comparisons. St Louis: Wolters Kluwer; 2004.

P450 enzyme (celecoxib through 2C9 and valdecoxib through both 2C9 and 3A4). As a consequence, both interact with many drugs that undergo metabolism through this mechanism. In addition, African Americans and the elderly are often deficient in 2C9, which may lead to elevated levels of the drug (43).

Opioids

The menu of opioids has not changed substantially in recent years. Morphine remains the standard against which all other opioids are measured. Morphine is inexpensive, has been used for as long as any other medicine in the pharmacopoeia, has well-characterized pharmacokinetics and pharmacodynamics, and is available in many dosage forms. In the United States other available opioids include meperidine, hydromorphone, codeine, oxycodone, propoxyphene, hydrocodone, methadone, and fentanyl.

Indications for Use

Opioids are considered the cornerstone of the analgesic regimen for major surgery, for any minor procedure expected to cause moderate-to-severe pain, or in disease states such as cancer, where moderate-to-severe pain is a potential side effect of the disease or its treatment. The use of opioids in chronic non-malignant pain conditions is still controversial. Chronic pain, particularly neuropathic pain, may be only partially responsive to opioid therapy. Adverse effects of chronic therapy have not been comprehensively established, but they may include hormonal changes, suppression of the immune system, and in some cases paradoxical hyperalgesia. On the other hand, the risk of addiction appears to be low (44). Consensus statements that guide physicians in prescribing opioids when treating chronic noncancer pain have been published by major medical groups (45,46).

Patients who initially present with moderate-to-severe pain should be started on the second or third step of the WHO ladder. Drugs that are morphine-like or mu-opioid agonists lack a ceiling to their acute analgesic efficacy and should be administered in increasing doses until pain relief is obtained or unacceptable side effects occur. It is suggested that opioids be administered along with non-opioids and/or adjuvant analgesics to provide additive analgesia (20,24). Often opioids are combined with NSAIDs or acetaminophen in single preparations. Maximum single or daily dose may be limited by the nonopioid component; for example, when oxycodone 5 mg is combined with acetaminophen 500 mg (Percocet 5/500), the maximum number of tablets that can be administered is eight in a 24-hour period (8 tabs = 4000 mg of acetaminophen). If the maximum daily number of doses is insufficient to manage a patient's pain, the opioid and non-opioid should be given as separate dosage forms to allow further upwards titration of the opioid.

Efficacy

The choice and dose of opioid depends on several factors including severity of pain, setting (outpatient or inpatient), route of administration, pharmacokinetics, patient preference, efficacy, side effect profile, and cost. There is little difference between opioids in speed of onset or duration of effect (47). Differences in kinetics are achieved by changing formulation or route of administration. A variety of oral controlled-release formulations of morphine and oxycodone are available, and approval of hydromorphone in a controlled-release form is expected soon. Transdermal fentanyl is another option to provide continuous analgesia. Each physician should familiarize himself or herself with the properties of morphine and two or three other opioids, and rely on those primarily.

There are limited data to support differences in efficacy when comparing opioids. The Oxford League table of analgesics (Table 6-3) rates analgesic efficacy by comparing results of single-dose RCTs in patients with acute moderate-to-severe pain (48). Efficacy is expressed in terms of the "number needed to treat" (NNT) in order to reduce pain by 50% in one patient with moderate-to-severe pain compared with placebo over a 4-6 hour period. The NNT of 2.9 for morphine translates to approximately 53% of patients having a 50% reduction in pain. NNTs for a 30% reduction in pain may be lower than those calculated for a 50% reduction (49,50). In addition, recent studies in both acute and chronic pain models have suggested that a reduction in pain of around 30%, in patients with moderate-to-severe pain, may be significant from the patient's point of view. Table 6-3 does

Table 6-3   Analgesic Efficacy of Selected Opioids

Analgesic (route and dose)	No. of Patients	Percentage of Patients with At Least 50% Pain Relief	NNT (95% CI)
Meperidine IM 100 mg	364	54	2.9 (2.3-3.9)
Morphine IM 10 mg	946	50	2.9 (2.6-3.6)
Tramadol oral 100 mg	882	30	4.8 (3.8-6.1)
Codeine oral 60 mg	1305	15	16.7 (11.0-48.0)
Oxycodone oral IR 5 mg/ acetaminophen 500 mg	150	60	2.2 (1.7-3.2)
Oxycodone oral IR 15 mg	60	73	2.3 (1.5-4.9)
Oxycodone IR 10 mg/ acetaminophen 650 mg	315	66	2.6 (2.0-3.5)
Dextropropoxyphene oral 130 mg	50	40	2.8 (1.8-6.5)

IM = intramuscular; IR = immediate release; NNT = number needed to treat.
Adapted from: Oxford Pain Internet Site:
www.jr2.ox.ac.uk/bandolier/booth/painpag/Acutrev/Analgesics/Leagtab.html. Accessed 6/13/04.

not take into account drug side effect profiles. It is interesting to note that the combination of oral acetaminophen 1000 mg with codeine 60 mg produced an NNT of 2.2, and that the oral NSAIDS naproxen and ibuprofen both produced lower NNTs than the above opioids, adding credence to the practice of multimodal analgesia.

Advantages/Benefits
Full opioid agonists have no dose ceiling effect. Unlike nonopioid analgesics, opioid doses can be titrated upwards until satisfactory pain control is achieved or side effects become intolerable. Opioids lack the GI ulcerative, renal, and anti-platelet effects of NSAIDs. There are several different classes of opioids and multiple choices within each class. Lack of success with one opioid does not preclude use of another opioid from the same class or from another class. In addition, opioids come in several dosage forms that can be optimized to meet the needs of the individual patient.

Mechanism of Action
Opioid receptors are expressed both centrally and peripherally (during the inflammatory response in injured tissue). Opioids bind to receptors of the mu, delta, and kappa classes and block the release of neurotransmitters such as substance P (51). Opioids are classified as full agonists (usually at mu-receptors), partial agonists, or mixed agonist/antagonists. Morphine, hydromorphone, methadone, fentanyl, and meperidine are all full opioid agonists at the mu-receptor. Buprenorphine is the only available partial agonist (active at the mu-receptor). Nalbuphine and butorphanol are agonist-antagonist opioids, a term that denotes their property of activating kappa-opioid receptors while simultaneously blocking mu-opioid receptors. Both agonist-antagonists and partial agonists have a ceiling effect to their analgesic properties and can precipitate reversal of analgesia or withdrawal if given to patients chronically taking morphine or other opioids that act upon the mu-receptor.

Toxicities and Adverse Effects
The most common side effects encountered with opioids given by any systemic route are constipation and sedation. Other side effects include nausea, vomiting, confusion, urinary retention, pruritus, myoclonus, dysphoria, euphoria, sleep disturbance, sexual dysfunction, respiratory depression, physiological dependence, tolerance, and inappropriate secretion of vasopressin (52). Different side effects often emerge and subside (due to tolerance) at different rates. Although many patients develop tolerance to certain side effects (e.g., respiratory depression) such adverse affects must still be treated aggressively. For other effects (e.g., constipation), patients do not develop tolerance and a prophylactic bowel regimen should be prescribed at initiation of therapy (30,53). Persistent respiratory depression, nausea, and vomiting are rare in opioid-tolerant individuals. A summary of

opioid-related side effects and methods to prevent or manage them is given in Table 6-4. Due to the great individual variation in the development of these side effects, clinicians need to inquire regularly about them, monitor them, and be ready to treat them quickly. In the absence of a history of substance abuse, addiction rarely occurs in patients with cancer or other illness who newly receive opioids.

Limited data exist to support differences in side effect profiles between opioids at equianalgesic doses. Study results are often confounded by the use of non-equianalgesic doses or by the fact that pain itself can cause side effects such as nausea (47). Differences in the incidence of side effects of opioids may be a consequence of individual characteristics (54). The elderly and the young are prone to exaggerated responses to meperidine, possibly due to decreased circulating levels of α-1 glycoprotein to which this drug is 70% bound. Opioid metabolites may also cause side effects. Adverse events attributed to the meperidine metabolite normeperidine are well documented, even with acute administration (55). Normeperidine, which has a half-life of approximately 40 hours, can accumulate causing dysphoria, excitation, and seizures, especially in the elderly or in patients with renal dysfunction. Although active metabolites of other opioids have been discovered, there is less evidence to support their being implicated in adverse events similar to those seen with normeperidine. The APS now states that meperidine should not be used for either acute or cancer pain (20).

Contraindications

Although genuine allergy to opioids is rare, the use of an opioid of the same chemical type as an opioid to which a patient has a documented allergy is contraindicated. Under these circumstances an opioid of another chemical structure should be chosen. Morphine, hydromorphone, hydrocodone, codeine, and oxycodone belong to the class of opioids known as phenanthrenes, whereas meperidine and fentanyl belong to the class known as phenylpiperidines. Methadone exists in a class by itself (56). In many cases, patients report having an opioid allergy when they have suffered from an opioid-related adverse effect, such as nausea or confusion. Diagnosis of allergy can be further confounded by the fact that many opioids cause release of histamine.

Meperidine is contraindicated in patients who have received a monamine oxidase (MAO) inhibitor within the previous two weeks. Even a single dose of meperidine, when combined with this class of drugs, can lead to serotonin syndrome, characterized by autonomic instability, behavioral changes, and neuromuscular changes. Several cases have been reported including two reports of patient death (57). In addition, it is suspected that concomitant use of meperidine and selective serotonin reuptake inhibitors (SSRIs), such as fluoxetine, may result in a similar catastrophic outcome (58).

Table 6-4   Prevention and Treatment of Opioid-Related Side Effects

Side Effect	Incidence/Frequency	Management
Constipation	Estimated to occur in 25%-50% of cancer patients. Constipation is an almost inevitable consequence of opioid use, and one of the side effects of opioids to which few patients develop tolerance.	*Pharmacological treatment* Initiate bowel regimen at commencement of opioid therapy: • Use both a stool softener and a stimulant: e.g., docusate sodium 100 mg (1 cap bid-tid) + senna 8.6 mg (1 tab daily up to 4 tabs tid) respectively. • Bulk laxatives such as psyllium and osmotic laxatives such as lactulose are also commonly employed. Psyllium requires that the patient maintain adequate fluid intake, lest fecal impaction occur. Metoclopramide may also improve symptoms for patients with depressed gastric motility.
Confusion and delirium	Mild cognitive impairment and hallucinations frequently occur when opioids are initiated or with significant dosage increase.	1. Rule out or eliminate other causes such as metabolic disturbances. 2. Reduce doses of, or discontinue nonessential, centrally acting medications. 3. If analgesia is satisfactory, reduce dose of opioid by 25% and add, if needed, an adjuvant analgesic. 4. Change the route of opioid administration (may be impracticable in a terminally ill patient). *Pharmacological treatment* • Haloperidol is considered first-line therapy for patients who have agitated delirium: 0.5-1 mg orally bid or tid or 0.25-0.5 mg IV or IM. • Chlorpromazine can be used if sedation is required, though hypotension may occur. • Addition of a benzodiazepine is another option, though in some patients, paradoxically, delirium may be exacerbated.

(cont'd)

Table 6-4   Prevention and Treatment of Opioid-Related Side Effects *(Cont'd)*

Side Effect	Incidence/Frequency	Management
Myoclonus	Myoclonus is an occasional side effect that can be precipitated by any opioid analgesic. Most commonly seen with use of meperidine due to accumulation of metabolite normeperidine. Tends to occur when patients are drowsy or entering light sleep.	1. Often resolves spontaneously with reduction in opioid dose and addition of, or increase in dose of, an adjuvant analgesic, or with rotation to a different opioid. 2. Eliminate other causes. *Pharmacological treatment* Low-dose benzodiazepine (e.g., clonazepam, midazolam) or skeletal muscle relaxants (e.g., dantrolene).
Nausea and vomiting	Estimated incidence is 10%-40%.	1. Gradual upward titration of opioid dose may prevent nausea from arising. May subside with chronic dosing. 2. Address reversible comorbidities, such as hypercalcemia, and raised intracranial pressure. 3. Taper or discontinue, if possible, emetogenic drugs such as digoxin, antibiotics, iron, and cytotoxics. 4. Add or increase dose of adjuvant analgesic. 5. If analgesia is satisfactory, reduce opioid dose by 25%. *Pharmacological treatment* Tailor specifically to the source, though antiemetic combinations are often necessary. Initially parenteral administration may be required, but the oral route should be reverted to as soon as possible. • If caused by stimulation of the chemoreceptor trigger zone (as is commonly the case with initial opioid dosing): the dopamine antagonists prochlorperazine (10 mg orally/IV every 6 hours) or haloperidol (0.5-1 mg every 8 hours) or the more costly serotonin antagonists such as ondansetron. • If caused by gastric stasis, the prokinetic metoclopramide 10 mg IV/orally tid prn.

(cont'd)

Table 6-4   Prevention and Treatment of Opioid-Related Side Effects *(Cont'd)*

Side Effect	Incidence/Frequency	Management
Nausea and vomiting (cont'd)		*Pharmacologic treatment (cont'd)* • If exacerbated by motion, diphenhydramine or transdermal scopolamine may be helpful. • Antiemetics themselves are associated with a number of side effects including sedation, confusion, and extrapyramidal symptoms, and for this reason are often only introduced once symptoms appear.
Pruritus	Occasional side effect of opioid use, most commonly when epidural or intrathecal routes of morphine administration are used.	1. Reduce opioid dose by 25% or increase dose of a non-opioid analgesic. 2. Non-pharmacological interventions such as cool compresses or moisturizers may offer some relief. *Pharmacological treatment* • Antihistamines still commonly used as first-line treatment. Diphenhydramine (25-50 mg IV/orally every 6 hours prn) employed with varying degrees of success. Its sedating effect may be as important in relieving symptoms as its antihistaminic properties. • Increased sedation may be a problem with patients who are already suffering from opioid-induced sedation. Under these circumstances a less-sedating antihistamine such as hydroxyzine or cyproheptadine may be employed. • Mixed agonist/antagonists, such as butorphanol, or pure opioid antagonists, such as naloxone (0.8 mg/1000 mL IV infusion), can reverse itching but at the risk of also reversing analgesia. Dosing must be carefully titrated to achieve an acceptable balance between reduced pain control and reduced itching.

(cont'd)

Table 6-4 Prevention and Treatment of Opioid-Related Side Effects (Cont'd)

Side Effect	Incidence/Frequency	Management
Respiratory depression	Tolerance usually develops within days to weeks. Respiratory depression is rare in patients who have been receiving opioids chronically.	1. Seek alternative explanation, such as pneumonia, pulmonary embolism, or cardiomyopathy, or the co-administration of another sedating medication such as a benzodiazepine. 2. Closely monitor and carefully treat possible high-risk patients. *Pharmacological treatment* Due to the risk of systemic opioid withdrawal, the opioid antagonist naloxone should only be used in impending or symptomatic respiratory depression (less than 8 breaths per minute), and small, titrated doses employed.
Sedation	Most frequently occurs at initiation of opioid therapy or with significant dose increase. Associated with transient drowsiness or cognitive impairment. Symptoms frequently resolve after a few days.	1. Many medications including antihistamines, antidepressants, and anxiolytics can contribute to sedation or reduce the metabolism and hence increase the effects of opioids. Discontinue or taper if possible. 2. Rule out comorbidities. 3. If analgesia is satisfactory, reduce opioid dose by 10%-25%. 4. Opioid rotation. *Pharmacological treatment* • Simple stimulant such as caffeine. • If unsuccessful, psychostimulant such as methylphenidate. • In refractory cases, consider neurosurgical procedures.

Adapted from McNicol E, Horowicz-Mehler N, Fisk R, et al. Management of opioid side effects in cancer-related and chronic noncancer pain: a systematic review. J Pain. 2003;4:231-56; with permission.

Drug Interactions

Many drugs interact with opioids causing changes in their metabolism, excretion, or both. Phenobarbital and phenytoin increase the metabolism of meperidine. Phenytoin and rifampin increase the metabolism of methadone. In all cases the increased metabolism of opioid may result in a reduced effect. Conversely, the tricyclic antidepressants, clomipramine and amitriptyline, may increase the bioavailability and half-life of morphine, resulting in an increase in both analgesic and side effects (59).

Other classes of drugs can cause additive analgesia or side effects when co-administered with opioids. Undesirable interactions caused by drugs such as antihistamines, benzodiazepines, and neuroleptics can lead to increased sedation. Conversely, positive interactions can be taken advantage of, such as the use of NSAIDs or adjuvant analgesics to increase analgesia, without a corresponding increase in side effects. Preliminary data suggest that co-administration of distinct mu-agonist opioids, such as oxycodone and morphine, may produce analgesic synergy (60,61).

The combination of meperidine and MAO inhibitors or SSRIs can cause fatal hyperpyrexia (see Contraindications above). Seizures have also been documented with the combination of tramadol and the aforementioned antidepressants.

Dosage
For pain that is always present, opioids should be administered around-the-clock and not on an "as-needed" basis. Opioid doses should be adjusted to allow for maximum pain relief with tolerable side effects for each patient. Breakthrough medication (supplemental doses of a short-acting opioid) is added to this regimen, ideally administered in advance of activities, such as movement, that predictably elicit pain. The breakthrough dose of the short-acting opioid should ordinarily equal 10%-15% of the total daily dose, and under optimal circumstances should not be required more than four times a day. Increments in total daily dosage in order to reduce the need for breakthrough doses are generally at least 25%.

Tolerance and physical dependence are common, even predictable, during chronic opioid administration. Tolerance to opioids is defined as an increase over the course of therapy in the dose required to produce analgesia. Tolerance may be heralded by a shortened duration of analgesia after a routinely administered opioid dose. The clinician must be aware that increasing analgesic dose requirements may also be a sign of disease progression or recurrence. Patients with stable disease on a regimen that has pain well controlled usually do not require increases in their doses. Physical dependence refers to the need for ongoing doses of an opioid in a subject who is chronically receiving an opioid, lest an abstinence syndrome be produced. Tolerance and physical dependence are often confused with psychological dependence ("addiction") manifested as drug abuse or drug seeking-behavior. This simple misunderstanding of nomenclature leads to unnecessary stigmatization of opioid requesting, dispensing, and administering for pain in patients who lack substance abuse issues, and hence fosters undertreatment.

Opioid Rotation and Equianalgesic Conversion
At equianalgesic doses full agonists have similar efficacy but may differ in their side effect profile for a given individual. When one opioid proves ineffective in achieving a satisfactory balance between analgesic effects and undesirable side effects, it is advisable to try other opioids before deciding

that the patient's pain is entirely refractory to opioids. This practice, known as *opioid rotation*, is supported by several clinical trials (52). While morphine is considered the standard of opioid analgesia, the selection of a different opioid may be appropriate when allergy, intolerance, or lack of efficacy occur. For example, patients who experience unmanageable dose-dependent sedation or nausea with oral morphine may be well managed with an equianalgesic dose of hydromorphone, fentanyl, or methadone. In addition to opioid rotation, it may be necessary to convert to a different route of the same opioid when, for example, a patient is unable to swallow and is administered opioid intravenously rather than orally. The clinician should be comfortable with the most commonly prescribed opioids and be competent at calculating doses when converting from one opioid to another. Equianalgesic tables commonly use an intramuscular dose of morphine 10 mg to compare alternative routes and opioids. It should be noted that conversions are based on limited data, are approximate, and that just as patients may vary in their response to a certain opioid, they may also require higher or lower conversion factors than those suggested (62). The conversion to alternative drug and/or route is a five-step process:

1. Total the 24-hour dose of current drug, including all breakthrough doses.
2. Convert 24-hour dose to new drug and/or route using an equianalgesic conversion table (Table 6-5).
3. Divide the total dose of new drug by the schedule of the new drug.
4. In opioid-tolerant patients, consider reducing calculated dose of the new drug by 33%-50% to account for incomplete cross-tolerance.
5. Calculate a breakthrough dose, either 10%-20% of the total daily opioid dose or 25%-30% of the single standing dose (20,63).

Table 6-5   Equianalgesic Doses and Duration of Action of Selected Opioids

Opioid	Parenteral Dose (mg)	Oral Dose (mg)	Duration (hours)
Morphine	10	30	2-4
Codeine	120	200	3-4
Fentanyl*	100 µg	NA	IV: 1 hr; TD: 48-72 hr
Hydromorphone	1.5	7.5	2-4
Meperidine	75	300	2-4
Methadone	10	20	6-8
Oxycodone	NA	20	2-4

TD = transdermal.
* The dose of transdermal fentanyl in micrograms/hour is approximately half the 24-hour dose of oral morphine.

Special Considerations

The manufacturer of transdermal fentanyl provides recommendations on converting to this system from oral or parenteral opioids, based on first converting the original opioid to an equivalent dose of oral morphine. Clinical practice, however, suggests that these recommendations under-dose the patient in over half of all cases and result in a titration period that is too long (64). A simpler and more accurate method, which has become common clinical practice, involves converting the original opioid to an equivalent dose of oral morphine (as with the manufacturer's recommendations) and then halving this dose (and converting to micrograms) to find an appropriate patch size. For example, if the conversion to oral morphine equivalents is 200 mg/day, the patient should be started on a 100 µg/hr patch. Patches are changed every 48-72 hours. Opioid-naïve patients should not be started on a patch size of greater potency than that which delivers 25 µg/hr.

Recent years have seen an upturn in the use of methadone. Proponents of its use point to its ready availability, low cost, naturally long plasma half-life, low risk of toxic metabolites, and efficacy in treating neuropathic pain. However, its complex pharmacokinetic properties make dose conversion challenging (56). Equianalgesic conversion tables routinely suggest a conversion of 30 mg of oral morphine to 20 mg of oral methadone. More recent evidence suggests that this conversion may grossly overestimate the equivalent dose of methadone in patients with chronic pain (65,66). In addition, methadone accumulates with repeated dosing, such that the drug is normally given twice daily with continued use, as opposed to the initial six-hourly dosing. It may be advisable for PCPs not to use methadone as a first-line drug, unless they have ample experience with its use.

Table 6-6 gives a sample equianalgesic conversion. A more comprehensive review of equianalgesic conversion can be found elsewhere (67).

Patient-Controlled Analgesia

In selected patients, patient-controlled analgesia (PCA) devices may be used to deliver intravenous (or occasionally subcutaneous, intrathecal or epidural) medication, primarily opioids. The subcutaneous route is a low-tech approach to PCA, because analgesics may be administered via a small butterfly catheter inserted at a sterile site that is then covered with a nonocclusive dressing. This route may not be feasible in cachectic patients. Two separate meta-analyses of RCTs concluded that patients using PCA obtained better pain relief than with conventional analgesia without an increase in most side effects (68,69). In addition, patient preference strongly favored PCA. Although initial studies of PCA showed a trend towards reduced hospital stay and opioid usage (68), these trends did not achieve statistical significance and were not supported by subsequent literature (69). PCA can promote patient independence and reduce the need for repeated pain assessment and titration of analgesics by health care providers.

Table 6-6   Equianalgesic Conversion Example

A patient is receiving IV morphine 2 mg/hour continuous infusion and has received six breakthrough doses of 1 mg within the last 24 hours. The patient is now able to tolerate oral medication. Convert the patient's opioid regimen to oral controlled-release oxycodone.

Step 1   Total the 24-hour dose of current drug, including all breakthrough doses:

- 2 mg × 24 hours = 48 mg
- Six breakthrough doses × 1 mg = 6 mg
- Total daily dose = 54 mg

Step 2   Convert 24-hour dose to new drug and/or route using an equianalgesic conversion table:

- 10 mg IV morphine = 20 mg oral oxycodone
- Multiply 54 mg × conversion factor of 2 (20/10)
- Total 24-hour dose of oxycodone = 108 mg

Step 3   Divide the total dose of new drug by the schedule of the new drug:

- Controlled-release oxycodone is usually dosed every 12 hours
- 108/2 = 54 mg every 12 hours
- Closest dose available is 40 mg tablet + 10 mg tablet = 50 mg

Step 4   In opioid-tolerant patients, consider reducing calculated dose of the new drug by 33%-50% to account for incomplete cross-tolerance:

- If situation warrants, reduce 54 mg by 33% to 50% = 27-36 mg
- We may choose 20 mg tablet + 10 mg tablet = 30 mg

Step 5   Calculate a breakthrough dose: either 10%-20% of the total daily opioid dose or 25%-30% of the single standing dose:

- If we choose the 50 mg dose, and decide to administer 20% of total daily dose, breakthrough dose = 20 mg.
- Oxycodone is usually scheduled every 6 hours.

New Regimen   Oxycodone controlled-release tablets 50 mg every 12 hours, plus oxycodone immediate-release tablets 20 mg every 6 hours as required for breakthrough pain

Appropriate patient selection is important. Patients who can tolerate oral medication may not require intravenous PCA. Patients should be able to understand the dosing principle, be fully oriented, and be able to push the button that administers medication. PCA has been used successfully in patients as young as 6 years of age (70). If a patient's mental or physical status should deteriorate, conversion of by-the-clock and breakthrough opioid doses from PCA to other routes and agents is relatively easy.

A new development in PCA involves the use of a patient-controlled transdermal system, which the patient activates by pressing a dosing button twice within three seconds. The system, which is about the size of a credit card, delivers a preset dose of fentanyl by use of a low-intensity direct current to move drug from a hydrogel reservoir into the skin, where it then diffuses into the local circulation and is transported to the central nervous system. A recent multi-center RCT concluded that this new system provided post-surgical pain control equivalent to that of a standard intravenous morphine regimen delivered by a PCA pump. In addition, the new system may offer advantages over conventional PCA in that the need for venous access and a programmable pump are avoided (71).

Spinal Opioids

The intrathecal and epidural routes, which are generally used perioperatively, are effective ways to provide analgesia. Opioids can be infused alone, in combination with each other, or in combination with other agents such as local anesthetics, or the α-2 agonist clonidine (72). Fentanyl and morphine are the most commonly used opioids, each having a different pharmacokinetic profile (20). Agents can be administered as a single bolus perioperatively, as a continuous infusion, or as a patient controlled device (see Patient Controlled Analgesia). In a meta-analysis of post-operative pain treatment regimens, patients who received epidural analgesia had improved pulmonary outcomes compared with those who received systemic opioids (73). The use of spinal opioids for patients with chronic pain, including cancer pain, may be considered when a sufficient trial of systemic opioid has failed to control pain or when unacceptable side effects arise (20).

Although spinal administration of analgesics is often used to avoid the side effects patients experience with systemic administration, the intrathecal and epidural routes are not without risk of side effects or adverse outcomes. Nausea, itching, and urinary retention are common (20) side effects. Serious adverse outcomes, though rare, include epidural hematoma, infection, and respiratory depression. Spinal administration requires a degree of expertise that may necessitate involvement of a dedicated pain service, including an experienced anesthesiologist.

Adjuvant Analgesics

Adjuvant drugs, including antidepressants, anticonvulsants, systemically administered local anesthetics, corticosteroids, N-methyl-D-aspartate (NMDA) antagonists, neuroleptics, and bisphosphonates can be used at any of the three steps of the analgesic ladder (see Fig. 6-1) (23). Adjuvant drugs enhance the analgesic efficacy of opioids or provide analgesia for specific types of pain (e.g., antidepressants for the treatment of neuropathic pain, bisphosphonates to alleviate malignant bone pain). Besides boosting analgesia, adding an adjuvant to an opioid regimen may decrease the incidence of side effects. Adjuvant analgesics have been studied predominately in the treatment of post-herpetic neuralgia, trigeminal neuralgia, and painful diabetic neuropathy (PDN). Despite a lack of high-quality evidence confirming efficacy in other models, the similarities between underlying mechanisms have led to the use of adjuvants for various peripheral and central neuropathies.

Indications for Use

Chronic pain (cancer and non-cancer) is often only partially responsive to treatment with opioids and/or NSAIDs. Most commonly this type of pain is a consequence of damage to the peripheral or central nervous system, or both. Such "neuropathic pain" is often described as burning, shooting, stabbing, or electric shock-like in nature. Because it is less likely than nociceptive pain to respond to monotherapy, co-administration of several medications or invasive techniques may be required to reduce it. Often, the extremely high doses of opioids required to treat neuropathic pain cause intolerable or unmanageable side effects. Tolerance to the analgesic effects of opioids also often becomes a management issue during treatment of neuropathic pain. Optimal treatment of neuropathic pain is aimed at the underlying mechanisms, rather than symptoms or etiology. However, diagnosis of such mechanisms can be complex and time consuming and often the physician may be forced into prescribing therapy empirically. At present the FDA has approved medications for only two specific neuropathic pain syndromes: trigeminal neuralgia (carbamazepine) and post-herpetic neuralgia (gabapentin and lidocaine 5% patch). Historically, however, clinicians have wide experience with, and RCTs support the use of, tricyclic antidepressants and antiepileptic drugs for neuropathic pain of varied etiologies (74,75).

Efficacy

Members of the faculty of the Fourth International Conference on the Mechanisms and Treatment of Neuropathic Pain recently developed treatment recommendations based upon best-available evidence (76). The faculty recommended five first-line medications for neuropathic pain, three of which are classed as adjuvants: gabapentin, 5% lidocaine patch, opioid analgesics, tramadol hydrochloride, and tricyclic antidepressants. All five have been shown to provide statistically and clinically significant benefits in treating neuropathic pain, compared with placebo (see Chapter 5 for a detailed discussion of these five medications). In addition, these medications are considered to have acceptable safety and tolerability profiles.

Selection of a first-line drug is dependent on many factors including cost, availability, diagnosis, and safety profile in specific populations. For example, both gabapentin and the lidocaine patch are still protected under patent (a generic version of gabapentin will be available shortly) and may be considerably more expensive than other therapies. Carbamazepine is considered by the authors to be a second-line drug, but it has been well-established for the treatment of trigeminal neuralgia. Tricyclic antidepressants should be used with caution in the elderly due to their potential for cardiotoxicity and their anticholinergic side effects. RCTs of combination therapy with of any of the first-line drugs are lacking. Therefore, although combination therapy may be required, it is unclear which combination will work best in a given population or what the adverse consequences of such polypharmacy are. Second-line drugs have either not demonstrated efficacy in multiple trials (i.e., tested only in a single trial or yielded conflicting results in multiple trials) or are less commonly used.

Advantages/Benefits

Adjuvants can be beneficial in conditions resistant to other drug regimens. As already mentioned, when added to an existing regimen, adjuvants can increase efficacy, reduce side effects by reducing the dose of opioid or NSAID required, or counteract/treat side effects of analgesic or disease-specific drug regimens.

Mechanisms of Action

The mechanisms of action of adjuvant analgesics have not been fully elucidated. As previously stated, therapies should be aimed at the underlying mechanisms perpetuating neuropathic pain, rather than symptoms or disease etiology. Multiple mechanisms perpetuate both peripheral and central pain. A change in the function, chemistry, and structure of neurons underlies the pathophysiology of neuropathic pain (77). A simplified approach to targeting treatment breaks down these mechanisms to three processes (78):

1. Increased primary afferent nociceptor firing due to, for example, de novo expression of phenotypically abnormal sodium channels on damaged peripheral nerve fibers

2. Decreased inhibition of central neuronal activity (e.g., due to loss of descending inhibitory neurons)

3. Central sensitization mediated through NMDA receptors

Anticonvulsants, tricyclic antidepressants, and local anesthetics at least partially exert their analgesic effects by blocking the sodium channels expressed on nociceptor sensory neurons in neuropathic pain states (77). Gabapentin may exert its analgesic effects by interaction with α-2–δ modulatory sites on neuronal calcium channels (78). Ketamine and dextromethorphan inhibit activity of the NMDA receptor complex. Adrenergic agents such as clonidine and prazosin may be targeted at the treatment of sympathetically maintained pain or may interact with receptors in the spinal cord.

Toxicities and Adverse Effects

Many of the side effects of adjuvant analgesics are a result of their nonspecific actions. For example, tricyclic antidepressants not only block sodium channels responsible for perpetuating peripheral neuropathy but also those involved in cardiovascular nerve conduction. Gabapentin has proven an attractive option due to its low incidence of, and generally mild, side effects (see also Chapter 5). The 5% lidocaine patch has a low incidence of side effects when limited to application of three patches for 12 hours or less each day. Antidepressants are often dose-limited by the incidence of anticholinergic, sexual, or cardiotoxic side effects, although for the treatment of pain, lower doses than those required to treat depression may suffice. Older anticonvulsants such as carbamazepine and phenytoin may not be suitable in many patients due to side effects such as sedation, agranulocytosis (carbamazepine), and gingival hyperplasia (phenytoin). Many of the side effects experienced with adjuvants are transitory and can be avoided or diminished by gradual upward titration of dose.

Contraindications

There are few absolute contraindications to the use of any of the adjuvants; however, they should be used with caution in certain populations or in patients with comorbidities. The elderly are more susceptible to both the therapeutic and adverse effects of drugs in general. They can be particularly susceptible to the anticholinergic side effects of tricyclic antidepressants and to the sedating effects of many of the anticonvulsants. In this population, it is advisable to use a tricyclic with a lower incidence of anticholinergic side effects, such as desipramine or nortriptyline. Tricyclics should be used with extreme caution in patients with suicidal ideation or who may accidentally overdose. The use of SSRIs concurrently or within two weeks of administration of an MAOI is contraindicated.

Drug Interactions

Adverse effects of adjuvants are compounded by the fact that patients are often taking multiple medications, either for pain itself or because of comorbidities. The addition of an anticonvulsant to an opioid regimen may result in increased sedation. All SSRIs inhibit cytochrome P4502D6 and may therefore increase concentrations of tricyclic antidepressants in addition to other classes of drugs.

Dosage

With most adjuvants, patients are started at a low dose that is then titrated upward, thus minimizing adverse effects. The elderly, in particular, should be started at the lowest dose possible. Lidocaine patches, due to their mild side effect profile, do not require titration. Dosing regimens for selected adjuvant drugs are shown in Table 6-7.

Local Anesthetics

Infiltration or topical application of local anesthetics is widely used for minor office procedures such as suturing lacerations (79). Simple techniques of neural blockade such as field infiltration, digital nerve block, and trigger point injection can be carried out by most physicians. Complex peripheral

Table 6-7   Dosing Regimens for Adjuvant Drugs

Medication	Starting Dose; Maximum Dose	Titration Schedule	Duration of Adequate Trial	Comments
Gabapentin	100-300 mg every night or 100-300 mg 3 times daily; 3600 mg (1200 mg 3 times daily)	Increase by 100-300 mg 3 times daily every 1-7 days as tolerated	3-8 wks for titration + 1-2 wks at maximum dose	Reduce dose for low creatinine clearance
5% Lidocaine patch	Maximum of 3 patches daily for a maximum of 12 hrs	None needed	2 wks	Patches can be cut to size
Tricyclic anti-depressants (e.g., amitriptyline, desipramine)	10-25 mg every night; 75-150 mg	Increase by 10-25 mg every 3-7 days as tolerated	6-8 wks with at least 1-2 wks at maximum tolerated dose	Start at lowest dose in elderly; consider agents with lower incidence of anti-cholinergic side effects (e.g., nortriptyline, desipramine); lower doses required than for depression

Adapted from Dworkin RH, Backonja M, Rowbotham MC, et al. Advances in neuropathic pain: diagnosis, mechanisms, and treatment recommendations. Arch Neurol. 2003;60:1524-34; with permission.

nerve blocks (intercostal, ankle, and brachial plexus) carry greater risks and benefits, and are best left to those with specialized training. Spinal administration of opioids with or without local anesthetics is also effective to control pain after operation or trauma, or during a variety of cancer-related or non-cancerous chronic diseases, but requires expertise and infrastructure to administer and monitor properly. The same cautions apply for neurolytic nerve block procedures that are proven to decrease distress from abdominal or otherwise localized cancer, and nitrous oxide inhalation as a means to control transient procedure-related pain (23).

Conclusion

Major changes have taken place in the attitudes of the public and medical profession towards pain control. Fatalism has been replaced by widespread acceptance of the importance of routine pain assessment and treatment, and by the institutionalization of this new view in clinical practice guidelines and quality assurance processes up to, and including, the most recent JCAHO standards. A list of relevant resources and guidelines can be found in Table 6-8.

This new outlook toward pain management extends across all aspects of medical care—from surgery and as a symptom of other underlying disease processes to end-of-life care. Increasingly, diagnostic and surgical procedures are being performed using "minimally invasive" techniques that minimize painful tissue injury and allow patients promptly to resume their previous level of function. As society faces its resource limits in providing medical care at the end of life, this interest in minimizing pain has extended further to palliative care. The control of pain and other symptoms appears likely to play a substantial role in 21st century medical practice, not only because of humanitarian considerations, but also because of economics. Inadequate pain control during the course of cancer, HIV/AIDS, sickle disease, or even readmission for pain control after major operations in too-quickly-discharged patients are, in aggregate, common causes of costly yet avoidable hospital admissions. Such admissions, and the suffering and inconvenience associated with them, could be averted if proactive planning and continuity of pain management across care settings (home, hospital, hospice...) were the rule.

The importance of educating patients, families, and health care providers to monitor and manage pain cannot be overemphasized. Patients should be taught to report any new pain or any changes in their pain so that these can be assessed and treatment adjusted or diagnostic studies arranged. Recently the concept of "disease management" has gained currency as a means to provide optimal, cost-effective care that involves an array of specialists during the course of an illness episode or chronically. Pain control, with pharmacotherapy as its cornerstone, has now become an integral part of the disease management process for many patients. The integration of pain control in such disease management may be summarized in the mnemonic "ABCDE" from the AHCPR clinical practice guideline on cancer pain control (30):

A Ask about pain regularly/Assess pain systematically

B Believe patient and family reports of pain and what relieves it

C Choose pain control options appropriate for the patient, family, and setting

D Deliver interventions in a timely, logical, and coordinated fashion

E Empower patients and families/Enable them to control their care to the greatest extent possible

Pharmacotherapy is "effective, relatively low risk, inexpensive, and usually of rapid onset" (30). It is an essential component of pain management, as reflected in the above AHCPR guidelines, and in the other guidelines referred to in Table 6-8. In addition, national and international organizations,

---

Table 6-8 Resources for Pharmacological Treatment of Pain

Useful Internet Sites
- **International Association for the Study of Pain (IASP)** www.iasp-pain.org
- **The American Pain Society (APS)** www.ampainsoc.org
- **The Oxford Pain Internet Site** www.jr2.ox.ac.uk/Bandolier/booth/painpag
- **Agency for Healthcare Research and Quality (AHRQ) Acute and Cancer Pain Guidelines** www.ahrq.gov/clinic/epcix.htm
- **Cochrane Collaboration Pain, Palliative Care and Supportive Care Group** www.jr2.ox.ac.uk/Cochrane
- **American Academy of Pain Medicine** www.painmed.org
- **American Pain Foundation** www.painfoundation.org
- **Beth Israel-Pain Medicine & Palliative Care** www.stoppain.org
- **Drug Enforcement Administration** www.usdoj.gov/dea
- **Federation of State Medical Boards of the United States** www.medsch.wisc.edu/painpolicy/domestic/model.htm
- **International Headache Society** www.i-h-s.org
- **Johns Hopkins Center for Cancer Pain Research/Pain Site** www.cancerpain.jhmi.edu/intro.htm
- **Joint Commission on Accreditation of Healthcare Organizations (JCAHO)** www.jcaho.org
- **Mayo Clinic Pain Management Center** www.mayoclinic.com/findinformation/diseasesandconditions/index.cfm
- **MD Anderson Pain Site** www.mdanderson.org/topics/paincontrol
- **MedlinePlus Pain** www.nlm.nih.gov/medlineplus/pain.html
- **National Foundation for the Treatment of Pain** www.paincare.org
- **National Pain Education Council** www.npecweb.org
- **National Pain Foundation** www.painconnection.org
- **Dannemiller Memorial Educational Foundation: Pain.com** www.pain.com
- **University of Wisconsin Pain and Policy Studies Group** www.medsch.wisc.edu/painpolicy
- **Partners Against Pain** www.partnersagainstpain.com
- **British Medical Journal collected papers on pain** http://bmj.com/cgi/collection/pain
- **American Academy of Pain Management** www.aapainmanage.org
- **American Chronic Pain Association** www.aapainmanage.org

Guidelines
- **Practice Guidelines for** Acute Pain Management in the Perioperative Setting: **An Updated Report by the** American Society of Anesthesiologists **Task Force on Pain Management. Anesthesiology. 2004;100:1573-81.**
- **Quality Improvement Guidelines for the Treatment of** Acute Pain and Cancer Pain. American Pain Society **Quality of Care Committee. JAMA. 1995;274:1874-80.**
- **Principles of Analgesic Use in the Treatment of** Acute Pain and Cancer Pain, 5th ed. **Glenview, IL:** American Pain Society; **2003.**
- **Jacox A, Carr DB, Payne R, et al. Management of** Cancer Pain. **Clinical Practice Guideline No. 9. AHCPR Publication No. 94-0592. Rockville, MD:** Agency for Health Care Policy and Research; **1994.**
- **Carr DB, Jacox AK, Chapman CR, et al.** Acute Pain Management: Operative or Medical Procedures and Trauma. **Clinical Practice Guideline No. 1. Rockville, MD:** Agency for Health Care Policy and Research; **1992.**

including government agencies, are recognizing the importance of drug therapy as a "mainstay of management for acute pain and cancer pain in all age groups" (20) and "an essential part of a pain management plan" for chronic pain (45).

REFERENCES

1. **Dunajcik L.** Chronic Nonmalignant Pain. In: Bowlus B, ed. Pain, 2nd ed. St. Louis: Mosby; 1999:471-521.
2. **Gureje O, Von Korff M, Simon GE, Gater R.** Persistent pain and well-being: a World Health Organization study in primary Care. JAMA. 1998;280:147-51.
3. **Nelson R.** Decade of pain control and research gets into gear in USA. Lancet. 2003;362:1129.
4. **Cleeland CS, Gonin R, Hatfield AK, et al.** Pain and its treatment in outpatients with metastatic cancer. N Engl J Med. 1994;330:592-6.
5. **Cleeland CS.** Undertreatment of cancer pain in elderly patients. JAMA. 1998;279: 1914-5.
6. **Donovan M, Dillon P, McGuire L.** Incidence and characteristics of pain in a sample of medical-surgical inpatients. Pain. 1987;30:69-87.
7. **Marks RM, Sachar EJ.** Undertreatment of medical inpatients with narcotic analgesics. Ann Intern Med. 1973;78:173-81.
8. **McGivney WT, Crooks GM.** The care of patients with severe chronic pain in terminal illness. JAMA. 1984;251:1182-8.
9. **Teno JM, Weitzen S, Wettle T, Mor V.** Persistent pain in nursing home residents [Letter]. JAMA. 2001;285:2081.
10. **Lasch KE, Greenhill A, Wilkes G, et al.** Why study pain? J Palliat Med. 2002;5:57-72.
11. **Weissman DE, Haddox JD.** Opioid pseudoaddiction: an iatrogenic syndrome. Pain. 1989;36:363-6.
12. **Furstenberg CT, Ahles TA, Whedon MB, et al.** Knowledge and attitudes of healthcare providers toward cancer pain management: a comparison of physicians, nurses and pharmacists in New Hampshire. J Pain Symptom Manage. 1998;15:335-49.
13. **Bressler LR, Geraci MC, Schatz BS.** Misperceptions and inadequate pain management in cancer patients. Drug Intel Clin Pharm. 1991;25:1225-30.
14. **Porter J, Jick H.** Addiction rare in patients treated with narcotics [Letter]. N Engl J Med.1980;302:123.
15. **Ward SE, Goldberg N, Miller-McCauley V, et al.** Patient-related barriers to management of cancer pain. Pain. 1993;52:319-24.
16. **Joranson DE, Berger JW.** Regulatory issues in pain management. J Am Pharm Assoc. 2000;40 (5 Suppl):S60-1.
17. **Smith G, Power I.** Audit and bridging the analgesic gap. Anaesthesia. 1998;53:521-2.
18. **Pasero C, McCaffery M.** The undertreatment of pain. Am J Nurs. 2001;101:62-5.
19. **Berman S, ed.** Approaches to Pain Management: An Essential Guide for Clinical Leaders. Oakbrook Terrace, IL: Joint Commission on Accreditation of Healthcare Organizations; 2003.
20. Principles of Analgesic Use in the Treatment of Acute Pain and Cancer Pain, 5th ed. Glenview, IL: American Pain Society; 2003.
21. **Loeser JD, Melzack R.** Pain: an overview. Lancet. 1999;353:1607-9.

22. **Wittink H, Wiffen P, Carr DB.** Evidence-based medicine in pain management. In: Berman S, ed. Approaches to Pain Management: An Essential Guide for Clinical Leaders. Oakbrook Terrace, IL: Joint Commission on Accreditation of Healthcare Organizations; 2003:21-34.

23. **Carr DB, Goudas LC, Balk EM, et al.** Evidence report on the treatment of pain in cancer patients. J Natl Cancer Inst Monogr. 2004;32:23-51.

24. **World Health Organization.** WHO Guidelines: Cancer Pain Relief, 2nd ed. Geneva: World Health Organization; 1996.

25. **Jadad A, Browman GP.** The WHO analgesic ladder for cancer pain management: stepping up the quality of its evaluation. JAMA. 1995;274:1870-3.

26. **Zech DFJ, Grond S, Lynch J, et al.** Validation of World Health Organization guidelines for cancer pain relief: a 10-year prospective study. Pain. 1995;63:65-76.

27. **McNicol E, Strassels S, Goudas L, et al.** Nonsteroidal anti-inflammatory drugs, alone or combined with opioids, for cancer pain: a systematic review. J Clin Oncol. 2004;22:1975-92.

28. **Goudas L, Carr DB, Bloch R, et al.** Management of Cancer Pain. Evidence Report/Technology Assessment No. 35 (prepared by the New England Medical Center Evidence-based Practice Center under Contract 290-97-0019). AHRQ Publication No. 02-E002. Rockville, MD: Agency for Healthcare Research and Quality; October 2001.

29. **Eisenberg E, Berkey CS, Carr DB, et al.** Efficacy and safety of nonsteroidal anti-inflammatory drugs for cancer pain: a meta-analysis. J Clin Oncol. 1994;12:2756-65.

30. **Jacox A, Carr DB, Payne R, al.** Management of Cancer Pain. Clinical Practice Guideline No. 9. AHCPR Publication No. 94-0592. Rockville, MD: Agency for Health Care Policy and Research; 1994.

31. **Hawkey CJ.** Cyclooxygenase inhibition: between the devil and the deep blue sea. Gut. 2002;50(Suppl 3):III25-30.

32. **Henry D, Lim LL, Garcia Rodriguez LA, et al.** Variability in risk of gastrointestinal complications with individual non-steroidal anti-inflammatory drugs: results of a collaborative meta-analysis. BMJ. 1996;312:1563-6.

33. **McCaffery M, Portenoy RK.** Acetaminophen and nonsteroidal anti-inflammatory drugs (NSAIDs). In: Bowlus B, ed. Pain, 2nd ed. St. Louis: Mosby; 1999:129-60.

34. **Fitzgerald GA, Patrono C.** The coxibs, selective inhibitors of cyclooxygenase-2. N Engl J Med. 2001;345:433-42.

35. **Graham DJ, Campen DH, Cheetham C, et al.** Risk of acute myocardial infarction and sudden cardiac death with use of COX-2 selective and non-selective NSAIDs. Presented at 20th International Conference on Pharmacoepidemiology & Therapeutic Risk Management; Bordeaux, France; 22-25 August 2004.

36. **Mukherjee D, Nissen SE, Topol EJ.** Risk of cardiovascular events associated with selective COX-2 inhibitors. JAMA. 2001;286:954-9.

37. **Konstam MA, Demopoulos LA.** Cardiovascular events and COX-2 inhibitors [Comment]. JAMA. 2001;286:2809.

38. **Merck Web site.** Merck Announces Voluntary Worldwide Withdrawal of Vioxx. Available at www.merck.com/newsroom/press_releases/product/2004_0930.html. Accessed 10/26/04.

39. **Fitzgerald GA.** Coxibs and cardiovascular disease. N Engl J Med. 2004;351:1709-11.

40. **Simon L, Lipman A, Caudill-Slosberg M, et al.** Guidelines for the Management of Pain in Osteoarthritis, Rheumatoid Arthritis, and Juvenile Chronic Arthritis, 2nd ed. APS Clinical Practice Guidelines Series, No. 2. Glenview, IL: American Pain Society; 2002.

41. Summary of Guidance Issued to the NHS in England and Wales. Issue 3. London: National Institute for Clinical Excellence; 2001.

42. **Spiegel BM, Targownik L, Dulai GS, Gralnek IM.** The cost-effectiveness of cyclooxygenase-2 selective inhibitors in the management of chronic arthritis. Ann Intern Med. 2003;138:795-806.

43. **Garnett WR.** Clinical implications of drug interactions with coxibs. Pharmacotherapy. 2001;21:1223-32.

44. **Ballantyne JC, Mao J.** Opioid therapy for chronic pain. N Engl J Med. 2003;349: 1943-53.

45. The use of opioids for the treatment of chronic pain: a consensus statement from the American Academy of Pain Medicine and the American Pain Society. Glenview, IL: American Academy of Pain Medicine and American Pain Society; 1997.

46. Model guidelines for the use of controlled substances for the treatment of pain: a policy document of the Federation of State Medical Boards of the United States. Dallas: Federation of State Medical Boards of the United States; 1998.

47. **McQuay H.** Opioids in pain management. Lancet. 1999;353:2229-32.

48. **Oxford Pain Internet Site:** http://www.jr2.ox.ac.uk/bandolier/booth/painpag/ Acutrev/Analgesics/Leagtab.html. Accessed 6/13/04.

49. **Farrar JT, Young JP Jr, LaMoreaux L, et al.** Clinical importance of changes in chronic pain intensity measured on an 11-point numerical pain rating scale. Pain. 2001;94:149-58.

50. **Cepeda MS, Africano JM, Polo R, et al.** What decline in pain intensity is meaningful to patients with acute pain? Pain. 2003;105:151-7.

51. **Cepeda MS, Carr DB.** Overview of pain management. In: Berman S, ed. Approaches to Pain Management: An Essential Guide for Clinical Leaders. Oakbrook Terrace, IL: Joint Commission on Accreditation of Healthcare Organizations; 2003:1-20.

52. **McNicol E, Horowicz-Mehler N, Fisk R, et al.** Management of opioid side effects in cancer-related and chronic noncancer pain: a systematic review. J Pain. 2003;4: 231-56.

52. Cancer pain. NCCN Practice Guidelines in Oncology, vol 1; 2001. www.nccn.org/ physician_gls/index.html. Accessed 7/9/2002.

54. **Kalso E, Vainio A.** Morphine and oxycodone hydrochloride in the management of cancer pain. Clin Pharmacol Ther. 1990;47:639-46.

55. **Kaiko RF, Foley KM, Grabinski PY, et al.** Central nervous system excitatory effects of meperidine in cancer patients. Ann Neurol. 1983;13:180-5.

56. **Fishman SM, Wilsey B, Mahajan G, Molina P.** Methadone reincarnated: novel clinical applications with related concerns. Pain Medicine. 2002;3:339-48.

57. **Latta KS, Ginsberg B, Barkin RL.** Meperidine: a critical review. Am J Therapeutics. 2002;9:53-68.

58. **Tissot, TA.** Probable meperidine-induced serotonin syndrome in a patient with a history of fluoxetine use. Anesthesiology. 2003;98:1511-2.

59. **Pasero C, Portenoy RK, McCaffery M.** Opioid analgesics. In: Bowlus B, ed. Pain, 2nd ed. St. Louis: Mosby; 1999:161-299.

60. **Lauretti GR, Oliveira GM, Pereira NL.** Comparison of sustained-release morphine with sustained-release oxycodone in advanced cancer patients. Br J Cancer. 2003;89:2027-30.

61. **Ross FB, Wallis SC, Smith MT.** Co-administration of sub-antinociceptive doses of oxycodone and morphine produces marked antinociceptive synergy with reduced CNS side effects in rats. Pain. 2000;84:421-8.

62. **Lipkowski AW, Carr DB.** Rethinking opioid equivalence. Pain: Clinical Updates. 2002;10:1-4.

63. **Levy MH.** Pharmacologic treatment of cancer pain. N Eng J Med. 1996;335:1124-32.

64. **Breitbart W, Chandler S, Eagel B, et al.** An alternative algorithm for dosing transdermal fentanyl for cancer-related pain. Oncology. 2000;14:695-705.

64. **Gammaitoni AR, Fine P, Alvarez N, et al.** Clinical application of opioid equianalgesic data. Clin J Pain. 2003;19:286-97.

65. **Lawlor PG, Turner KS, Hanson J, Bruera ED.** Dose ratio between morphine and methadone in patients with cancer pain: a retrospective study. Cancer. 1998;82:1167-73.

66. **Ripamonti C, Groff L, Brunelli C, et al.** Switching from morphine to oral methadone in treating cancer pain: what is the equianalgesic dose ratio? J Clin Oncol. 1998;16:3216-21.

68. **Ballantyne JC, Carr DB, Chalmers TC, et al.** Postoperative patient-controlled analgesia: meta-analyses of initial randomized control trials. J Clin Anesth. 1993;5: 182-93.

69. **Walder B, Schafer M, Henzi I, Tramer MR.** Efficacy and safety of patient-controlled opioid analgesia for acute postoperative pain: a quantitative systematic review. Acta Anaesthesiol Scand. 2001;45:795-804.

70. **Berde CB, Lehn BM, Yee JD, et al.** Patient-controlled analgesia in children and adolescents: a randomized, prospective comparison with intramuscular administration of morphine for postoperative analgesia. J Pediatr. 1991;118:460-6.

71. **Viscusi ER, Reynolds L, Chung F, et al.** Patient-controlled transdermal fentanyl hydrochloride vs. intravenous morphine pump for postoperative pain: a randomized controlled trial. JAMA. 2004;291:1333-41.

72. **Walker SM, Goudas LC, Cousins MJ, Carr DB.** Combination spinal analgesic chemotherapy: a systematic review. Anesth Analg. 2002;95:674-715.

73. **Ballantyne JC, Carr DB, de Ferranti, S, et al.** The comparative effects of postoperative analgesic therapies on pulmonary outcome: cumulative meta-analyses of randomized, controlled trials. Anesth Analg. 1998;86:598-612.

74. **Sindrup SH, Jensen TS.** Efficacy of pharmacological treatments of neuropathic pain: an update and effect related to mechanism of drug action. Pain. 1999;83: 389-400.

75. **Wiffen P, Collins S, McQuay H, et al.** Anticonvulsant drugs for acute and chronic pain (Cochrane Review). The Cochrane Library. 2001;4:Update Software, Oxford.

76. **Dworkin RH, Backonja M, Rowbotham MC, et al.** Advances in neuropathic pain: diagnosis, mechanisms, and treatment recommendations. Arch Neurol. 2003; 60:1524-34.

77. **Woolf CJ, Mannion RJ.** Neuropathic pain: aetiology, symptoms, mechanisms, and management. Lancet. 1999;353:1959-64.

78. **Backonja M.** Use of anticonvulsants for treatment of neuropathic pain. Neurology. 2002;59(Suppl 2):S14-S17.

79. **Eidelman A, Weiss J, Enu I, et al.** Comparative efficacy and costs of various topical anesthetics for repair of dermal lacerations: a systematic review of randomized, controlled trials. J Clin Anesth (in press).

7

■ ■ ■

Injection-Based
Analgesic Therapies

Lana Wania-Galicia, MD

Gagan Mahajan, MD

Scott M. Fishman, MD

hen primary care physicians decide that a patient should be referred to a pain specialist, a variety of treatments may be recommended: physical therapy, psychosocial support, cognitive-behavioral interventions, alternative and complementary approaches, medications, injections, or surgery. The recommended treatment often relates to the background of the specialist more than to the identified medical problem. How does one decide where to send a patient who is not responding to routine care? Many pain specialists are trained to offer various analgesic procedures. Of the many tools used for pain management, injection-based therapies have been among the most specialized. These procedures range from minor office-based myofascial or peripheral injections to neuraxial injection or instrumentation, which involve significant risk. The field of interventional pain management is complex and ever changing, with many new procedures being developed annually.

Interventional procedures such as injections are often used not only for therapeutic purposes but also to clarify certain diagnoses (i.e., by immediate symptom relief from the local anesthetic or delayed relief from the anti-inflammatory properties of the corticosteroid). The procedural approach to pain management can be invaluable but is rarely curative in longstanding complex pain problems. Nevertheless, improving pain even for a short time may allow the patient to start an exercise program or become involved in psychological strategies that may have been resisted when pain levels were intolerable. Usually these therapies are used in conjunction with pharmacotherapy and physical therapy, not as stand-alone treatments.

With the exception of trigger-point injections, the procedures described in this chapter are reserved for practitioners with specialized training and are most accurately performed under fluoroscopic guidance in an effort to maximize efficacy and minimize complications. Contraindications to performing any injection include a patient's refusal to consent to the procedure, coagulopathy, local infection at the site of injection, sepsis, or true allergy to any component of the injectate. Pregnancy is an absolute contraindication to fluoroscopy due to the teratogenicity associated with radiation exposure.

This chapter is intended as an introduction to some of the most common analgesic procedures: it is not comprehensive. It may serve as a reference to what an interventional pain specialist may offer your patients. The complexity of these techniques is impressive, and detailed instruction on performing them is beyond the scope of this chapter. Additionally, the following information on procedures is not intended to make you an interventionalist or to identify which specific procedure you should ask the pain specialist to perform; rather, it provides the curious reader with a better understanding of what these procedures entail, how they may help, and when a pain specialist is indicated.

Trigger-Point Injections

Trigger-point injections are used to decrease painful muscle contraction by eliminating foci of pain generation called myofascial trigger points. Therapeutic effect typically lasts only a few days. Local anesthetics such as 1% lidocaine or 0.25% bupivicaine are commonly injected; however, it may be the effect of needling that is most therapeutic.

Any area of muscle may possess a trigger point. Trigger points are discrete areas overlying muscles and their ligaments, often about the size of the examiner's finger pad. When palpating a trigger point, do not be confused by the much more common tender points. True trigger points have features beyond tenderness. They may present as small palpable collections, usually located within taut bands of muscle, which can be rolled between the examiner's fingers. Palpation or injection of a trigger point may produce tenderness as well as a local muscle twitch that may be felt and occasionally seen. Trigger points may be within the region of the patient's reported pain, but sometimes they are not. Palpation of true trigger points should reproduce the patient's typical pain. Radiation patterns have been well described. The radiation of pain should be regional and nondermatomal. If the radiation pattern of peripheral nerve or root is observed, other causes such as radiculopathy or other nerve lesion should be sought and excluded.

Using a 25-gauge, 1.5-inch needle, inject into and around the trigger point. With proper administration, patients typically report pain during the initial injection, with typical radiation and subsequent relief of pain post-injection. Many physicians inject local anesthetic, but some opt to use corticosteroids instead of or in addition to anesthetics. Others use saline or no injectate, the latter resulting in what is termed dry needling: the needle is manipulated at the trigger point to disrupt the trigger point.

Epidural Steroid Injection

Epidural steroid injections are commonly used for palliation of radiculopathy or radiculitis, spondylosis, stenosis, and post-laminectomy syndrome. Less-common uses include management of cancer pain, phantom limb pain, peripheral neuropathy, post-herpetic neuropathy, and complex regional pain syndrome. More specific indications for each type of epidural steroid injection (e.g., cervical, thoracic, lumbar, and caudal injections) are shown in Table 7-1.

The epidural space lies between the osseoligamentous structures lining the vertebral canal and the dural membrane surrounding the spinal cord and nerve roots (1,2). Epidural steroid injections may be administered at the cervical, thoracic, or lumbar levels, as well as through the sacral caudal canal. Two common means of accessing the epidural space include the translaminar and the transforaminal approach. While the transforaminal approach is only recommended with the aid of fluoroscopy due to its increased relative risk (cerebral vascular accident due to the close proximity of the vertebral artery at the cervical level, pneumothorax due to the proximity of the pleura at the thoracic level, and spinal cord ischemia due to the proximity of radicular arteries at the lumbar level), the translaminar approach can be

Table 7-1 Indications for Epidural Steroid Injections

Cervical epidural steroid injection	Cervical radiculopathy, cervical post-laminectomy syndrome, management of cancer pain involving the cervical dermatomes, phantom limb pain, peripheral neuropathy, post-herpetic neuralgia, complex regional pain syndrome involving the upper extremity, cervicogenic, or tension-type headache (5)
Thoracic epidural steroid injection	Thoracic radiculopathy or radiculitis, thoracic spondylosis, thoracic post-laminectomy syndrome, management of cancer pain involving the thoracic dermatomes, acute pain from herpes zoster, post-herpetic neuralgia, peripheral neuropathy, complex regional pain syndrome involving the trunk
Lumbar epidural steroid injection	Lumbar radiculopathy or radiculitis, spondylosis, stenosis or post-laminectomy syndrome, management of cancer pain involving the lumbar dermatomes, phantom limb pain, peripheral neuropathy, post-herpetic neuralgias, complex regional pain syndrome involving the lower extremities
Caudal epidural steroid injection	Palliation or treatment of the same acute and chronic pain syndromes as for a lumbar epidural steroid injection

executed with or without fluoroscopy. Nonetheless, use of fluoroscopy has been advocated for all epidural injections, based in part on the finding of a greater than 25% false injection rate by experienced clinicians performing fluoroscopically guided translaminar lumbar epidural steroid injections (3).

The transforaminal epidural steroid injection (also known as a selective epidural steroid injection or selective nerve root block) is indicated in cases of radiculopathy or radiculitis secondary to neuralforaminal stenosis, perineural fibrosis, or a disc pathology (lateral disc bulge, protrusion, or extrusion) involving the cervical, thoracic, or lumbar spine. Less common indications for sacral transforaminal epidural steroid injections include palliation for neuropathic pain in the feet and bladder dysfunction following cauda equina injury. Technically, the procedure is termed a selective nerve root block when the clinician is attempting to isolate involvement of a single nerve root by using only a small volume of local anesthetic and no corticosteroid. If the patient reports immediate analgesia, this precisely targeted procedure can help a surgeon identify the level(s) involved in the patient's pain syndrome. If a therapeutic result is desired, a higher volume of injectate containing corticosteroid may be used.

Epidural steroid injections include a corticosteroid, which may be combined with local anesthetic, normal saline, contrast, or a combination of these. The primary active ingredient, the corticosteroid, works by reducing perineural inflammation, stabilizing neural membranes and modulating peripheral nociceptor input, thereby relieving symptoms of pain, numbness, or weakness. Depending on the volume injected, inflammatory mediators may also get diluted. Though usually not curative, epidural steroid injections may complement other non-injection strategies (e.g., medications, physical therapy, and psychological therapy) with resultant longer-term efficacy, which may facilitate rehabilitation and performance of activities of daily living.

In general, epidural-steroid injection seems to be most effective in patients with acute (less than 3 month's duration) rather than chronic pain. Seventy percent to 80% of patients with acute pain may experience improvement, compared with only 40% to 50% of those with chronic pain (4). A history of previous back surgery may be another predictor of outcome, with only about 30% to 40% improving after an epidural steroid injection (4). For those that respond to an injection, onset of relief can occur within hours, though this is typically due to the anesthetic. In most cases it takes 1 to 3 days for the effect of the steroid to declare itself. Exact details for performing these injections are beyond the scope of this chapter.

Translaminar Approach

Positioning for this procedure is dependent upon the spinal level being injected, the patient's position of maximal comfort, and the practical limitations imposed by positioning of the fluoroscope. At the cervical level the patient is placed in a seated or prone position, while at the thoracic and lumbar levels the patient can be placed in the seated, prone, or lateral decubitus position. For purposes of this discussion, the technique used during prone or lateral decubitus positioning will be described.

After identifying the level to be injected by fluoroscopy and palpation, an 18- or 20-gauge, 3.5-inch or 6-inch Touhy needle is carefully advanced towards the epidural space using a loss-of-resistance to air or saline technique. After injecting contrast to confirm an epidurogram, corticosteroid mixed with local anesthetic, normal saline, and/or contrast is administered.

Transforaminal Approach

Positioning for this procedure is also dependent upon the spinal level being injected and the practical limitations imposed by positioning of the fluoroscope. At the cervical level the patient is placed in a supine or lateral decubitus position, while at the thoracic and lumbar levels the patient is placed in a prone position. A 22- or 25-gauge, 3.5-inch spinal needle is advanced towards the foraminal space. After injecting contrast to confirm a neurogram and epidurogram, a small volume of corticosteroid mixed with local anesthetic, normal saline, and/or contrast is administered.

Facet Joint Procedures

Facet joint procedures (intra-articular facet joint injections, medial branch nerve blocks, and radiofrequency lesioning of the medial branch nerves) are typically performed for patients whose neck and low back pain may be due to facet joint arthropathy. In addition to arthritis, facet joint pain can be secondary to trauma or inflammatory changes. Patients with cervical facet joint pain typically describe neck pain that may radiate to the scalp or top of the shoulders. Those with lumbar facet joint pain typically describe low back pain that radiates to the hips, buttocks, and posterior thighs. Decreased range of motion and increased pain with cervical or lumbar hyperextension, oblique extension, and/or lateral bending on physical exam are suggestive of facet pain. Unfortunately, there have not been convincing studies that evaluated the specificity and sensitivity of these exam maneuvers. (Because pain from thoracic facet joint arthropathy is not a common occurrence, it is not covered in this section.)

The facet joint is formed by the articulating surfaces of the superior and inferior articular processes of adjacent vertebrae. Because the facet joint is a true diarthrotic joint with a synovial lining and joint capsule, intra-articular joint injections can be performed using local anesthetic as a diagnostic maneuver to determine whether a facet joint is the pain generator and adding corticosteroid as a potential therapeutic maneuver if the diagnosis is positive. If the duration of analgesia from the intra-articular facet joint injection lasts only as long as the pharmacological effect of the anesthetic or the degree of analgesia is equivocal, a medial branch nerve block may be considered. If the patient obtains 50% or greater pain relief from both the facet joint injection and medial branch nerve block, the patient may be a candidate for radiofrequency lesioning (RFL) of the medial branch nerves.

At the cervical level, the C4-C7 medial branch nerve wraps around the articular pillar of its respective vertebra. At the lumbar level, the L1-4 medial branch nerves run in a groove between the junction of the superior articular process and transverse process of the vertebra one level below the numbered nerve. At the L5 level, however, it is the dorsal ramus that runs in the groove of the sacral ala before giving off the L5 medial branch nerve.

Because each joint is innervated by two medial branch nerves, completely anesthetizing (medial branch nerve block) or denervating (radiofrequency lesioning) a joint requires treating two nerves, one above and one below the involved joint. A medial branch nerve block is considered positive if the patient reports 50% or greater concordant pain relief shortly after anesthetizing the nerves. If the patient has not previously had a diagnostically positive intra-articular facet joint injection, the medial branch nerve block is repeated on a different date to see if the patient again receives 50% or greater concordant pain relief. Because only a local anesthetic is used during a medial branch nerve block, it is strictly a diagnostic injection that rarely gives greater than 24 hours of pain relief. However, for patients who have diagnostically "positive" medial branch nerve blocks performed on two separate occasions (or one diagnostically positive intra-articular facet joint injection and one medial branch nerve block), RFL of the affected nerves may potentially offer longer-term relief on the order of months.

In general, the advantages of RFL include relatively durable analgesia, relatively precise lesions, and the ability to stimulate nervous system elements before ablating, thus avoiding targeting the wrong tissue. Patients should be informed that it can take up to 1 week after the procedure to determine its efficacy.

Intra-Articular Facet Joint Injection

Due to the small size of the facet joint, an intra-articular facet joint injection (IAFJ) is most accurately performed under fluoroscopy using a 22- or 25-gauge, 3.5- or 6-inch spinal needle. After confirming an arthrogram with a small volume of contrast, a local anesthetic with or without corticosteroid can be injected.

Medial Branch Nerve Block

For the purposes of accuracy, this procedure is best performed under fluoroscopy. A 22- or 25-gauge, 3.5-inch spinal needle is advanced towards the affected medial branch nerve as it courses over the middle of the cervical spine's trapezoid-shaped articular processes or at the junction of the superior articular process and transverse process and the sacral ala of the lumbosacral spine. After confirming needle placement, a small volume of local anesthetic is injected.

Radiofrequency Lesioning of the Medial Branch Nerves

Radiofrequency lesioning (RFL) requires special (22-gauge, 10-cm SMK or RFK) needles and a radiofrequency machine capable of ablating the nerve. The target sites of injection for RFL are the same as those described above for medial branch nerve blocks. Once needle positioning is confirmed, sensory and motor stimulation are sequentially performed in an attempt to get as close as possible to the medial branch nerve without being near any motor nerve roots that innervate the upper or lower extremities. Upon affirming the dissociation between sensory and motor stimulation, each affected nerve is ablated at a temperature of 80°C for 90 seconds.

Sacroiliac Joint Injection

Patients with sacroiliac joint (SIJ) pain describe a deep, aching pain in the buttock, which may radiate to the posterior thigh and lower back. The implication of SIJ dysfunction as a significant source of low back pain remains controversial. The precise diagnosis of SIJ dysfunction can be made difficult by the associated presence of myofascial pain, disc herniation, spinal stenosis, or facet arthropathy. Furthermore, many of the physical exam maneuvers (Patrick's test; FABER [acronym for Flexion, ABduction, and External Rotation of the hip]; Gaenslen's test; Fortin's finger test; lateral compression test; anteroposterior pelvic compression test; SIJ compression test; distraction test; thigh thrust [or fade] test; passive straight-leg raising test; one-legged stork test; standing or seated flexion test) lack sufficient specificity due to poor inter- and intra-rater reliability, with some maneuvers demonstrating positive results in as many as 20% of asymptomatic individuals (5-8). Using multiple tests, however, has been shown to give a sensitivity range of 77% to 87% (9).

Many practitioners, however, believe an intra-articular injection with local anesthetic is the best way to confirm SIJ dysfunction (10). Reproduction of pain upon injection of the medication may occur and may be secondary to joint capsule distension, whereas post-injection analgesia is most likely due to the effect of the local anesthetic. Sequential occurrence of these two symptoms further suggests the diagnosis, though one cannot eliminate concomitant response of the surrounding soft tissues to the local anesthetic (11,12). Injection of corticosteroid into the SIJ is a standard therapeutic maneuver. Because repeated injections are not recommended as a long-term treatment plan due to potential steroid-related side effects, other promising treatments of SIJ pain include viscosupplementation with agents

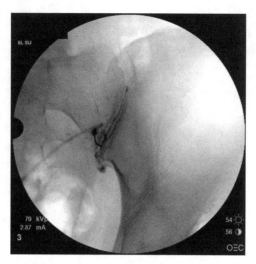

Figure 7-1   Sacroiliac joint arthrogram.

such as hyaluronic acid (Hylan) or radiofrequency (RF) lesioning of the nerves innervating the SIJ (13,14).

Considered a true synovial joint, the SIJ is a C-shaped, diarthrodial structure located between the sacrum and the ilium. While SIJ mobility exhibits a few millimeters of glide and 2-3 degrees of rotation, the SIJ is instead designed for stability (7). Muscles and numerous ligaments (iliolumbar, interosseous, anterior and superior sacroiliac, sacrospinous and sacrotuberous ligaments) are between the spine, sacrum, iliac bones, and pubic symphysis to stabilize the SIJ, which still allow for a small amount of gliding and rotation. In addition to the wide individual variation in innervation of the SIJ, its vast nerve supply helps explain why there are inconsistencies in pain referral patterns, limiting consistent diagnosis of SIJ pain.

While some practitioners perform SIJ injections in an office-based setting without fluoroscopy, it is more safely and accurately performed under fluoroscopic guidance, given the slender oblique nature of the joint which is potentially made even narrower if significant arthropathy is present. The patient is placed in a prone position, followed by advancement of a 22- or 25-gauge, 3.5-inch or 6-inch spinal needle towards the posteroinferior one-third of the SIJ. After injecting a small volume of contrast to confirm intra-articular placement (Fig. 7-1), a mixture of local anesthetic and/or corticosteroid is injected (11-14).

Piriformis Injection

Patients with piriformis syndrome describe a deep, aching pain in the buttock, which may radiate to the hip, lower back, and posterior thigh but rarely below the level of the knee. The syndrome is essentially a true sciatica. Various physical exam maneuvers and findings (Freiberg's sign, Pace's maneuver, Lasègue's sign, Beatty's maneuver, rectal exam, gluteal atrophy) in combination may help confirm the diagnosis (15-19). If the patient fails conservative management with physical therapy and medications, a piriformis injection with local anesthetic and steroid can be considered for treating potential inflammation and irritation of the surrounding neuromuscular structures.

Innervated by branches off the ventral rami of the first and/or second sacral nerves, the piriformis muscle is one of six short, external rotator muscles (superior and inferior gemmeli, obturator internus and externus and quadratus femoris) located below the posteroinferior edge of the gluteus medius muscle (20,21). However, external rotation is only with the hip and knee extended, whereas with standing, the piriformis muscle externally rotates the hip. When the hip is flexed to 90 degrees, as with sitting, contraction of the piriformis muscle abducts the hip.

The piriformis muscle occupies most of the greater sciatic foramen as it passes from its origin along the anterior surface of the second, third, and fourth sacral foramina and inserts on the greater trochanter. Upon active contraction, the muscle's diameter may significantly increase and potentially lead to compression of the accompanying sciatic nerve, depending on its course through the greater sciatic foramen (22). It is the compression of the sciatic and accompanying nerves (branches of the sacral plexus; superior and inferior gluteal nerves; pudendal nerve; posterior femoral cutaneous nerve; and nerves to the gemelli, obturator internus and quadratus femoris muscles) that pass through the foramen that cause symptoms of buttock, inguinal, posterior thigh, and calf pain (22).

The piriformis injection is most safely performed under fluoroscopic guidance, with the optional addition of EMG guidance for increased accuracy. With the patient placed in a prone position, a 22- or 25-gauge, 3.5-inch to 6-inch spinal needle is advanced under fluoroscopic guidance from the buttock to the piriformis muscle (Fig. 7-2). A mixture of corticosteroid with local anesthetic and/or normal saline is injected. Because repeated steroid injections are not recommended as a long-term treatment plan due to potential steroid-related side effects, injection of botulinum toxin may be efficacious in some cases (23,24).

Sympathetic Blocks

The autonomic nervous system, composed of the sympathetic (SNS) and parasympathetic (PNS) nervous systems, can be involved in pain modulation (25). The SNS controls and regulates functions like regional blood flow to the extremities, sweating, and glandular function. Certain pain states, such as complex regional pain syndrome types 1 (reflex sympathetic dystrophy)

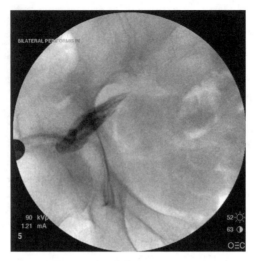

Figure 7-2   Piriformis myogram.

and type 2 (causalgia), certain types of neuropathic pain (e.g., postradiation neuritis, herpes zoster, postherpetic neuralgia, phantom limb pain, post-stroke pain), vascular disorders (e.g., intractable angina pectoris, Raynaud's disease, frostbite, occlusive vascular disease, vasospasm, embolic vascular disease, scleroderma), Paget's disease, hyperhidrosis, Meniere's disease, and vascular headaches may involve malfunction of the SNS (26). Some of these indications, such as post-stroke pain, phantom limb pain, vascular occlusion of large vessels, and Meniere's disease, are controversial, and efficacy is based largely on case reports instead of large studies.

Blockade of the appropriate sympathetic ganglion with local anesthetic can help determine the presence or absence of a sympathetically maintained pain (SMP) state. A sympathetic block that produces immediate, complete pain relief, which persists for hours to weeks or even longer, suggests sympathetically maintained pain. For some, the local anesthetic may lead to a reduction of pain far in excess of the anesthetic's pharmacological duration of action and facilitate the patient's ability to participate in physical therapy and a daily exercise program.

Stellate Ganglion Block

The stellate ganglion block (SGB) is most commonly performed in patients with SMP involving the face, neck, upper extremities, or upper thoracic region. The stellate ganglion lies anterior to the cervical spine, along the prevertebral fascia of the seventh cervical and first thoracic vertebrae. The stellate ganglion is composed of the lower cervical and first thoracic ganglia. The bony landmark for performing an SGB, the anterior tubercle of C6 (Chassaignac's tubercle), is easily palpated with one's finger. Because vital structures, such as the vertebral and carotid arteries, jugular vein, brachial plexus, and pleura, lie in close proximity, there is a risk of inadvertent intra-arterial, epidural, or intrathecal injection resulting in cardiovascular (hypotension, arrhythmia, or cardiovascular collapse) or central nervous system (seizure or loss of consciousness) complications, or inadvertent lung puncture resulting in a pneumothorax.

Skin temperature monitors or strips are applied on both upper extremities prior to performance of the block. The patient is placed in a supine position with the cervical spine in a neutral position. A 25-gauge, 3.5-inch spinal needle is advanced to the junction of the C7 vertebral body and uncinate process. After injection of contrast to demonstrate prevertebral fascial spread, the local anesthetic is administered. Technically, the SGB is considered successful if there is a greater than 1 degree centigrade rise in temperature in the ipsilateral upper extremity and an ipsilateral Horner's sign (ptosis, miosis, unilateral nasal congestion or stuffiness, and conjunctival injection). Clinically, the SGB is successful if the patient experiences a reduction in pain.

Celiac Plexus Block

The celiac plexus block (CPB) is used to differentiate visceral SMP from somatic pain originating from abdominal structures (pancreas, liver, gallbladder, mesentery, omentum, and the gastrointestinal tract from the stomach to the transverse colon), the retroperitoneum or flank (27). Most commonly, CPB is performed for patients with abdominal pain secondary to pancreatic cancer. The patient's life expectancy, analgesic response, and tolerance of potential side effects to the CPB will dictate whether chemical (phenol or alcohol) neurolysis should be performed (12). Chemical neurolysis may also be considered for malignancies of the retroperitoneum and abdomen and, in selected patients, for chronic pancreatitis (27). Finally, CPB has also been shown to relieve pain and reduce morbidity and mortality associated with acute pancreatitis, visceral vascular insufficiency, and arterial embolization of the liver for cancer therapy (12,27-29).

The celiac plexus lies at the level of the L1 vertebra, just anterior or anterolateral to the aorta and epigastrium and inferior to the level of the celiac artery. The preganglionic fibers of the celiac plexus, also known as the greater, lesser, and least splanchnic nerves, arise from T5-T10, T10-11, and T11-12, respectively. Their postganglionic fibers innervate the distal esophagus, stomach, duodenum, small intestine, ascending and proximal transverse colon, adrenal glands, pancreas, spleen, liver, and the biliary system.

Although there are multiple techniques for performing a CPB, the two most common involve either the "classic" retrocrural (also known as a splanchnic nerve block) or the "true" anterocrural approach. Because the anterocrural approach is the more common technique, this is the one that will be described. After placing the patient in a prone position, a 22-gauge, 6-inch spinal needle is advanced to the anterior surface of the L1 vertebral body until arterial pulsations are felt. The needle is carefully advanced until removal of the stylet from the needle reveals free flow of blood. The needle is advanced slightly further until the anterior aortic wall is reached and aspiration for blood is negative. A syringe with saline is then attached to the needle as it is advanced with positive pressure applied to the plunger. Passage into the preaortic tissue is confirmed by a relative loss of resistance to the saline-filled syringe. After contrast is injected under live fluoroscopy to confirm placement, a local anesthetic is given. Successful blockade is confirmed with the relief of pain.

Lumbar Sympathetic Block

The lumbar sympathetic block (LSB) is most commonly performed on patients with SMP involving the lower extremities, although it has also been beneficial for treating erythromelalgia, pain associated with vascular insufficiency, phantom limb pain, frost bite, trench foot, and urogenital pain.

The cell bodies of the lumbar sympathetic chain are located in the lower three thoracic and first three lumbar segments and synapse in ganglia located anterolateral to the vertebral bodies at the L2-3, L3-4, and L4-5 levels. Therefore classic approaches for an LSB are at the L2, L3, and L4 levels. Vital structures located in close proximity to the lumbar sympathetic ganglion include the anteromedially placed aorta on the left and inferior vena cava on the right (30).

Skin temperature monitors or strips are applied on both lower extremities before starting the LSB. After placing the patient in a prone position, a 22-gauge, 6-inch spinal needle is advanced towards the anterolateral aspect of the L2, L3, or L4 vertebral body. After injecting contrast under live fluoroscopy to confirm placement, local anesthetic is injected. An increase in skin temperature in the ipsilateral lower extremity combined with analgesia indicates a successful block.

Superior Hypogastric Block

The superior hypgastric block (SHB) is a diagnostic injection performed to address SMP involving the pelvis. In addition to being diagnostic, it can be potentially therapeutic in cases of intractable visceral pelvic pain of either neoplastic or non-malignant origin (31,32).

The superior hypogastric plexus innervates the ureters, sigmoid colon, uterus, bladder, vagina, prostate, testicular plexus, ovarian plexus, and the plexus surrounding the common and internal iliac arteries. Located in the retroperitoneum, the superior hypogastric plexus is composed of fibers from the aortic plexus and the L2 and L3 splanchnic nerves and extends from the inferior third of the fifth lumbar vertebral body to the superior third of the first sacral vertebral body, bilaterally.

After placing the patient in a prone position, a 22-gauge, 6-inch spinal needle is directed towards the anterolateral aspect of the L5-S1 vertebral interspace. After injecting contrast to confirm placement, local anesthetic is given. If bilateral coverage is desired, the procedure may be repeated on the contralateral side. For patients with a terminal illness, further palliation can be achieved with the addition of a neurolytic agent.

Ganglion Impar Block

The ganglion impar block may be effective in treating visceral pain or SMP involving the perineal area due to neoplasm or chronic benign conditions. Patients usually present with vague, poorly localized pain associated with sensations of burning or urgency.

The ganglion impar (ganglion of Walther) is a retroperitoneal structure that represents the most caudal ganglion of the sympathetic trunk. It is a single ganglion formed by the fusion of the ganglia from both sides and is located anterior to the sacrococcygeal junction. The ganglion impar innervates the perineum, distal rectum and anus, vulva, distal third of the vagina, and the distal urethra.

With the patient in a prone position, a 25-gauge, 1.5-inch needle is advanced through the sacrococcygeal ligament, until the needle lies just anterior to the anterior surface of the sacrococcygeal junction. After injecting contrast to confirm placement, local anesthetic is given. For patients with a terminal illness, further palliation can be achieved with the addition of a neurolytic agent.

REFERENCES

1. **Hogan QH.** Epidural anatomy examined by cryomicrotome section: influence of age, vertebral level, and disease. Reg Anesth. 1996;21:395-406.

2. **Sitzman B.** Epidural injections. In: Fenton DS, Czervionke LF, eds. Image-Guided Spine Intervention. Philadelphia: WB Saunders; 2003:99-126.

3. **Renfrew DL, Moore TE, Kathol MH, et al.** Correct placement of epidural steroid injections: fluoroscopic guidance and contrast administration. Am J Neuroradiol. 1991;12:1003-7.

4. **Ho AM.** Epidural-steroid injections. In: Warfield CA, Fausett HJ, eds. Manual of Pain Management. Philadelphia: Lippincott Williams & Wilkins; 2002:407.

5. **Waldman S.** Interventional Pain Management. Philadelphia: WB Saunders; 2001: 535-40.

6. **Reider B.** The Orthopaedic Physical Examination. Philadelphia: WB Saunders; 2001:195-7.

7. **Slipman CW, Patel RK, Shin CH, et al.** Studies probe complexities of sacroiliac joint syndrome. BioMechanics. 2000:67-78.

8. **Dreyfuss P, Dryer S, Griffin J, et al.** Positive sacroiliac screening tests in asymptomatic adults. Spine. 1994;19:1138-43.

9. **Broadhurst NA, Bond MJ.** Pain provocation tests for the assessment of sacroiliac joint dysfunction. J Spinal Disord. 1998;11:341-5.

10. **Wallace M, Staats P.** Pain Medicine: Just the Facts. New York: McGraw-Hill; 2004.

11. **Lennard T.** Pain Procedures in Clinical Practice. Philadelphia: Hanley & Belfus; 2000:265-75.

12. **Freburger JK, Riddle DL.** Using published evidence to guide the examination of the sacroiliac joint region. Phys Ther. 2001;81:1135-43.

13. **Srejic U, Calvillo O, Kabakibou K.** Viscosupplementation: a new concept in the treatment of sacroiliac joint syndrome—a preliminary report of four cases. Reg Anesth Pain Med. 1999;24:84-8.

14. **Fortin JD, Aprill CN, Ponthieux B, Pier J.** Sacroiliac joint: pain referral maps upon applying a new injection/arthrography technique. Part II: clinical evaluation. Spine. 1994;19:1483-9.

15. **Freiburg AH.** Sciatic pain and its relief by operations on muscle and fascia. Arch Surg. 1937;34:337-50.

16. **Pace JB, Nagle D.** Piriformis syndrome. West J Med. 1976;124:435-9.

17. **Beatty RA.** The piriformis muscle syndrome: a simple diagnostic maneuver. Neurosurgery. 1994;34:512-4; discussion, 514.

18. **Kaul M, Herring SA.** Functional rehabilitation of sports and musculoskeletal injuries. In: Kibler WB, Herring SA, Press JM, eds. The Rehabilitation Institute of Chicago Publication Series. Gaithersburg, MD: Aspen; 1998:209.

19. **Thiele GH.** Coccydgodynia and pain in the superior gluteal region. JAMA. 1937;109:1271-5.

20. **Perotto AO, Delagi EF, Perotto A.** Anatomical Guide for the Electromyographer: The Limbs and Trunk, 3rd ed. Chicago: Charles C Thomas; 1996:218-9.

21. **Jenkins DB.** Hollingshead's Functional Anatomy of the Limbs and Back, 7th ed. Philadelphia: WB Saunders; 1998:274-5.

22. **Travell JG, Simons DG.** Myofascial Pain and Dysfunction: The Trigger Point Manual, vol 2. Baltimore: Williams & Wilkins; 1992:186-214.

23. **Fishman LM, Zybert PA.** Electrophysiologic evidence of piriformis syndrome. Arch Phys Med Rehabil. 1992;73:359-64.

24. **Childers MK, Wilson DJ, Gnatz SM, et al.** Botulinum toxin type A use in piriformis muscle syndrome: a pilot study. Am J Phys Med Rehabil. 2002;81:751-9.

25. **Haugen F.** The autonomic nervous system and pain. Anesth Analg. 1968;47:283-4.

26. **Raj P.** Interventional pain management. In: Waldman S, ed. Stellate Ganglion Block. Philadelphia: WB Saunders; 2002:363.

27. **Bell SN, Cole R, Roberts-Thomson IC.** Coeliac plexus block for control of pain in chronic pancreatitis. Br Med J. 1980;281:1604.

28. **Dale WA.** Splanchnic block in the treatment of acute pancreatitis. Surgery. 1952;32:605-14.

29. **Waldman S.** Innovations in pain management. In: Weiner RS, ed. Celiac Plexus Block. Orlando, FL: PMD; 1990:10-15.

30. **Raj P.** Interventional techniques. In: Raj P, ed. Pain Medicine: A Comprehenisve Review. St. Louis: Mosby; 2003:255-65.

31. **Plancarte R, Amescua C, Patt RB, Aldrete JA.** Superior hypogastric plexus block for pelvic cancer pain. Anesthesiology. 1990;73:236-9.

32. **Lee RB, Stone K, Magelssen D, et al.** Presacral neurectomy for chronic pelvic pain. Obstet Gynecol. 1986;68:517-21.

8

■ ■ ■

Treating Pain Without Pills: An Integrative Approach to Complementary and Alternative Modalities

Maureen A. Flannery, MD

O ver the past 10 years, a number of studies have documented increasing use of complementary and alternative therapies in the United States and worldwide (1-4). In the majority of these surveys, pain is the most common reason for seeking alternatives to mainstream medicine. Because most users of complementary and alternative medicine (CAM) also receive care from conventional physicians, primary care clinicians should be familiar with alternative approaches to pain management.

CAM therapies have been defined as "interventions neither taught widely in medical schools nor generally available in U.S. hospitals" and as "those healing therapies that typically fall outside the Western biomedical model of disease, diagnosis, and treatment"(1,5). As more medical schools develop CAM curricula and more hospitals and conventional practitioners offer CAM therapies, "complementary" becomes a more accurate descriptor than "alternative". Among both consumers and the institutions and individuals who represent mainstream medicine, there is increasing acceptance of the idea that "unconventional" modalities may be useful adjuncts to standard medical and surgical practices.

Indicative of the increased legitimization of CAM in the United States, Congress funded the National Center on Complementary and Alternative Medicine (NCCAM) in 1998 as a center within the National Institutes of Health, replacing the Office of Alternative Medicine established earlier in the decade. The NCCAM mission statement acknowledges that for most CAM therapies, as for many conventional treatments, there are key questions that are yet to be answered through well-designed scientific studies: questions such as whether they are safe and whether they work for the diseases or medical conditions for which they are used. It also recognizes that what is considered to be CAM changes continually. Most surveys of CAM therapies in the United States have covered 15 to 20 representative modalities. Table 8-1 describes two approaches to categorization of these therapies, the classification of the "major domains of CAM" utilized by NCCAM and a "taxonomy of unconventional healing practices" in common use in the United States today (6,7).

The value of combining multiple modalities is well established in conventional pain management. Whether inclusion of CAM therapies is initiated by patients or by their physicians, the incorporation of CAM treatments into usual care may be understood as an extension of this accepted approach to the treatment of pain. As in conventional multidisciplinary pain

Table 8-1   Complementary and Alternative Medicine: Two Classification Systems

	Category	*Examples*
NCCAM *	Alternative medical systems	Homeopathy, naturopathy, traditional Chinese medicine, Ayurveda
	Mind-body interventions	Meditation, prayer, mental healing, creative therapies (art, music, dance)
	Biologically based treatments	Herbal therapy, dietary supplements, vitamins
	Manipulative and body-based methods	Chiropractic, osteopathic manipulation, massage therapy
	Energy therapies	Therapeutic touch, Qi Gong, Reiki, biomagnetic field therapies
Kaptchuk and Eisenberg**	Professional systems	Chiropractic, acupuncture, homeopathy, naturopathy, massage, dual-trained MDs
	Popular health reform	Mega-vitamins, nutritional supplements, botanicals; macrobiotic, vegan, organic, and other special diets
	New Age healing	Esoteric energies, crystals and magnets, spirits and other mediums, Reiki, Qi Gong
	Mind-body	Mind-cure approaches, biofeedback, hypnosis, guided imagery, relaxation response
	Non-normative	Chelation therapy, anti-neoplastics, iridology

* From National Center for Complementary and Alternative Medicine. Major Domains of Complementary and Alternative Medicine. Available at http://nccam.nih.gov/fcp/classify/index.html.
** From Kaptchuk T, Eisenberg DM. Varieties of healing. 2. A taxonomy of unconventional healing practices. Ann Intern Med. 2001;135:196-204; with permission.

management, accurate assessment is critical, individualization of treatment is important, and communication and coordination among all the practitioners caring for patients are essential.

The widespread use by patients of pain treatments that developed and continue to exist outside the conventional medical system raises many issues for the physicians who care for them. This chapter reviews what is known about CAM in terms of their implications in the primary care setting. From the perspective of evidence-based medicine (EBM), this chapter also discusses issues related to research on CAM modalities and describes useful resources for evaluating the state of knowledge about the safety and efficacy of CAM modalities commonly used for pain treatment. While clinicians await conclusive evidence that any given CAM modality is more effective than placebo, patients continue to choose CAM therapies to treat their pain. By exploring the way in which a physician might approach a patient who wants to use acupuncture treatment for low back pain, for example, this chapter suggests methods that balance rigor and pragmatism. It concludes with a review of research in progress on CAM approaches to pain and a discussion of issues related to the integration of CAM into primary care practice.

Which Patients Use Complementary and Alternative Medicine and Why

A review of the history of medicine reminds us that "medical pluralism" is not a new phenomenon, in the United States or elsewhere (8). However, it is clear that there has been a marked increase in the past 50 years in the percentage of the population who utilize therapies not considered part of conventional mainstream medicine, both in the United States and in other industrialized counties (3). According to longitudinal data from a large random telephone survey of U.S. households, the percentage of individuals who reported use of least one of 15 CAM modalities in the past 12 months increased from 34% to 42% between 1990 and 1997 (2). In 1997, the total number of visits to CAM providers exceeded total visits to all primary care physicians for that year; and that year consumers paid more out-of-pocket for CAM than for conventional health care.

While population-based surveys provide useful information for health planners and policy makers, information on the use of CAM in patient populations may be more relevant to clinicians. Studies of family practice clinic patients have shown between 28% and 47% utilization of CAM (5,9-10). A survey of patients attending clinics that belong to a practice-based research network in southern California focused on use of CAM related to specific health problems that also precipitated visits for conventional care. Including both practitioner-based and self-care-based therapies, this survey found an overall CAM utilization rate of 21% (11). Among patients with certain common health problems, the prevalence of CAM use is strikingly high. For instance, in various surveys, 60%-94% of patients with rheumatic disease report CAM use (12). Between one third and two thirds of all patients with cancer report CAM use; women with breast cancer are especially likely to be consistent users of CAM compared with patients with other cancer sites (13,14). Whether for treatment of symptoms or enhancement of health, desire for wellness and interest in prevention were strong predictors of frequent CAM use in a recent national survey (15).

Surveys of general populations suggest that as much as half of all CAM use is related to prevention. In research on patients in practice settings, however, pain emerges as the most common reason for CAM use. In one study, pain was the primary complaint of nearly all CAM users at one time or another, with back pain accounting for 56% (5). In another study, musculoskeletal and connective tissue ICD-9 diagnostic codes accounted for about one third of all CAM use (11).

The profile of the typical CAM user that emerged from research in the early 1990s was of a well-educated, middle-income, white female. Recent, more representative, surveys demonstrate that CAM use exists within all segments of the U.S. population. Patterns of CAM utilization vary with the type of therapy used. For instance, it seems that self-care-based therapies are more likely to be used by well-educated patients, and traditional folk remedies are more likely to be used by immigrants with low levels of education (11). Use of practitioner-based therapies correlates with income but not with education This is not surprising given that lack of coverage for CAM modalities by government-funded medical insurance and even by private insurers restricts its availability to those with sufficient resources to explore and pay for non-funded services. While the popular media report that increasing numbers of insurers are offering coverage for CAM, the results of actual surveys indicate that the current status of CAM coverage remains quite limited (15). This leads to a paradoxical situation. While alternative therapies cost society less than conventional ones, for individuals with insurance coverage the direct costs associated with CAM modalities are greater than those of mainstream treatments. At the same time, those who are uninsured or underinsured may find CAM treatment less costly than conventional care (24).

Studies suggest that frustration over the shortcomings of conventional treatment, concern over adverse side effects, and skepticism over the tenets of western biomedicine may be more common among users than non-users of CAM (20). While these beliefs may reflect an "alternative treatment ideology", it seems that most individuals embrace CAM therapies because of the perception that the combination of CAM and conventional treatments are superior to either alone (21). In countries in which CAM modalities are integrated with conventional care and CAM modalities are covered by government insurance, there is less marked income differentiation between CAM users and nonusers (16). And, of course, in many parts of the world, therapies NCCAM considers within the domain of CAM may comprise usual care. Indeed, the focus of the 2002-2005 World Health Organization Policy and Strategy on Traditional Medicine is on modalities considered alternative in the United States (17).

In the United States both self-care and practitioner-based CAM therapies are more likely to be utilized in addition to conventional treatment than as an alternative to conventional medicine (18). Dissatisfaction with mainstream medical care predicts CAM use only in the small percentage of the population who rely exclusively upon alternative medicine. In a 1996 survey, for instance, only 1.8% of the population made visits to unconventional practitioners in the absence of visits for conventional health care. Indeed, in this population, use of CAM was actually associated with increased likelihood and number of physician visits (19).

It is important to note that individual differences in CAM treatment utilization may stem in part from systemic differences across racial and ethnic groups in perceptions of the risks and benefits of interventions. As a recent review pointed out, patient "preferences" for unconventional, and often less intensive, treatment may be indicative of the actual outcome of care in underserved communities. This may reflect resignation to the perceived status quo, a belief that certain interventions are "unavailable, unaffordable, ineffectual, or unduly risky, even if those perceptions are not accurate" (22). A better understanding of reasons for preferences for CAM or conventional treatments is critical if we are to find effective ways to address disparities in access to health care.

Practitioners of Complementary and Alternative Medicine

While many forms of CAM are variations of self-care, other CAM modalities are quite as practitioner-based as conventional medicine, among them a number of "professional systems" (7). Given the diversity of modalities within the domain of CAM, generalization about CAM practitioners is impossible. An attempt at a summary of the characteristics of alternative CAM practitioners in the United States, Canada, and the United Kingdom suggests that their perspectives and backgrounds are similar to and as varied as those of people who seek CAM (23).

A qualitative study of non-physician CAM practitioners in a Midwestern urban community identified a number of themes (24). CAM practitioners stressed the holism of their approach, distinguishing it from that of biomedicine, which they characterized as mechanistic and reductionist. They emphasized their role in empowering patients and encouraging personal responsibility for health. Practitioners were concerned about justice issues related to access to CAM and conventional treatments. Their philosophical orientation suggested that they might be characterized, as Astin described CAM users, as "cultural creatives" in terms of values and beliefs (19).

Training programs for CAM practitioners vary widely in prerequisites; in the quality, intensity, and length of educational program; and in requirements for credentialing. Experience and apprenticeship are often valued as alternatives or adjuncts to formal education. Most CAM training programs take place in relative isolation and without the infrastructure provided by conventional medical and academic institutions. In many cases, there are different "schools" within a particular field and more than one internal accrediting body or member organization for a given CAM profession.

In contrast to the relatively standard approach to regulation of most biomedical occupations, countries and states vary widely in their approach to CAM modalities. All states in the United States license chiropractors, for instance, and more than half of the states license non-physician acupuncturists. Some states recognize and regulate practitioners of other CAM modalities such as massage therapy, herbal medicine, naturopathy, and homeopathy (25). Although there is a trend towards more licensing and accreditation of CAM practitioners, controversy abounds about the appropriateness of such regulation, both within mainstream medicine and among CAM practitioners. Advocates of CAM are wary of control by mainstream medicine, and conventional physicians worry about the implications of incorporating practitioners of therapies that lack an evidence base (23). Meanwhile, this chaos results in confusion for consumers, for mainstream physicians, and often for CAM practitioners themselves.

Both worldwide and in the United States, far more nonphysicians than physicians practice CAM. Over the past 20 years or so, increasing numbers of conventionally trained physicians have themselves become CAM practitioners. For some physicians, training in a CAM therapy is not unlike learning a new technique or seeking subspecialty certification; for others, embracing CAM represents a radical and often transformative process (26). Physician-acupuncturists provide good examples of dual-trained MDs. Over 4000 physicians have completed the acupuncture program sponsored by the University of California at Los Angeles since it began training physicians in 1983. The current program includes two pathways, one with a pain management focus (27). In 2000 the American Board of Medical Acupuncture instituted a board examination and certification process for physician acupuncturists (28). The American Board of Holistic Medicine provides board certification to licensed physicians who demonstrate knowledge and skills about the spectrum of complementary and alternative therapies (29).

Communicating with Patients About Complementary and Alternative Medicine

The first large national survey of CAM use in the United States served as something of a wake-up call for mainstream medicine. Not only did the report disclose that large numbers of patients were seeking and obtaining care outside the conventional medical system, but it also demonstrated that physicians were apt to be quite unaware of what their patients were doing. In population-based studies, 40%-70 % of CAM users report that they have not mentioned their CAM use to their physicians (21). Again, surveys in practice settings may have more clinical relevance. Of the 28% of patients in a family practice clinic population who reported use of some form of CAM as a adjunct to physician-prescribed care for the same problem, 63% reported that they had not disclosed their CAM use to their primary care physician (5). Patients indicate that they do not reveal their use of unconventional therapies for a variety of reasons. Not being asked and belief that CAM use was insigificant in terms of conventional care are more common explanations than concerns about physician lack of understanding or disapproval (21).

Studies of patient-physician communication about pain reveals some similarities. For instance, we know that older patients often under-report pain, even when it interferes significantly with the quality of their lives and that conventional medical providers are often unaware of the level of pain of patients with cancer (30,31). As with CAM use, patients often indicate that they do not report the level of their pain simply because no one posed the appropriate questions.

With communication about CAM as with inquiry about pain, there is a consensus that health care and patient satisfaction are best when physicians "ask the unasked questions" and their patients answer honestly. Physicians now have several models for initiating discussions about use of CAM and for advising patients who seek alternative treatments (32-34). Eisenberg provides an especially useful strategy, and includes recommendations for dealing with patients who choose to utilize unconventional treatment while rejecting a medical evaluation. Table 8-2 summarizes these guidelines for communicating with patients about CAM.

Another important issue concerns the primary care physician's bounds of professional responsibility regarding awareness of patients using unconventional treatments. Recent reviews suggest that the same ethical principles that apply to conventional care are relevant to physician-patient communication about CAM, including respect for patient autonomy and requirement for informed consent. When a patient discloses CAM use to a primary care physician who is not involved in referring or providing services, it appears that risks of liability are low. However, when the primary care physician considers that the information available on a particular CAM modality does not meet the standards required for informed consent, that fact should be communicated and documented (35).

A possible side-effect of enhanced communication about CAM in clinical encounters is a deepening of physician-patient relationships as patients feel more "cared for" and better "listened to" and as physicians learn more about their patients' preferences and values. Opening up communication about CAM may make it easier for patients to share and seek medical counsel

---

Table 8-2   Guidelines for Physician Communication with Patients About Complementary and Alternative Medicine

1. Always ask an open-ended question such as "What else are you doing to take care of your health?"
2. Convey an open and nonjudgmental attitude.
3. Listen for and respond to nondisclosing cues, which may indicate a patient's interest in discussion of CAM use.
4. Ensure that medical evaluation is complete and that patient is aware of conventional options for treatment. Reassess as needed.
5. Discuss patient's preferences and expectations and encourage use of a symptom diary to monitor results.
6. Review issues of safety and efficacy.
7. If appropriate and desired by patient, arrange to release and request records in order to coordinate conventional and CAM treatments.
8. Be honest about your lack of knowledge about particular modalities and be open to new information and education.
9. Monitor results of treatment and arrange follow-up.
10. Document all discussions and advice in medical records.

Adapted from Eisenberg DM. Advising patients who seek alternative medical therapies. Ann Intern Med. 1997;127:61-9; and Pappas S, Perlman A. Complementary and alternative medicine: the importance of doctor-patient communication. Med Clin N Amer. 2002;86:1-10; with permission.

---

about other aspects of their lives that affect their health. Especially for patients with chronic pain, the "nonspecific effects" of improved physician-patient relationships may be in themselves therapeutic.

Communicating with Complementary and Alternative Medicine Practitioners

Advances in pain management over the past decade have highlighted the importance of communication not only between physicians and patients but also among physicians and other members of multidisciplinary teams involved in comprehensive care. Although there is similar value in communication between conventional physicians and CAM practitioners caring for the same patient, a number of factors make its occurrence less likely. CAM practitioners operate primarily outside the mainstream medical network of referrals and consultations in which reciprocal exchanges of information is expected. Perhaps more importantly, unlike members of allied health disciplines that have developed within the context of western biomedicine, often CAM practitioners and conventional physicians do not even "speak the same language" (36). When communication is impossible, collaboration is unlikely, and patient care suffers.

Education is needed to provide both conventional medicine and CAM practitioners with an understanding of each other's vocabulary and concepts. In a recent survey of the extent to which physicians communicated with their patients about CAM use, an overwhelming majority of physicians expressed a need for more education about CAM (37). Both undergraduate and continuing medical education programs have been developed to respond to this need (38). NCCAM has promoted the concept of including CAM practitioners in these efforts by providing them with the information they need to communicate with conventional medical providers.

Evidence-Based Medicine and Complementary and Alternative Medicine

Any discussion of the efficacy of CAM modalities for pain management must take into account the lively discussions in the medical literature over the past decade about EBM and its relevance for the evaluation of complementary and alternative modalities (39,40). It must also acknowledge that the "persuasive appeal" of alternative medicine often has little to do with efficacy as understood by biomedicine and much to do with "nonspecific effects" related to the patient-practitioner relationship, nature of the illness, and characteristics and setting of the intervention (41). What we understand about the biopsychosocial characteristics of patients with chronic pain suggests that these nonspecific effects may be important determinants of the results of treatment.

EBM has been described as "the integration of best research evidence with clinical expertise and patient values" (42). Thus understood, EBM aims to combine the proficiency and judgment that clinicians acquire through experience and practice with clinically relevant research while taking into account the unique preference and expectations each patient brings to the clinical encounter. Basic to the debate about EBM and CAM is a difference of opinion about what constitutes "good evidence". EBM is based upon a "hierarchy of evidence". Information from objective randomized controlled clinical trials (RCCTs) represents the best evidence. Meta-analyses or systematic reviews of a series of RCCTs are considered the most authoritative for clinicians, planners, and policymakers. Results of observational studies, case series, reports of individual experiences, and qualitative research studies are distinctly less compelling.

After a decade of attempts to provide a solid research grounding for CAM within this framework, it has become clear that there are fundamental conceptual barriers to evaluating CAM with EBM, in addition to problems related to lack of attention and resources. CAM presents both philosophical and methodological challenges to EBM (43). Among the questions CAM researchers ask are

- How relevant are population-based methods of assessment for the evaluation of CAM practices which understand illness and healing only in the context of particular individuals?

- Is it useful or even possible to adapt methods used for evaluating drug therapies to the study of physical and manipulative interventions?

- How feasible is it to attempt to double-blind interactive therapies?

- Are the scales and checklists used to assess RCCTs (which use completeness of double-blinding, for instance, as an index of quality) valid for research on CAM?

Researchers actively involved in investigating CAM support "methodological pluralism". Rather than the "pyramid" of evidence that EBM offers, Jonas offers the model of an "evidence house" with rooms for different types of evidence (44). For exploration of the efficacy of CAM modalities, a balanced research strategy that incorporates qualitative case reports, epidemiological outcomes studies, and health services research, alongside the research approaches valued by EBM, seems most likely to yield data that will be clinically useful as well as scientifically sound.

Complementary and Alternative Medicine Resources

CAM remains a hot topic in the popular press. Lately there has been an explosion of information in the medical literature as well. More than 1500 CAM-related articles are added to the MEDLINE database annually. Fortunately, a number of excellent resources are available for physicians and patients seeking clinically relevant information about the CAM modalities (Table 8-3).

Among many excellent overviews, *The Desktop Guide to Complementary and Alternative Medicine,* which includes a searchable CD-ROM, provides the most practical text for busy clinicians. Jonas and Levin's *Essentials of Complementary and Alternative Medicine* includes excellent reviews of the most commonly used CAM modalities.

Besides the increased attention being paid to CAM in mainstream medical journals and newsletters, many peer-reviewed specialty journals publish both original research and reviews of CAM modalities. As with conventional EBM searches, the most efficient way to access information is to use one of several large computer databases. Table 8-3 lists several of these. Particularly useful for exploring CAM pain management options are CAMPAIN and ARCAM, two databases which focus on pain and arthritis and rheumatic disease, both maintained by the University of Maryland Complementary Medicine Program. The International Cochrane Collaboration registry has had a Complementary Medicine Field since 1996, and the

Table 8-3   Resources for Evidence-Based and Complementary/Alternative Medicine

References for Clinicians

Ernst E, Pittler MH, Stevinson C, et al. The Desktop Guide to Complementary and Alternative Medicine: An Evidence-Based Approach. St. Louis: Mosby; 2001.

Jonas WB, Levin JS, eds. Essentials of Complementary and Alternative Medicine. Philadelphia: Lippincott Williams & Wilkins; 1999.

Databases

CAM on PubMed: www.nlm.nih.gov/nccam/camonpubmed.html

Cochrane Collaboration: www.cochrane.org

CAMPAIN and ARCAM: www.compmed.ummc.umaryland.edu/InformaticsDatabases.html.

Guides for Patients

Fugh-Berman A. Alternative Medicine: What Works. Philadelphia: Lippincott Williams & Wilkins; 1997.

Pelletier KH. The Best Alternative Medicine. New York: Fireside; 2002.

NCCAM: http://nccam.nih.gov

Cochrane database provides links to completed reviews and protocols. In addition to a direct link to CAM on PubMed, the NCCAM Web site maintains a list of open and ongoing clinical trials.

Physicians who wish to assist patients in sorting through the almost unlimited quantity of CAM-related information available through the internet can recommend the NCCAM Web site as a place to start. Especially useful sections of the NCCAM site provide information on evaluating CAM practitioners and on determining the quality of internet CAM sources. It is helpful for physicians to remind their patients the extent to which purveyors of CAM-related products and services may influence reports of safety and efficacy, just as the pharmaceutical industry may bias reports about conventional treatments.

Applying Complementary and Alternative Medicine Research to Clinical Care: One Approach

One useful approach to determining what evidence is available and relevant for decision making in a primary care setting utilizes five questions that Linde and Jonas propose for clinically relevant research (Table 8-4). Using this framework, the following sections show how a conventionally trained clinician who desires to practice EBM might respond to a patient who inquires about a particular CAM treatment.

Table 8-4   Applying CAM Research to Clinical Care: Five Questions for Physicians

---

1. Is the treatment effective for this patient for this condition?

2. Is this treatment effective on average for patients with similar conditions?

3. Is an aspect of this treatment effective on average for patients with conditions like this?

4. For patients with conditions like this, is this a more effective treatment on average than another treatment?

5. Is there biological evidence for the effectiveness of this treatment for this condition?

From Linde K, Jonas WB. Evaluating complementary and alternative medicine: the balance of rigor and relevance. In: Jonas WB, Levin JS, eds. Essentials of Complementary and Alternative Medicine. Philadelphia: Lippincott Williams & Wilkins; 1999:57-71; with permission.

Is This Treatment Effective for This Patient?

When a patient inquires about acupuncture as a treatment for low back pain, this, of course, is the question that usually matters to the patient. Often a patient becomes interested in a CAM modality such as acupuncture as a result of reports from other individuals who have benefited from acupuncture, perhaps also as treatment for back pain. However, like many other CAM approaches, traditional Chinese medicine (TCM) focuses on underlying causes rather than on presenting symptoms. As a consequence, the same conventional diagnosis, low back pain, may lead to various TCM diagnoses and to quite dissimilar treatments in different patients (45). Although individual testimonials, the physician's clinical observations of other patients, or case reports in the literature may suggest that acupuncture may be useful for patients who present with certain types of problems, among them back pain, it is only within the context of a particular individual that a determination can be made.

To answer this first question, a therapeutic trial is an obvious approach, in practice as in research. The widespread use of CAM modalities can be seen as a proliferation of therapeutic trials, in large part undocumented and unmonitored. A physician can look upon a patient's disclosure of use or intention to use a CAM treatment as an opportunity to become an observer, if nothing else. However, as Chez, Jonas, and Eisenberg caution, with CAM as with conventional treatments, the physician's first obligation is to protect patients from harm (25). While most CAM interventions are low risk, there is potential for harm as a direct consequence of the CAM treatment, as a result of interaction with other conventional or CAM treatments, or because other more effective treatments are neglected. In the case of a patient interested in acupuncture for low back pain, the physician's foremost obligation is to ensure that an adequate diagnostic evaluation has been performed to eliminate sources for the back pain that suggest the need for conventional medical intervention and to be certain that no contraindications to acupuncture exist.

Given a patient for whom conservative medical treatment is appropriate, the physician may assist the patient in assessing the safety of acupuncture as a possible alternative. A quick review of information available using the resources listed in Table 8-3 is reassuring.

Contraindications for acupuncture are few. While the early literature on the safety of acupuncture consisted entirely of isolated case reports, both extensive reviews and several large prospective studies now provide reassurance that acupuncture is safe in the hands of competent practitioners (46). A physician can direct the patient to the NCCAM Web site for information on evaluating the competence and training of acupuncture practitioners.

If the patient has no contraindications to acupuncture and wishes to pursue treatment, the physician may document the patient's decision in the chart, observe for changes that indicate a need for re-evaluation, monitor for adverse effects, and assist the patient in evaluating outcomes.

Is This Treatment Effective for Patients with Similar Conditions?

For the physician who wishes to generalize experience from one patient to others who present with the same problem, this question is relevant. A patient who is hesitant to try an unfamiliar approach or concerned about cost or other factors may be interested in the answer as well. A research response to this question requires randomized controlled trials in which acupuncture is compared with no treatment for patients with back pain.

A 1999 Cochrane review of the effectiveness of acupuncture in the management of acute and chronic low back pain identified 11 randomized trials (47). In three studies, acupuncture was compared with no treatment. While the reviewers noted serious methodological problems with the design of each of these studies, each one suggested that acupuncture was more beneficial than no treatment.

Experience with CAM research over the past few years has heightened the awareness of the role of "nonspecific effects. As a treatment that combines novelty, ritual, relationship with a practitioner, and a palpable physical intervention, acupuncture may lead to a host of these effects. Given the influence of patient expectations of benefit, it is difficult for studies comparing acupuncture to no treatment for back pain to demonstrate that acupuncture itself is responsible for the therapeutic effect.

From the perspective of EBM, studies without controls for nonspecific effects do not lead to reliable conclusions. And because in actual experience patients with pain problems do not consider "no treatment" an acceptable option, these studies provide little guidance for clinical decisions.

Is a Particular Aspect of This Treatment Effective?

An answer to this question requires a reliable control for "nonspecific effects", generally a sham or placebo control. Research on many CAM modalities has been stymied because of the challenges of designing trials with appropriate controls. Acupuncture research provides a good example of the difficulties CAM investigators encounter. Considerable effort has gone into devising a placebo control that effectively simulates acupuncture treatment—for example, using "sham" needles cleverly crafted like stage daggers, needling at non-acupuncture points or at points not known to influence the symptom or condition being studied, and utilizing mock electro-stimulation units. All of these strategies have shortcomings. Practitioner blinding is even more problematic (48).

Two recent and thorough reviews of randomized sham-controlled trials of acupuncture for back pain led to different conclusions. A meta-analysis by Ernst and White considered 12 studies deemed adequate (though not excellent) in terms of acupuncture technique, follow-up, and sample size. (Another 16 studies of acupuncture for low back pain were excluded for various reasons.) The reviewers concluded that the combined results of all studies indicated that acupuncture was superior to various control interventions for the treatment of back pain, though evidence was not considered sufficient to determine that acupuncture was more effective than placebo (49). A systematic review within the framework of the Cochrane Collaboration included many of the same studies, using a "best evidence synthesis" approach (47). The conclusion of this second review was that there is no convincing evidence that acupuncture is effective in the management of acute or chronic low back pain.

Both of these reviews criticized the poor methodological quality of most of the studies and made specific recommendations for further research. Of three RCCTs published since these reviews were completed, two showed benefit of acupuncture over placebo, and one concluded that improvement in pain was due to placebo (50-52). An international group recently developed a set of guidelines for reporting interventions in controlled trials of acupuncture that will hopefully lead to more rigorous trial design, more robust conclusions, and clearer conclusions (53).

Is This Treatment More Effective Than Another Treatment?

Investigations to answer this question must involve one modality compared with either standard care and/or one or more other active treatments. Given the widespread use of a variety of CAM modalities for low back pain, and the current lack of evidence that any one conventional treatment is best, this is a relevant question for patients and their physicians. CAM presents patients with a range of options for pain treatment that vary in availability, cost, and degree of patient involvement in the intervention. While most CAM options are far less costly and less invasive than conventional choices, it is useful for patients, physicians, insurers, and health planners to be able to determine the relative efficacy and cost-effectiveness of different approaches to the treatment of pain problems.

A recent large randomized trial of patients with chronic low back pain compared TCM acupuncture with therapeutic massage and self-care education (54). The study did not include a "no treatment" or "usual care" control group. Active treatment included up to ten massage or acupuncture treatments over a 10-week period, with follow-up for a year. This study demonstrated that neither acupuncture nor massage was conclusively superior to self-care, although there was a suggestion that massage might be somewhat more efficacious.

A secondary analysis of the data in this study examined the relationship between patients' expectations of benefit from specific treatments and their self-reported outcomes (55). The study demonstrated improved outcomes when patients had higher expectations of the treatment they received, independent of which treatment it was. As the authors point out, these findings indicate the importance of assessing patient expectations in the design and interpretation of clinical trials of conventional and CAM modalities.

In addition to highlighting the importance of nonspecific effects, research on CAM has emphasized the need to consider treatment preferences in clinical decisions. For a physician faced with a patient who wants to try CAM treatments for a pain problem, among the most important questions to ask may be "What do you think might be helpful?" and "What approach would you like to try?" If acupuncture is the patient's answer, research suggests that it may be more likely to benefit the patient than another modality, apart from the presence or lack of evidence for its effectiveness in general.

Is the Effect Biologically Demonstrated?

Although this question is of concern to scientists, it is not always relevant to others. Individual patients and physicians vary in the extent to which theoretical plausibility determines what treatments they will try, permit, or promote. In the case of acupuncture, basic neurophysiologic research over the past 25 years has identified many explanations for analgesic responses to acupuncture, among them the activation of endogenous opioids. The recent development of devices to measure biomechanical responses to needling in humans and the use of functional magnetic resonance imaging to link clinical effects to specific brain structures has led to explanations that are convincing to scientists and skeptics. Indeed, as one researcher points out, the mechanism of acupuncture analgesia is better understood than that of many medications routinely used for pain management (56).

Should You Recommend or Approve the Use of a Particular Complementary or Alternative Therapy?

After utilizing the framework of the foregoing five questions to review the medical literature, how does a physician ultimately respond to a patient's inquiry about a particular CAM therapy? Let us turn again to our example of the patient who inquires about acupuncture for low back pain. Certainly there is reassuring evidence of safety and interesting information on the presumed neurophysiologic basis for acupuncture effects. Nevertheless, for a physician or patient looking for clinically relevant research to guide clinical decisions, the search yields few data that are reliable and useful. Even though acupuncture has been the subject of more clinical research than many other CAM modalities, the medical literature provides no definite evidence firm enough to promote acupuncture for low back pain, one of the conditions for which it is commonly used.

The current state of knowledge (and lack of knowledge) about acupuncture treatment for low back pain is, unfortunately, typical. Review of the available research on this topic illustrates many of the problems faced by physicians who wish to apply EBM to CAM. Lack of good-quality evidence and uncertainty about whether the results of research have relevance for clinical care complicate the evaluation of almost any CAM modality for any particular pain problem.

Many conventional pain treatments have been adopted without good quality research to support their effectiveness. Among the accepted interventions for common pain problems are many that are costly, invasive, likely to have adverse effects, and provide inadequate relief for substantial numbers of patients. While most CAM interventions presently lack an evidence base, they are generally low-cost, low-risk, and free of serious side-effects, and extensively used. There is an urgent need for larger and better trials of CAM therapies that are already widespread.

While the original Office of Alternative Medicine funding in FY 1992 was $2 million, anticipated appropriation for NCCAM for FY 2003 is $113.2 million. This represents a significant increase in funding for research into CAM modalities. At this point clinical trials are in progress for evaluation of the efficacy and safety of CAM approaches to most of the pain problems commonly seen in primary care practice. Already there are some promising results suggesting the efficacy of certain CAM modalities for the pain of osteoarthritis, fibromyalgia, and chronic back pain.

Biologically Based Therapies

Considerable research effort is going into the study of therapies that NCCAM categorizes as biologically based: herbal and botanical medicine, nutritional approaches, and dietary supplementation. Although the understanding of pain that underlies these therapies is often consistent with the biomedical model, use of these CAM therapies generally reflects a preference for "natural" rather than chemical or synthetic products, with the assumption that these alternative treatments are safer or at least less likely to result in adverse effects than conventional therapies.

Many biologically based treatments have a long history of use, but recent reports of severe adverse effects suggest that caution is necessary in the widespread use of products that are neither tested with the rigor of conventional drugs nor regulated in terms of quality and purity (57). Even pure single-entity herbal products may contain a number of naturally occurring chemicals, any one of which may interact with conventional over-the-counter and prescription medications (58). It is particularly important for conventional physicians to be aware of patients' use of these substances. Several large clinical trials are planned or in progress investigating herbal therapy interactions with medications commonly used for pain, including opioids.

A good example of a promising biologically based CAM approach to pain is the use of glucosamine hydrochloride and chondroitin sulfate, two nutritional supplements derived from animal products, for the treatment of arthritic pain. Over the past 5 years, use has become widespread. A recent systematic quality assessment and meta-analysis of 15 RCCTs of these products suggests some evidence of efficacy in treating the pain of osteoarthritis (59). A large multi-site clinical trial, NIH-GAIT, is now underway to determine whether glucosamine, chondroitin, and/or glucosamine/chondroitin combined are more effective than placebo in the treatment of knee pain associated with osteoarthritis (60).

For modalities within this domain of CAM, as the NIH-GAIT study demonstrates, research on safety and efficacy can often proceed using models developed for the evaluation of pharmaceuticals. If research demonstrates effectiveness, an "alternative" treatment may quickly and easily become incorporated into conventional medicine.

Mind-Body Medicine

Neither investigation or incorporation is as straightforward within other domains. Mind-body medicine, for instance, includes a number of modalities widely utilized for pain management. Challenging the dualistic thinking characteristic of western biomedicine, mind-body approaches consider pain as a physical sensation that is potentially modifiable by various techniques that alter an individual's attention and awareness. Some mind-body techniques that were considered alternative in the past have become mainstream approaches to pain management, among them clinical hypnosis and cognitive-behavioral therapy.

A current focus of research on mind-body approaches to pain management involves various forms of meditation (transcendental meditation, relaxation response, and mindfulness meditation). A recent Cochrane systematic review of a variety of these therapies for fibromyalgia concluded there is evidence for the effectiveness of mind-body techniques in outcomes such as perceived self-efficacy, even without demonstrable pain reduction (61). Given the low risk of these interventions and their potential value in terms of improving overall well-being, there is need for research to suggest which approaches might be most effective for particular patients and conditions.

Manipulative Modalities

Among the most utilized practitioner-based CAM modalities are therapies that utilize manipulation and/or movement of one or more parts of the body for therapeutic effect. Although there is tremendous variation in derivation and orientation of these treatments, they are all based on the belief that correction of the dysfunction of one body part may have positive effects on pain and on overall health and well-being. Chiropractic and massage are among the manipulative modalities commonly used for pain management.

Although considered within the domain of CAM, chiropractic is probably the most mainstream of the professional systems or practitioner-based therapies. Despite vigorous opposition from conventional medicine, chiropractors are licensed in all states, and chiropractic care is covered by major insurance carriers and by Medicare. In surveys of CAM use, chiropractic visits account for as much as a third of all visits. Treatment of pain, particularly musculoskeletal pain, is the primary reason that individuals seek chiropractic care (62).

Even though chiropractic is more amenable to evaluation by evidence-based methods than some other CAM modalities, high-quality research is lacking. Even for back pain, the most common symptom for which individuals seek chiropractic care, research has not shown clear evidence that chiropractic manipulation, either alone or with myofascial therapy, improves outcomes over a standard care or a back education self-care program (63). Given chiropractic's extensive use, evidence regarding safety is needed. A recent systematic review of the literature on the risks associated with spinal manipulation concluded that direct serious adverse effects are rare and most often associated with cervical manipulation, but that indirect and less serious complications are frequent (64). Clearly there is a need for more large-scale prospective studies on safety and efficacy. Current clinical trials of chiropractic are evaluating the usefulness of chiropractic manipulation for chronic neck pain (compared with medication and self-care) and for low back pain (when chosen in an expanded benefits package that includes acupuncture and massage).

Massage therapy includes a variety of approaches that address pain as a physical and psychological sensation caused by or reflected in the soft tissues of the body (65). Relatively few RCCTs of massage therapy have been published. In addition to the large study mentioned earlier, which compared acupuncture, massage, and self-care education for treatment of low back pain, a recent Cochrane review of massage for subacute and chronic low back pain concluded that there was some evidence that massage might be useful, especially when combined with education and exercise (54,66). Like mind-body modalities, massage therapy is a low-risk intervention that has the potential to maximize a number of positive nonspecific effects. The benefits that patients with pain experience with massage may include decreased anxiety and improved sleep patterns as much as measurable pain reduction.

Traditional Chinese Medicine

Among the modalities that NCCAM classifies as alternative medicine systems, TCM is the one most used for pain management in the United States and perhaps worldwide. TCM is an integrated and coherent system that includes herbal medicine, acupuncture, mind-body exercise, and dietary therapy. Of these components, acupuncture is probably the most common approach to pain. Within TCM, pain is understood as a result of obstruction in the flow of vital energy, or *qi,* and the aim of interventions is to restore this free flow and balance.

The only pain problem for which the 1997 NIH consensus development conference concluded that acupuncture was clearly efficacious was postoperative dental pain (67). For a number of other pain problems, the NIH panel found the evidence for acupuncture effectiveness equivocal but promising. In the 5 years since the NIH conference, systematic reviews have been published of research on acupuncture for headaches and fibromyalgia (68,69). As is the case with acupuncture for low back pain, there is no firm evidence for acupuncture's efficacy, either in the treatment of these specific conditions or for chronic pain (70). Large-scale clinical trials are presently recruiting patients for the investigation of acupuncture treatment of fibromyalgia, osteoarthritic knee pain, arm pain related to repetitive stress disorder, and temporomandibular joint pain.

Among CAM approaches commonly used for pain are several modalities that present major challenges for researchers. Recently NCCAM initiated the Frontier Medicine Research Program to encourage research on extensively used CAM practices for which there is no plausible biomedical explanation. Included are a variety of energy therapies, all of which involve the use of biofields and electromagnetic fields; alternative medical systems that seem to contradict rational scientific principles, like homeopathy; and such mind-body approaches as prayer and spiritual healing. For all these CAM modalities, there is an urgent need to determine whether there are research designs that will yield meaningful clinical data.

Integrating Complementary and Alternative Therapies into Your Practice

Several years ago, an eminent gastroenterologist declared (not so happily) that "now only a leaky, semipermeable membrane separates alternative practices from mainstream orthodoxy" (71). The current status of CAM therapies for pain management demonstrates how leaky, and how impenetrable, the barrier between unconventional and accepted therapies may be.

Patients have at their disposal a whole range of CAM treatments for pain, in addition to the various modalities and treatments that are part of the conventional approach to pain management. Studies show that CAM treatments are widely used for pain. Increasingly, knowledge of the use of CAM modalities is considered important for physicians to provide competent and comprehensive care in a primary care setting. At the same time, physicians need to be aware of issues related to integrating CAM approaches in patient care. In a recent review of potential physician malpractice liability associated with complementary and integrative therapies, Cohen and Eisenberg discuss the problems that changing standards of care related to CAM therapies create for physicians (72). They propose that physicians adopt different stances towards patient CAM use depending upon an assessment of evidence for safety or efficacy. The strategies they propose for physicians to minimize the risk of liability related to CAM incorporate the communication guidelines summarized in Table 8-2. Although surveys indicate that large numbers of mainstream physicians are referring to CAM practitioners, Cohen and Eisenberg advise caution regarding referrals to and collaboration with nonphysician CAM providers (72,73). Strategies for physicians to minimize liability are less clear-cut in this area.

The Federation of State Medical Boards recently approved model guidelines for the use of complementary and alternative therapies in medical practice (74). These guidelines include recommendations regarding patient evaluation, treatment planning, consultation and/or referral to CAM practitioners, medical record documentation, and training. Recommendations regarding sale of goods from a physician's office and involvement with clinical investigation are similar to those for conventional practice. For physicians who wish to integrate CAM treatments into their practices and for physicians who wish to enter into relationships with nonphysician CAM providers, review of these guidelines is essential.

As defined by NCCAM, integrative medicine represents a combination of mainstream medical therapies and CAM therapies for which there is some high-quality scientific evidence of safety and effectiveness. More than simply combining approaches, however, practicing integrative medicine requires a paradigm shift from the disease-centered approach of conventional biomedicine to one in which the healing relationship is central and the values and participation of patients become as significant in treatment planning as research evidence and clinical judgment (75). The satisfaction that patients report from relationship-centered and individualized CAM therapies serve to remind us that we can never know with certainty what therapy, alternative or otherwise, will work for an particular patient, no matter what randomized controlled clinical trials indicate.

Conclusion

From the perspective of integrative medicine, the phenomenon of widespread use of complementary and alternative modalities invites primary care physicians to listen to patients, to contribute what evidence-based medicine has to offer, to advocate for better research, and to acknowledge the existence of other types of information that may be more relevant to a given individual or for a particular clinical situation. Physicians able to respond to their patients' interest in complementary and alternative approaches to pain may discover benefits for themselves as well as for their patients:

> The integration of complementary and alternative medicine gives doctors and the health profession an opportunity to bring together the strengths and to balance the weaknesses inherent in the different systems of health care, representing a coming together of heart, head, and hand. Could this be a healing process in itself? (76)

REFERENCES

1. **Eisenberg DM, Kessler RC, Foster C, et al**. Unconventional medicine in the United States: prevalence, costs, and patterns of use. N Engl J Med. 1993;328:246-52.

2. **Eisenberg DM, Davis RB, Ettner SL, et al.** Trends in alternative medicine use in the United States, 1990-1997: results of a follow-up national survey. JAMA. 1998; 280:1569-75.

3. **Kessler RC, Davis RB, Foster DF, et al.** Long-term trends in the use of complementary and alternative medical therapies in the United States. Ann Intern Med. 2001;135:262-8.

4. **Ernst E.** Prevalence of use of complementary/alternative medicine: a systematic review. Bull World Health Org. 2000;78:252-7.

5. **Drivdahl CE, Miser WF.** The use of alternative health care by a family practice population. J Am Board Fam Pract. 1998;11:193-9.

6. **National Center for Complementary and Alternative Medicine.** Major Domains of Complementary and Alternative Medicine. Available at http://nccam.nih.gov/fcp/classify/index.html.

7. **Kaptchuk T, Eisenberg DM.** Varieties of healing. 2. A taxonomy of unconventional healing practices. Ann Intern Med. 2001;135:196-204.

8. **Kaptchuk T, Eisenberg DM.** Varieties of healing. 1. Medical pluralism in the United States. Ann Intern Med. 2001;135:189-95.

9. **Elder NC, Gilchrist A, Mintz R.** Use of alternative health care by family practice patients. Arch Fam Med. 1997;6:181-4.

10. **Del Mundo WFB, Shepherd WC, Marose TD.** Use of alternative medicine by patients in a rural family practice clinic. Fam Med. 2002;34:206-12.

11. **Palinkas LA, Kabongo ML, and the SURF*NET Study Group.** The use of complementary and alternative medicine by primary care patients. J Fam Pract. 2000;49:1121-30.

12. **Ramos-Remus C, Gutierrez S, Davis P.** Epidemiology of complementary and alternative practices in rheumatology. Rheum Dis Clin North Am. 1999;25:789-804.

13. **Cassileth BR.** Complementary and alternative cancer medicine. J Clin Onocl. 1999;17:44-52.

14. **Morris KT, Johnson N, Horner L, Walts D.** A comparison of complementary therapy use between breast cancer patients and patients with other primary tumor sites. Am J Surg. 2000;179:407-11.

15. **Wolsko PM, Eisenberg DM, Davis RB, et al.** Insurance coverage, medical conditions, and visits to alternative medicine providers. Arch Intern Med. 2002;162: 281-7.

16. **MacLennan AH, Wilson DH, Taylor AW.** Prevalence and cost of alternative medicine in Australia. Lancet. 1996;347:569-73.

17. World Health Organization, Traditional and alternative medicine: facts and figures. June 2002. Available at www.who.int/medicines/organization/trm/orgtrmmain.html.

18. **Druss BG, Rosenheck RA.** Association between use of unconventional therapies and conventional medical services. JAMA.1999;282:651-6.

19. **Astin JA.** Why patients use alternative medicine: results of a national study. JAMA. 1998;279:1548-53.

20. **Kelner M, Wellman B.** Health care and consumer choice: medical and alternative therapies. Soc Sci Med. 1997;45:203-12.

21. **Eisenberg DM, Kessler RC, Van Rompay MI, et al.** Perceptions about complementary therapies relative to conventional therapies among adults who use both: results from a national survey. Ann Intern Med. 2001;135:344-51.

22. **Katz JN.** Patient preferences and health disparities. JAMA. 2001;286:1506-9.

23. **Ernst E, Fugh-Berman A.** Complementary and alternative medicine needs an evidence base before regulation. West J Med. 1999;171:149-50.

24. **Barrett B, Marchand L, Scheder J, et al.** Bridging the gap between conventional and alternative medicine: results of a quantitative study of patients and providers. J Fam Pract. 2000;49:234-9.

25. **Chez RA, Jonas WB, Eisenberg D.** The physician and complementary and alternative medicine. In: Jonas WB, Levin JS, eds. Essentials of Complementary and Alternative Medicine. Philadelphia: Lippincott Williams & Wilkins; 1999:31-45.

26. **Davis-Floyd R, St. John G.** From Doctor to Healer: The Transformative Journey. New Brunswick, NJ: Rutgers University Press; 1998.

27. Medical Acupuncture for Physicians, Office of Continuing Medical Education, UCLA School of Medicine, 10920 Wilshire Boulevard, Suite 1060, Los Angeles, CA 90024-6512. Web site: www.medsch.ucla.edu/cme/.

28. American Board of Medical Acupuncture, 4929 Wilshire Boulevard, Suite 428, Los Angeles, CA 90010. Web site: www.medicalacupuncture.org/cme/cme/abma.

29. American Board of Holistic Medicine, 14 Daniels Drive NE, East Wenatchee, WA 98802. Web site: www.amerboardholisticmed.org.

30. **Reyes-Gibby CC, Aday L, Cleeland C.** Impact of pain on self-rated health in community-dwelling older adults. Pain. 2002;95:75-82.

31. **Abraham JL.** A Physician's Guide to Pain and Symptom Management in Cancer Patients. Baltimore: Johns Hopkins University Press; 2000.

32. **Eisenberg DM.** Advising patients who seek alternative medical therapies. Ann Intern Med. 1997;127:61-9.

33. **Lazar JS, O'Connor BB.** Talking with patients about their use of alternative therapies. Prim Care Clin North Am. 1997;24:6699-714.

34. **Pappas S, Perlman A.** Complementary and alternative medicine: the importance of doctor-patient communication. Med Clin North Am. 2002;86:1-10.

35. **Ernst E, Cohen MH.** Informed consent in complementary and alternative medicine. Arch Intern Med. 2002;161:2288-92.

36. **Caspi O, Bell IR, Rychener D, et al.** The tower of Babel: communication and medicine. Arch Intern Med. 2000;160:3193-4.

37. **Winslow LC, Shapiro H.** Physicians want education about complementary and alternative medicine to enhance communication with their patients. Arch Intern Med. 2002;162:1176-81.

38. **Berman B.** Complementary medicine and medical education. BMJ. 2001;322:121-2.

39. **Tonelli MR, Callahan TC.** Why alternative medicine cannot be evidence-based. Acad Med. 2001;76:1213-20.

40. **Bloom BS.** What is this nonsense that complementary and alternative medicine is not amenable to controlled evaluation of population effects? Acad Med. 2001;76:1221-3.

41. **Kaptchuk TJ, Eisenberg DM.** The persuasive appeal of alternative medicine. Ann Intern Med. 1998;129:1061-5.

42. **Sackett DL, Straus SE, Richardson WS, et al.** Evidence-Based Medicine: How to Practice and Teach EBM, 2nd ed. Edinburgh: Churchill-Livingstone; 2000.

43. **Lewith G, Jonas WB, Walach H.** Clinical Research in Complementary Therapies: Principles, Problems, and Solutions. Edinburgh: Churchill Livingstone; 2002.

44. **Jonas WB.** The evidence house: how to build an inclusive base for complementary medicine. West J Med. 2002;175:79-80.

45. **Sherman KJ, Cherkin DC, Hogeboom CJ.** The diagnosis and treatment of patients with chronic low-back pain by traditional Chinese medical acupuncturists. J Altern Complement Med. 2001;7:641-50.

46. **Vincent C.** The safety of acupuncture. BMJ. 2001;323:467-8.

47. **Tulder MW van, Cherkin DC, Berman B, et al.** Acupuncture for low back pain (Cochrane Review). In: The Cochrane Library, Issue 3, 2002. Oxford: Update Software.

48. **White AR.** Acupuncture research methodology. In: Lewith G, Jonas WB, Walach H, eds. Clinical Research in Complementary Therapies: Principles, Problems, and Solutions. Edinburgh: Churchill Livingstone; 2002:307-23.

49. **Ernst E, White AR.** Acupuncture for back pain: a meta-analysis of randomized controlled trials. Arch Intern Med. 1998;158:2235-40.

50. **Carlsson CP, Sjoulund BH.** Acupuncture for chronic low back pain: a randomized placebo-controlled study with long-term follow-up. Clin J Pain. 2002;17:296-305.

51. **Ceccherelli F, Rigoni MT, Gagliardi G, Ruzzante L.** Comparison of superficial and deep acupuncture in the treatment of lumbar myofascial pain: a double-blind randomized controlled study. Clin J Pain. 2002;18:149-53.

52. **Leibing E, Leonhardt U, Koster G, et al.** Acupuncture treatment of chronic low back pain: a randomized, blinded, placebo-controlled trial with 9-month follow-up. Pain. 2002;96:189-96.

53. **MacPherson H, White A, Cummings M, et al.** Standards from reporting interventions in controlled trials of acupuncture. ACP Med. 2002;20:22-5.

54. **Cherkin DC, Eisenberg DM, Sherman KJ, et al.** Randomized trial comparing traditional Chinese medical acupuncture, therapeutic massage, and self-care education for chronic low back pain. Arch Intern Med. 2001;161:1081-8.

55. **Kalauokalni D, Cherkin DC, Sherman KJ, et al.** Lessons from a trial of acupuncture and massage for low back pain: patient expectations and treatment effects. Spine. 2001;26:1418-24.

56. **Stux G, Hammerschlag R, eds.** Clinical Acupuncture: Scientific Basis. Berlin: Springer; 2001.

57. **Favreau JT, Ryu ML, Braunstein G, et al.** Severe hepatotoxicty associated with the dietary supplement LipoKinetix. Ann Intern Med. 2002;136:590-5.

58. **Hardy ML.** Herb-drug interactions: an evidence-based table. Altern Med Alert. 2000;64-9.

59. **McAlindon TE, LaValley MP, Gulin JP, Felson DT.** Glucosamine and chondroitin for treatment of osteoarthritis: a systematic quality assessment and meta-analysis. JAMA. 2000;283:1469-75.

60. NIH-GAIT (Glucosamine-Chondriotin Arthritis Intervention Trial). Web site: www.nihgait.org/.

61. **Hadhazy VA, Ezzo J, Creamer P, Berman BM.** Mind-body therapies for the treatment of fibromyalgia: a systematic review. J Rheumatol. 2000;27:2911-8.

62. **Meeker WC, Haldeman S.** Chiropractic: a profession at the crossroads of mainstream and alternative medicine. Ann Intern Med. 2002;136:216-27.

63. **Hsieh CY, Adams AH, Tobis J, et al.** Effectiveness of four conservative treatments for subacute low back pain: a randomized clinical trial. Spine. 2002;27:1142-8.

64. **Stevinson C, Ernst E.** Risks associated with spinal manipulation. Am J Med. 2002;112:566-71.

65. **Field T.** Massage therapy. Med Clin North Am. 2002;86:163-71.

66. **Furlan AD, Brosseau L, Imamura M, Irvin E.** Massage for low back pain. (Cochrane Review). In: The Cochrane Library, Issue 3, 2002. Oxford: Update Software.

67. Acupuncture. NIH Consensus Statement. 1997 November 3-5;15:1-34.

68. **Melchart D, Linde K, Fischer P, et al.** Acupuncture for idiopathic headache (Cochrane Review). In: The Cochrane Library, issue 3, 2002. Oxford: Update Software.

69. **Berman B.** Is acupuncture effective in the treatment of fibromyalgia? J Fam Pract. 1999;48:213-8.

70. **Ezzo J, Berman B, Hadhazy VA, et al.** Is acupuncture effective for the treatment of chronic pain? A systematic review. Pain. 3000;86:217-25.

71. **Spiro H.** The Power of Hope: A Doctor's Perspective. New Haven, CT: Yale University Press; 1998:139.

72. **Cohen MH, Eisenberg DM.** Potential physician malpractice liability associated with complementary and integrative medical therapies. Ann Intern Med. 2002;136:596-603.

73. **Astin JA, Marie A, Pelletier KR, et al.** A review of the incorporation of complementary and alternative medicine by mainstream physicians. Arch Intern Med. 1998;158:2303-10.

74. **Federation of State Medical Boards of the United States.** New model guidelines for the use of complementary and alternative therapies in medical practice, adopted April 2002. Altern Ther. 2002;8:44-7.

75. **Maizes V, Caspi O.** The principles and challenges of integrative medicine: more than a combination of traditional and alternative therapies. West J Med. 1999;171:148-9.

76. **Owen DK, Lewith G, Stephens CR.** Can doctors respond to patients' increasing interest in complementary and alternative medicine? BMJ. 2001;322:154-7.

9

▪ ▪ ▪

Motivating Behavior Change in Patients with Chronic Pain

Antoine B. Douaihy, MD

Mark P. Jensen, PhD

Roger J. Jou, MD

Primary care is the port of entry for most patients seeking medical attention for chronic pain conditions. It is a setting that provides easy access to the many pain interventions, and primary care physicians (PCPs) are in the best position to provide the bulk of chronic pain care.

However, management of chronic pain can pose significant challenges in primary care settings. For example, patients with chronic pain are sometimes perceived by physicians as difficult and poorly motivated individuals who "don't want to change". PCPs have been criticized for their use of pain medications (sometimes for providing too many, sometimes for providing too few medications) and for failure to enhance patient self-care by implicitly (or explicitly) promising a medical cure for chronic pain. Other challenges faced by PCPs include difficulties engaging patients in treatment and poor patient adherence to treatment recommendations.

A major difficulty with chronic pain management in any medical care setting is that it depends more on what the patients do than on what the physician does to them. The patient's readiness to accept and adopt a self-management approach is therefore a key issue in the primary care consultation. For this reason, a central task for the PCP is to understand and build motivation in patients for pain self-management.

The good news for the PCP is that there are interventions that he or she can implement to enhance patient motivation. Moreover, although motivational strategies and interventions may require some study and practice before they are effectively incorporated into patient consultations, they do not necessarily require that physicians take more time with patients. If anything, these approaches can actually save time by reducing patient resistance to the idea of pain self-management.

This chapter describes a general ("patient-centered") approach that can be used to help motivate patients with chronic pain to take more responsibility for pain management. The approach goes far beyond traditional advice-giving but is a framework rather than an absolute methodology for enhancing motivation. Because clinicians and patients are infinitely diverse, the skills and strategies recommended are designed for adaptation and refinement.

What is Patient-Centered Medicine?

A patient-centered approach has been conceptualized in many fields of health care, including medicine. It emphasizes the importance of considering the patient's perspective when giving recommendations and making decisions about treatment and behavioral change.

Stewart and colleagues have formulated a patient-centered approach which focuses on the importance of understanding the patient as a whole in the context of disease and illness (1). Their formulation considers the patient's ideas and feelings about illness and their expectations from the physician. Each contact between patient and physician is an opportunity for health promotion and for developing a therapeutic relationship. Assessing patient goals and goal-setting are also important. There is significant evidence showing the effectiveness of this approach (1,2).

The goals of a patient-centered approach are

1. To assess and address patient's worries and concerns
2. To enhance a collaborative relationship
3. To provide information that patients are interested in (i.e., ready to hear)
4. To change the focus of the visit from treatment recommendation to supporting and enhancing patient self-care practices
5. To foster greater patient control of decision-making and responsibility for self-care.

The Role of the Patient

Recognizing that it is the patient who has the primary responsibility for carrying out pain management requires reorientation to the patient-physician relationship. Patients must be viewed as autonomous and equal members of the health care team whose expertise (knowledge of self) is central to the management of pain. Because the locus of control and decision-making concerning pain management is in the patient, the physician's role should ideally be that of advisor and coach, rather than a person "in charge" of patient care.

Giving Advice and Reflective Listening

Although a patient-centered approach may be more successful than directed advice alone, advice-giving remains an important part of many aspects of health care consultations. If advice is provided with compassion and clarity, it can also be effective. In fact, there is evidence that simple advice can promote behavior change in the fields of smoking and excessive drinking (3). When provided without sensitivity or knowledge of patient concerns, however, advice can disrupt the process of behavior change. By its very definition, advice consists of telling others what you think they should do and how they should do it. Very frequently, this undermines patient autonomy and limits options and choices, while potentially damaging the therapeutic relationship.

One of the main determinants of whether advice is taken or rejected is the manner in which the advice is given. Here is a typical exchange between doctor and patient:

PCP. You need to lose weight; otherwise your back pain will get worse. You need to exercise daily.

Patient. I'm not sure if I have enough spare time for exercise.

PCP. Well, you should find the time. I can't help you unless you help yourself.

Patient. Yes, but I'm concerned that exercise will make the pain worse. I wonder if there are any other ways to decrease the pain.

PCP. Exercise is the best thing you can do. You should start exercising at least twice a week, and then we can discuss other options.

Patient. I know I should do that, but . . . .

Reflective listening is a therapeutic technique which involves making statements that indicate you understand what the patient is saying (4). The goals of reflective listening include demonstrating empathy, affirming the patient's thoughts and feelings, and helping the process of information exchange. There are several types of reflective statements:

- Repeating what the patient has said
- Rephrasing or paraphrasing what the patient has said
- Continuing the patient's thoughts (e.g., saying the next sentence that you anticipate the patient might say rather than repeating the last one)
- Reflection of feelings

The following dialogue illustrates some reflective statements:

PCP. You might consider some ideas to help you reduce your pain. Maybe you could think about taking more exercise.

Patient. I'm not sure if I have enough spare time for exercise.

PCP. So you find exercise hard to fit it into your schedule [reflective statement].

Patient. Right. If I could find a way to make exercise a priority, I would.

PCP. You are interested in exercise, but you have a lot of other responsibilities as well. You'd exercise much more than you do now if you could find the time [reflective statement].

What makes reflective listening work is not any one technique or strategy, but rather the spirit of the collaborative discussion about self-care behavior change. This in turn encourages the patient to be an active participant in decisions concerning his or her pain management.

Basis of a Motivational Approach: Patient Readiness

The trans-theoretical model of behavior change and its potential relevance to chronic pain management has recently been receiving more attention (5). The Pain Stages of Change Questionnaire proposes that individuals experiencing chronic pain vary in their readiness to adopt a self-management approach (6). According to this model, people who strongly believe that their pain problem is purely a biological problem that requires only medical intervention are not ready or willing to accept a self-management approach. Others, believing that medical interventions can provide only limited assistance, are more likely to perceive self-management skills as potentially helpful. Still other patients may be actively engaged in developing self-management strategies for coping with chronic pain. Therefore readiness to change varies among individuals and over time.

Readiness to self-manage pain is not an either-or phenomenon and should be assessed along a continuum across each different self-management strategy. For example, a patient may be very willing to engage in regular exercise but not yet ready to manage the negative impact of chronic pain on relationships. The Stages-of-Change model (Figure 9-1 and Table 9-1) provides a natural fit within the context of the patient-centered framework that we have suggested (5). To optimize the outcome of a consultation, interventions should be tailored to the individual patient's readiness to change (see below).

The patient's understanding of the importance of behavior change and his or her self-confidence contribute to this state of readiness. Understanding the importance of change entails exploring "Why I should change" and the pros and cons of change. Self-confidence is a reflection of self-efficacy, which determines whether behavior change will be initiated, how much effort will be expended, and for how long effort will be maintained in the face of obstacles and adverse experiences.

Motivation-Enhancement Strategies

There are a number of specific strategies that the PCP can use to build and enhance patient motivation for pain self-management. These are discussed

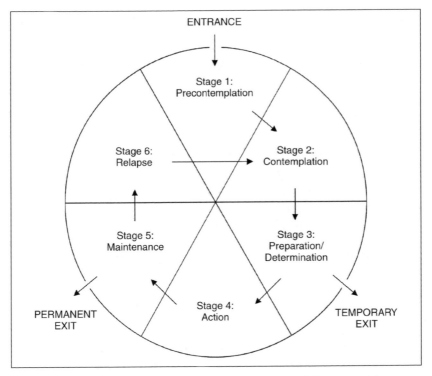

Figure 9-1   Prochaska-DiClemente-Norcross Stages-of-Change model.

Table 9-1   Description of Prochaska-DiClemente-Norcross Stages-of-Change Model

Stage	Description
(1) Precontemplation	The person is not yet considering changing a target behavior.
(2) Contemplation	The person is considering changing the behavior.
(3) Preparation/Determination	The person is making plans to change the behavior.
(4) Action	The person has begun to change the behavior.
(5) Maintenance and relapse prevention	The person works toward preventing relapse (Stage 6) and maintaining those changes made in the Action stage (#4).

in detail elsewhere (7-9). Almost all of these strategies involve first eliciting from the patient reasons for pain self-management and then reflecting back those statements that self-management is possible ("motivational statements" or "change talk").

To elicit motivational statements from the patient, the clinician must first learn to listen more and speak less. Although the prospect of allowing or even encouraging patients to speak more may seem daunting to some clinicians, the fact is that when patients are encouraged to speak in a focused way about a specific problem, the consultation time is usually more efficient. (There are fewer arguments and "Yes, but . . ." statements from patients in response to advice.) A treatment plan that the patient endorses can be negotiated much more quickly. In this way, patient-centered interactions can actually save time in the office.

Before the Consultation: Identifying Self-Management Goals

Most PCPs agree on the important general health care goals: Patients should be encouraged to stop smoking, maintain adequately low blood pressure, and control blood sugar appropriately. However, the important goals for pain self-management are not as readily agreed upon. In general, pain specialists would likely agree that the following pain self-management goals are of importance:

1. Begin or maintain a regular exercise program
2. Use medications as prescribed (some pain specialists argue that it is best if patients with chronic pain use no or minimal amounts of opioid or sedative medications, whereas others believe that these medications are appropriate for some patients)
3. Return to or maintain normal daily activities
4. Practice appropriate pain and stress coping strategies (e.g., relaxation, reassuring self-talk, identifying and eliminating negative or "catastrophizing" cognitions)
5. Return to or sustain normal work activities
6. Pace activities appropriately
7. Monitor and manage symptoms of depression and anxiety as appropriate
8. Practice appropriate eating habits (e.g., to reduce or maintain weight if needed)
9. Engage in other healthy lifestyle behaviors as needed and appropriate (e.g., reduce alcohol use or stop drinking, quit smoking)

Keeping these pain self-management goals in mind, the PCP is in a position to begin to motivate the patient.

Establishing Rapport and Setting the Agenda

A patient-centered approach assumes that little progress can be made until there is adequate rapport between the patient and physician and an agenda has been selected for pain self-management on which both agree. Often, establishing rapport and setting an agenda can be accomplished at the same time and in short order. A good way to accomplish both is to elicit from the patient his or her greatest concerns early in the session or encounter, then to select one of more of these concerns as the agenda for the session. More often then not, the patient's concerns will relate to one or more of the pain self-management goals given above.

Asking Open-Ended Questions

One simple way to get started is to ask a general, open-ended question about the patient's concerns. Open-ended questions are questions that cannot easily be answered with one or just a few words. For example, for a first encounter with a patient:

> I understand you have had chronic pain now for over 10 years. I have had a chance to review the medical records, and at some point we will need to go over some medical questions that I have concerning your pain problem. But before we do that, I want to understand your primary concerns. What concerns you most about your pain problem? How would you like to see us work together to address these concerns?

Setting the Agenda

Usually, unless the patient's response to the initial open-ended question requires additional follow-up, this response can be used to develop an agenda for pain self-management. This is a critical point in the encounter, and one that requires a great deal of physician sensitivity and judgment. Perhaps the patient raises a single issue that he or she feels needs to be addressed immediately ("I am here because I am in pain and I cannot get any doctor to believe me! I need surgery to fix my back!"). Perhaps the patient expresses multiple issues and concerns that will require some sorting out before a specific agenda can be selected ("I do not know where to begin. I can't work because of the pain. All I can do is lie down all day. I am angry a lot. My life is a mess!").

Depending on the amount of time allowed for the encounter, the physician may have the luxury of exploring the patient's concerns in depth, using further open-ended questions and "reflections" of patients responses (see above), and helping the patient select a primary issue to focus on. However, many PCPs have only between 5 and 10 minutes allotted for each encounter. In this case, the physician may select a single concern or issue to focus on (but be ready to switch gears if the patient shows little interest) or provide the patient with a few issues to discuss and let the patient choose the important one. Either approach fits well within the patient-centered model, since ultimately the physician is asking for patient endorsement of the agenda item.

> Although there are other issues important to back pain management that we can, and at some point should, discuss, it seems as if you really want us to

focus on getting an answer about whether back surgery can help your pain. Is that correct?

or

Although every person is unique, you've raised a lot of issues that I've often discussed with patients with chronic pain. You are not able to work because of pain, and you are now extremely inactive, often because it hurts just to move. The pain is affecting you emotionally. I would not be surprised if there are people who are very worried about you because of the pain problem. I think there are some changes that can be made so that you can do more and hurt less. These may include increasing your strength and flexibility, making changes in your pain medications, and pacing your activities. You may need treatments to improve your mood. I do not think we should or can make changes in everything all at once. We only have about 10 minutes now, but that's enough time to start to develop a plan. Let's focus on an appropriate exercise program. What do you think?

Both of these approaches suggest an agenda but importantly ask the patient for permission to proceed with that agenda. Assuming that care of the patient's pain problem will occur over the course of many weeks, months, and perhaps years, it is not necessary to select any one agenda over the others. In fact, unless there is an immediate medical need to address a specific agenda (e.g., the patient's presentation suggests the possibility of a life-threatening illness that must be ruled out), from the patient-centered perspective it is more important that the patient endorse the agenda for the encounter than that any one agenda be selected over others.

Helping Patients Understand the Importance of Change

People change behaviors only when they believe that it is important to do so and when they believe that they are capable of doing so. People with significant pain will therefore only exercise regularly if they view exercise as being more beneficial than harmful. Even then, however, they must also see themselves as having the resources (time, skill, endurance) to be able to exercise regularly before they will begin an exercise program. The same concepts hold true for any pain self-management behavior: understanding the importance of behavior change and then having confidence that this change is possible form the foundation of motivation.

Rating Self-Management Strategies

One way of assessing this foundation is to use "importance" and "confidence" scales (9). The physician first asks the patient to rate the importance of using a pain self-management strategy, then asks the patient to rate his or her confidence that he or she can engage in this strategy, both on a scale of 0 to 10.

Let us consider the case of the patient who is asked his or her views on exercise. High ratings (7-10) on both scales would obviously suggest high motivation. Low ratings (0-3) on the importance of exercise, but high ratings on the belief that it could be done if necessary, would indicate that work is needed to increase the patient's views of the importance of (or confidence in) exercise before any adherence to an exercise program can reasonably be expected. On the other hand, for those patients who rate the importance of change to be high but for whom the confidence rating is low, brainstorming for solutions may prove helpful (see below).

Low ratings on both scales would indicate minimal motivation for exercise and that any efforts to develop an exercise program would be premature (and probably doomed to failure until and unless motivation can be enhanced). In this case, it may be best to encourage consideration of other self-management strategies that patients may believe are more important to them and then go back to approach the topic when they have greater confidence in their abilities. It is with patients who describe "moderate" levels (4-6) of importance and confidence that clinicians have the greatest opportunity to increase motivation in the short run.

Enhancing Communications

Often, as an initial strategy to increase patient motivation, the temptation for clinicians is to lecture patients, to "sell" patients on the importance of the self-management strategy, and perhaps to reassure patients that they are able to learn to use the strategy. A major drawback to lecturing patients is that information and advice presented in this way often leads patients to give "Yes, but . . ." responses. In this situation, precious consultation time is wasted and patients end up verbalizing the reasons against trying a new approach. Social-psychological research tells us that people are much more likely to believe what they themselves say over what is said to them. Hence this approach may *decrease* patient motivation for pain self-management. If the physician finds that the patient is arguing against pain self-management, it is almost certain that the physician has been arguing for self-management. In such a situation, the physician should stop lecturing or "pushing" so hard for change, regroup, and ask an open-ended question that will elicit from the patient reasons for change.

Four simple strategies are given below that help patients understand the importance of change and increase their confidence to make that change (8). These strategies are effective because they provide the opportunity for patients to talk themselves into using pain self-management practices. These strategies include 1) eliciting positive statements from the patient, 2) examining the pros and cons of behavior change, 3) eliciting concerns about the status quo, and 4) brainstorming for solutions.

Strategy 1: Eliciting Positive Statements from the Patient
Assuming that the patient scored at least 5 (out of 10) on the importance and confidence scales, the clinician can ask two questions that will almost

always elicit positive reasons for change: "Why so high?" and "How can you go higher?" The physician can then encourage continued discussion of the importance of behavior change and confidence by "reflecting" patients' responses back to them. An example of the "Why so high?" question concerning importance is

> *PCP.* How important do you think it is that you exercise regularly as one way to deal with your pain and its effects on your life? Put it on a scale of 0 to 10, where 0 means 'Not important' and 10 means 'Very, very important'.
>
> *Patient.* About a 5.
>
> *PCP.* So it is of medium importance. Why did you give it a 5 instead of a 1?
>
> *Patient.* Well, everyone knows that exercise is good for you.
>
> *PCP.* You see exercise as helping you with your pain problem.
>
> *Patient.* I used to love exercising. I was a marathon runner. But now it hurts anytime I try to run.
>
> *PCP.* You used to be a very good runner, and you seem to miss being able to exercise every day. So you'd like to be able to exercise again but in a way that did not hurt so much.

In this dialogue, the "Why so high?" question elicited statements that reflect the importance of exercise for the patient. The clinician effectively used reflective listening to elicit further statements and to reflect the reasons that the patient wants to exercise back to the patient. Below is an example of an interaction in which the physician uses a "How can you go higher?" question to increase patient confidence in exercise:

> *PCP.* How confident are you about exercising regularly as one way to deal with your pain and its effects on your life? Put it on a scale of 0 to 10, where 0 means 'Not confident' and 10 means 'Very, very confident'.
>
> *Patient.* About a 6.
>
> *PCP.* So you seem to be somewhat confident that you can do this. What would it take for this 6 to become an 8, a 9, or even a 10?
>
> *Patient.* Well, I used to exercise 5 days a week. That was before I was injured. I know a lot of exercises, and I have a lifetime membership in a gym. What really stops me now is the pain. I think I could work through the pain if I knew that I was not injuring myself. But I don't want to make things worse.
>
> *PCP.* So if you were confident that you were not damaging yourself with exercise, you feel you could do it nearly every day, even if it hurt sometimes.
>
> *Patient.* Yes, I am not as much afraid of the pain as I am of hurting myself.
>
> *PCP.* What if I told you that I think it *is* possible for you to exercise in a safe way? A way to make you stronger and able to do more and that would improve your back pain in the long run even if it might be more uncomfortable in the short run?

The idea here is to ask specific questions, and then use reflective listening, to get the patient talking about the importance of pain self-management and gaining confidence that self-management of pain is possible, thereby increasing both. Once importance and confidence are raised, the physician can then propose a specific plan (e.g., for exercise or for learning a specific pain self-management skill) or, better yet, provide the patient with a menu of potential plans that the patient can select and follow through on.

Strategy 2: Examining the Pros and Cons of Behavior Change

More likely than not, the patient will feel ambivalent about each of the self-management strategies. It is the rare person who does not feel ambivalent about engaging in healthy behavior regularly; even people who do not have the added burden of a chronic pain problem may feel that regular exercise takes up too much time or that rich food tastes too good to give up. Asking follow-up questions to the importance and confidence scales, as described above, is one way to elicit positive comments about change. However, these questions do not directly address the problem of ambivalence; even "motivated" patients very likely feel two ways about each self-management strategy.

Again, when faced with a patient who is ambivalent about some aspect of pain self-management, the temptation is to start arguing for change, to perhaps make the patient feel frightened or guilty by reviewing all the negative consequences of the status quo ("Your pain has gotten worse despite your remaining inactive and taking more pain-killers. I see no reason that it will not continue to get worse if you stay on this path.") However, pushing hard for a decision to self-manage pain will almost always result in patients arguing against change, and patients tend to be more convinced by their own arguments than by yours.

For this reason, a more effective strategy, at least for encouraging motivation, is to ask questions and make comments that allow the patient to consider the pros and cons of change in a judgment-free environment, which is an environment where the physician is not pushing for one decision over the other. If the patient is allowed to carefully think through the pros and cons of pain self-management, he or she will most likely come to the conclusion themselves that pain self-management is the best way for them to address their pain problem. This strategy can be particularly useful with patients who rate importance or confidence as being relatively weak.

With this strategy, the physician is not necessarily expecting to see a quick change in motivation (although this is certainly possible) in a single consultation. Rather, the goal is to help the patient think about the possibility of change and the reasons that pain self-management may be worthwhile and possible. The role of the physician in this process is easy to describe, but it can be difficult to do. The physician mostly provides the structure, listens carefully (without judgment or pushing for one decision over the other), and then provides a summary at the end of the consultation.

Two simple questions can be used to initiate a pros and cons discussion. First, the physician can ask about the benefits of the self-management behavior (e.g., "What would be the benefits of regular exercise for you?"). The patient's response to this question should be followed by a brief discussion of each benefit raised by the patient, and then a summary of all the benefits raised by the patient if appropriate. After this question, patients should then be asked to describe the cons of the self-management behavior (e.g., "What are the less good things about regular exercise?"), again followed by a brief discussion of each "less good" thing and a summary. The clinician can then end this interaction with a brief summary of the pros and cons of the self-management strategy raised by the patient, without suggesting necessarily that the patient do anything about the self-management strategy at this time. Of course, if it is clear that the pros outweigh the cons, it would be appropriate for the physician to gently encourage consideration of behavior change by asking a "Where does this leave you now?" question. Any statements indicating intent to change at this point could then be quickly summarized and followed by appropriate encouragement and support of action towards pain self-management.

Strategy 3: Eliciting Concerns about the Status Quo

As indicated earlier in this chapter, for patients who rate the importance of pain self-management as being particularly low and who are not at all concerned about how they are choosing to manage their pain, efforts to instill concern about what the consequences will be if change is not made can backfire and "push" patients into being even more resistant to the idea of pain self-management. Merely raising the question about pain self-management may be enough for these patients to consider such an approach sometime in the future when (and if) other more medically focused (e.g., interventional approaches) have proven to be of little help for their pain problem.

Patients who rate the importance of pain self-management as at least weak (e.g., 2-4 on the 0-10 scale) may be experiencing some preliminary concerns about their current situation. While the follow-up on the importance scale may not be appropriate in such patients ("Why did you say '2' instead of '0'?" may not elicit much in the way of positive comments), they may have enough concern about the status quo that a brief discussion could lead to more serious consideration of behavior change.

Successful use of this strategy involves three steps:

- *Step 1*—The physician asks a question that elicits concerns from the patient about the consequences of not making change. In this step, it is very important that the patient, not the physician, raise the concern(s).

- *Step 2*—Once the patient has come up with as many concerns as he or she can think of, the clinician summarizes these concerns, using the patient's words if possible. Summarizing patient concerns allows patients to hear and endorse their own reasons for making a change. Because they had already expressed these concerns, it is highly likely that they will endorse the physician's summary as their own idea. This strategy can effectively increase the patient's perception of the importance of behavior change. Sample questions for eliciting concern are "What concerns you most about your level of inactivity?" and "What concerns do you have about your level of inactivity?"

- *Step 3*—After this discussion, the physician should ask the patient "Where does that leave you now?" There should be no physician agenda; let the patient take the lead here. The patient may want to change the status quo and, for example, increase his or her tolerance for activity. In this case, the physician can explore options for doing so. However, the patient may indicate that this leaves him or her with few options, given the perceived difficulties of changing activity level. In this case, the physician *should not* demand change (e.g., "Now that you have told me your concerns, aren't you ready to do something about it?"). Such pushing could undo the benefits (for motivation) accomplished by this strategy: the development in the patient's mind of reasons for change. Raising concerns about the status quo and bringing them out in the open is sufficient. It may be enough that the patient ponders these concerns after the session so that he or she is more amenable to change at the next encounter.

It is important, in all of these strategies, to understand that the patient must set the pace. Although it can be difficult to watch a patient make decisions about pain management that contribute to suffering and greater pain, pushing patients to make adaptive decisions will only decrease the chances that such decisions will be made and acted on. The physician's responsibility is to create an environment that maximizes the chances for adaptive change; it is the patient's decision to make the change.

Strategy 4: Brainstorming for Solutions

For patients who rate the importance of change to be high, but whose motivation for action may be constrained by a relative lack of confidence, brainstorming can help them identify a means of achieving a goal that they rate as being very important. Again, it is important to avoid specifically giving advice. Rather, it is the physician's job to remind the patient that there are usually many ways to achieve self-management goals and to encourage him or her to come up with a number of possibilities.

If asked by the patient, the physician can of course mention some strategies that have worked in the past for other patients. But the physician should clearly stress that the patient probably knows what will work best for himself or herself and that any suggestions should only be considered as such; they may not necessarily work for this particular patient. Questions such as "What ways have you tried so far to [reach some self-management goal]?", "What ways have others that you know used to [reach the same or similar self-management goal]?", and "Can you think of any other ways that might work for you?" can all be asked to help the patient devise a list of potential plans for reaching his or her self-management goals.

Once a complete list has been developed, it is very likely that some options will be perceived as being more possible than others for the patient. In this way, the patient can see that his or her confidence level can vary to some degree depending not only on the final goal but on the strategy chosen to reach a goal. Once a complete list of possible options for achieving a valued goal has been developed, the next step is to let the patient decide which, if any, of the approaches he or she wishes to use: "Which option suits you best?" and "Are any of these options something that interests you at this time?" Then the physician can work with the patient to develop the plan further.

Progress Reports

There are several approaches to motivating the patient to talk about his or her progress:

- "At our last visit, we spent some time talking about changes you were thinking about making in your exercise regimen. How has this been going?"

- "The last time we met you were thinking about increasing the number of times you practiced relaxation every week. I would be interested in hearing how this went and the changes, if any, you have noticed in your ability to manage your pain."

- "We spent a lot of time at our last meeting talking about activity pacing. At that time, you came up with a plan for pacing your activities in a way that allowed you to get more done. How did that go?"

These, and similar types of open-ended questions, communicate an interest in the patient's perspective on his or her problem. Not only does this allow for an informal assessment of the patient's readiness, but open-ended questions such as these are an excellent way to build rapport with patients.

Open-ended questions can be contrasted to closed-ended questions. The latter elicit very brief responses (often either "yes" or "no"), limit rapport, and provide little information about the patient's readiness to engage in self-management practices. Examples of closed-ended questions are "Did you take the medications as I prescribed them?", "Are you exercising every day like we talked about at our last appointment?", and "How often did you practice your relaxation strategies this week?"

Conclusion

In patient-centered care, the patient with chronic pain assumes primary responsibility for the management of his or her pain problem, while the physician serves as an advisor and a collaborator in care. As such, the physician can help the patient by motivating him or her to engage in self-care. Patients are motivated when they 1) understand the importance of self-care and 2) when they believe that they are capable (i.e., have confidence) of performing self-care. Furthermore, patients are more likely to be motivated when they arrive at decisions on their own than when they are given advice by the physician. Strategies that PCPs can use to increase this understanding and self-confidence therefore focus on empowering the patient to address his or her concerns, consider the pros and cons of changing self-care behaviors, and create the pain management agenda.

Although the effectiveness of these strategies among patients with chronic pain have not been tested empirically, wide-range support for their use and effectiveness is promising (8). Moreover, there is a considerable shift towards incorporating motivational strategies in the multidisciplinary pain treatment practice. The strategies we have suggested should be considered guidelines that can help PCPs switch from the more prescriptive, expert-driven, practitioner-centered techniques traditionally used to the spirit of negotiation in structuring the conversation with the patient about behavior change.

REFERENCES

1. **Stewart MA, McWhinney IR, Weston WW, et al.** Patient-Centered Medicine: Transforming the Clinical Method. Thousand Oaks, CA: Sage Publications; 1995.
2. **Kaplan SH, Greenfield S, Ware JE.** Assessing the effects of physician-patient interactions on the outcomes of chronic disease. Med Care. 1989;27:S110-27.
3. **Ashenden R, Silagy C, Weller D.** A systematic review of the effectiveness of promoting lifestyle change in general practice. Fam Pract. 1997;14:160-76.
4. **Miller WR, Rollnick S.** Motivational Interviewing: Preparing People to Change Addictive Behavior. New York: Guilford Press; 1991.
5. **Prochaska JO, DiClemente CC, Norcross JC.** In search of how people change: applications to addictive behaviors. Am Psychol. 1992;47:1102-14.
6. **Kerns RD, Rosenberg R, Jamison RN, et al.** Readiness to adopt a self-management approach to chronic pain: the Pain Stages of Change Questionnaire (PSOCQ). Pain. 1997;72:227-34.
7. **Miller WR, Rollnick S.** Motivational Interviewing: Preparing People for Change. New York: Guilford Press; 2002.
8. **Rollnick S, Mason P, Butler C.** Health Behavior Change: A Guide for Practitioners. Edinburgh: Harcourt Publishers; 1999.
9. **Jensen MP.** Enhancing motivation to change in pain treatment. In: Turk DC, Gatchel RJ, eds. Psychological Approaches to Pain Management: A Practitioner's Handbook, 2nd ed. New York: Guilford Press; 2002:71-93.

10

■　■　■

Disability Management
in Primary Care

James P. Robinson, MD, PhD

P hysicians often have to manage disability for patients whom they are treating for chronic pain. Many physicians find disability manage- ment at least distasteful and often stressful. But society gives physi- cians little choice in the matter. If you are treating a patient who is applying for disability or is receiving disability benefits, you will almost certainly be contacted by the agency that administers the disability program. You will be asked questions about your patient's medical condition and the extent to which he or she is disabled by it. If you do not respond to the questions, the disability agency will typically reject your patient's claim or terminate his or her benefits.

The purpose of this chapter is to describe strategies that will help you manage disability in patients who have sustained work injuries and are re- ceiving benefits through a workers' compensation system. The chapter as- sumes that a patient who has been under your care for general health presents with recent onset of a work-related disabling low back injury. The focus is on four areas:

1. Evaluating the risk of long-term disability
2. Establishing a treatment contract with a patient who has had a disabling injury
3. Intervening in ways that reduce the likelihood of long-term disability
4. Interfacing with agencies that administer disability benefits

Unfortunately, there is no step-by-step "cookbook" for evaluating and managing disability. The question "How do you manage disability in a patient with chronic pain?" is just as complex as the question "How do you provide medical or surgical care for a patient with chronic pain?" In both instances general principles can be described, but the application of these principles to specific patients requires a good deal of clinical judgment.

Basic Issues

When people are unable to perform tasks because of a medical condition, they often seek disability benefits from various agencies. Disability can take many forms, and the benefits dispensed by disability agencies vary accordingly. For example, a person who is unable to perform self-care activities (e.g., a quadriplegic) might apply for financial support to hire an attendant, a person with limited walking tolerance might apply for a disabled parking sticker, etc. Individuals who are work disabled (i.e., unable to work because of a medical condition) may apply for wage replacement (also called time-loss) benefits so that they can maintain a reasonable standard of living even though they are not earning wages. Many receive these benefits through the workers' compensation (WC) system.

Workers' compensation systems provide medical benefits, time loss payments, and vocational rehabilitation for individuals who develop injuries or illnesses that arise "out of and in the course of employment". Each of the 50 states administers its own WC program, and there are also federally administered programs (1). There is considerable variation in WC law from one jurisdiction to another (2), but several common threads exist:

1. WC programs are no-fault. *The injured worker forgoes the right to sue his or her employer. In return, the employer assumes financial liability for medical costs and lost wages incurred by a worker as a result of an industrial injury or illness.*

2. WC programs provide benefits only for work-related conditions. *Thus, when a worker reports symptoms, a judgment must be made not only about the nature of the underlying medical problem but about causation (i.e., whether or not the problem arose "out of and in the course of employment") (1).*

3. WC programs distinguish between industrial injuries, in which there is a clear precipitant for a medical condition, and occupational illnesses, in which a medical condition arises from activities or exposures over extended time periods.

4. WC programs assume responsibility not only for medical care of an injured worker but for his or her inability to work. *Thus they provide time-loss payments for workers who are temporarily incapacitated because of injury and, sometimes, vocational services after the workers have reached maximal medical improvement.*

*They also provide pensions for workers who remain incapaci-
tated after maximal improvement has been achieved.*

Informal observation suggests that WC programs embody two important assumptions:*

The first, fundamental, assumption made by WC agencies is that impairment and disability should be "transparent" to an experienced physician; that is, activity limitations as described or demonstrated by patients
should be highly correlated with evidence of tissue damage or organ dysfunction that can be objectively assessed by a physician. This assumption
underlies the routine demand that claims managers make for physicians to
base their conclusions about activity limitations of patients on "objective
findings".

The assumption that impairment and disability can be objectively assessed is so pervasive that most physicians—and essentially all disability
adjudicators—accept it without question. The assumption indeed works
well for certain medical conditions, especially those associated with severe
biological insult and complete loss of function of an organ or body part.
For example, physicians have tools to quantify impairment stemming from
amputations or complete spinal cord injuries. However, in many medical
conditions, including most chronic pain syndromes, physicians cannot objectively identify impairments that rationalize the activity limitations that patients report. In a monograph on the disability programs administered by
the Social Security Administration, Osterweis et al. summarized the problem as follows:

> The notion that all impairments should be verifiable by objective evidence is
> administratively necessary for an entitlement program. Yet this notion is fun-
> damentally at odds with a realistic understanding of how disease and injury
> operate to incapacitate people. Except for a very few conditions, such as the
> loss of a limb, blindness, deafness, paralysis, or coma, most diseases and in-
> juries do not prevent people from working by mechanical failure. Rather,
> people are incapacitated by a variety of unbearable sensations when they try
> to work. (3)

A second assumption is that recovery after an injury follows a fairly predictable course, such that an injured worker (IW) initially shows progressive improvement and then reaches a plateau (Fig. 10-1; see Need for
Further Treatment below). In compensation law, a worker is said to "medically stable" or to have reached "maximal medical improvement" when he
or she plateaus. At this juncture, compensation law generally dictates that
medical treatment be terminated and that either a definitive vocational plan
be developed or the patient be pensioned. Also, the patient is entitled to a
cash settlement based on her permanent partial impairment when she
reaches maximal medical improvement.

---

* The conceptual models on which WC procedures are based are often implicit, so a discussion of them is of necessity speculative.

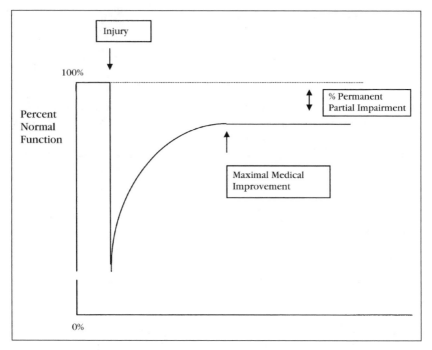

Figure 10-1   Hypothetical recovery curve after a work injury.

Disabling Work Injuries

When you treat injured workers, it is important to have some basic knowledge about the natural history of disabling injuries in the WC system. This permits you to assess the risk of chronic disability in IWs you treat.

Table 10-1 and Figure 10-2 are based on data from the Washington State Department of Labor and Industries for the years 1987-89 (4). The following conclusions may be drawn:

1. Most work injuries do not lead to any time loss.

2. For injuries that do lead to time loss, the time lost is usually short; 55% of workers who sustain injuries requiring time loss return within a month.

3. It is feasible to designate workers as having prolonged time loss if the time loss exceeds 120 days. By this point, the recovery curve has flattened significantly, so that if an IW has been on time loss for more than 120 days, he or she has more than a 50% chance of still being work disabled at 12 months.

4. The costs associated with prolonged time loss are exceedingly high. DLI data indicate that about 5% of all claims are associated with prolonged time loss, but that these 5% account for

Table 10-1   1988 Washington State Injury Profile by Nature of Injury

Nature of Injury	All Claims	Percent of Claims That Produce Time Loss >120 Days	No. of Claims with Time Loss >120 Days (% of All Claims with >120 Days Time Loss)
Contusions, bruises, cuts, lacerations, punctures, scratches, abrasions	75,713 (47.6%)	0.8	644 (9.6)
Sprains, strains	59,729 (37.6%)	7.5	4456 (66.1)
Fractures	424 (4.7%)	11.9	882 (13.1)
Burns	5777 (3.6%)	0.6	38 (0.6)
Multiple injuries	2689 (1.7%)	10.2	273 (4.0)
Dislocations	1483 (0.9%)	19.0	282 (4.2)
Amputations	237 (0.1%)	18.1	43 (0.6)
Other	5918 (3.7%)	2.1	123 (1.8)
Total	158,970 (100%)	—	6741 (100)

Source: Washington State Department of Labor and Industries data (unpublished).

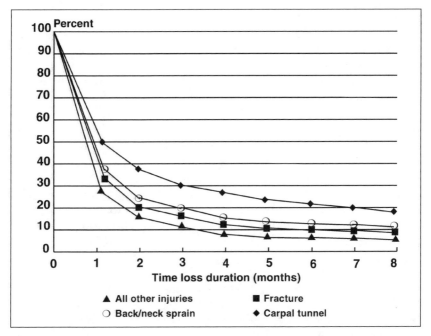

Figure 10-2 Percentage of workers receiving disability payments after the indicated number of months since injury, by injury. *Note:* Values were derived from "reference case" model (male, <30 years old, unmarried, not hospitalized).

approximately 85% of the indemnity and medical payments that DLI makes (5).

5. A fairly high proportion (11.9%) of workers with fractures are work disabled for more than 120 days.

6. Sprains and strains are particularly problematic from a disability standpoint. They occur commonly, and because 7.5% of workers with these conditions go on to have more than 120 days of time loss, sprains and strains represent fully 66% of all conditions associated with prolonged time loss. Among the sprains and strains that lead to prolonged time loss, the most common by far are those of the low back (4).

Should You Get Involved?

Assume that an established patient of yours, Jane Robinson, reports that she recently injured her lower back at work and is now unable to work. You evaluate her and find that she appears to have an axial, mechanical spine problem with no evidence for a lumbar radiculopathy and no Red Flags for a serious medical condition underlying her LBP (6). She asks you to manage her new problem and gives you a Report of Industrial Injury or Occupational Disease form to complete (Fig. 10-3). Should you get involved?

You should recognize at the outset that managing Ms Robinson's back problem will be a challenge. In addition to the generic difficulties associated with managing LBP, there are special difficulties associated with managing the problem in the context of a WC claim.

The generic difficulties include interpreting patient reports about pain and deciding how much weight to give those reports (7,8). Many patients with LBP report severe functional limitations in the absence of clear-cut physical findings that make these limitations inevitable. A treating physician thus constantly faces the issue of whether to take the reports at face value or to discount them in some way. A related dilemma is that the physician needs to decide how aggressively to treat a patient with LBP. Some observers have recommended that when primary care physicians treat LBP, they should generally focus on information, reassurance, and encouragement of self-management. But if a patient reports incapacitating pain, and if you rely heavily on her reports when making treatment decisions, you will almost certainly feel pressured to move to more aggressive approaches (e.g., advanced spinal imaging, invasive procedures such as epidural injections, opiate medications for pain control, surgical consultation).

The treatment of an IW is complicated by several factors, including time pressures, the inflexibility of return-to-work (RTW) options, and the requirement of the WC system that you play an adjudicative role rather than simply a clinical role. These additional complications accentuate the uncertainties and pressures that are inherently associated with the treatment of

DOCTOR INFORMATION

41. Diagnosis	42. ICD Diag. codes	43. Date you first saw patient for this condition
		Month–day–year

44. Subjective complaints supporting your diagnosis

45. Objective findings supporting your diagnosis   Include physical, lab and X-ray findings

46. Treatment and diagnostic testing recommendations

47. Was the diagnosed condition caused by this injury or exposure?
Circle one of four
PROBABLY (50% or more)   YES
POSSIBLY (Less than 50%)   NO

48. Will the condition cause the patient to miss work?
Circle one; if YES, estimate no. of days
NO   YES _____ days

49. Is there any pre-existing impairment of the injured area?
NO   Circle one; if YES, describe briefly or attach report
YES

50. Has patient ever been treated for the same or similar condition?
NO   Circle one; if YES, give year, name of physician and city of treatment
YES

51. Are there any conditions that will prevent or retard recovery?
NO   Circle one; if YES, describe briefly or attach report
YES

52. Referral physician Complete if you refer patient to another doctor for follow-up
Name   Telephone
                                                  (   )
Address

53. Name of hospital or clinic
Name   Telephone
                              (   )
Address
City   State   ZIP code

55. Place of service
Select one
Inpatient   ER   Outpatient

Dr.'s
Office   Clinic

56. Provider number
For billing purposes

54. Attending physician
Name   Telephone
                              (   )
Address

57. Signature
Licensed physician must sign report
X   Today's
                               date _____

L&I USE ONLY

Figure 10-3   Report of Industrial Injury or Occupational Disease (detail). (Courtesy of Washington State Department of Labor and Industries.)

LBP. When you treat an IW with LBP, special problems that you are likely to encounter include ambiguity about the factors underlying the pain and its treatment, conflict of interests between the patient and insurance carriers and consequent (possible) disruption of your relationship with your patient; lack of familiarity with the regulations and policies of the WC system with which you must interact; and time demands. (Even if you are knowledgeable about the WC system, you will almost certainly find that treating IWs takes much more of your time than treating patients with comparable medical conditions but without WC claims.)

All of these potential problems should give you pause as you consider whether or not to assume responsibility for treating your patient's low back problem. There are, however, considerations on the other side of the equation. One is that the WC system requires the attending physician for an IW to perform at least minimal disability management services. If, for example, the attending physician refuses to fill out appropriate forms, the IW might have her benefits terminated. Thus someone needs to take responsibility for both supervising the medical care that your patient receives for her LBP and managing the associated disability. If you have a good working relationship with the patient, you may be able to perform these services better than any other physician.

Another consideration is that the stakes for your patient may be very high. Many disabled workers experience significant anxiety about their ability to return to the work force and provide economically for themselves and their families. The vast majority of individuals who file WC claims have uneventful recoveries from their injuries, with little or no time off work. Primary care physicians are usually the most appropriate professionals to treat these uncomplicated injuries. In contrast, patients with prolonged work disability are likely to present significant disability management challenges. For physicians who are uncomfortable treating these IWs, it is perfectly appropriate to provide initial management after injuries but to then refer patients if they demonstrate delayed recovery and/or difficulty returning to work.

Disability Management

There are four main components to a successful strategy for managing disability: 1) disability evaluation, 2) assuming care and contracting with a patient, 3) interventions to reduce the risk of prolonged disability, and 4) interfacing with disability agencies.

Disability Evaluation

Is Workmens' Compensation Likely To Be an Issue?
When evaluating a patient shortly after the onset of LBP, you may be unsure whether work disability is likely to be an issue (9). At one extreme,

you might evaluate a homemaker who experienced onset of LBP while lifting her child. This individual will not become a disabled worker within the WC system because she is not entitled to any WC benefits. At the opposite extreme, your patient may have filed a WC claim and be receiving time-loss benefits by the time of your first evaluation. Ask the patient questions similar to those given in Table 10-2. Based on the answers, you can broadly place the patient into one of the following groups:

1. *Work disability within the WC system is impossible.* The patient is not eligible for a WC claim.

2. *Work disability within the WC system is possible but highly unlikely.* For example, a patient is eligible for a WC claim but has chosen to get medical help for her LBP under her private insurance and convincingly states that she is able to continue working despite her LBP.

3. *Patient has filed a WC claim, is getting medical benefits under the claim, is continuing to work, and indicates that the LBP is unlikely to interfere with her work.*

4. *Patient has filed a WC claim, is getting medical benefits under the claim, is continuing to work, but is having great difficulty and is considering going off work.*

5. *Patient is off work.* She has filed a WC claim and is receiving both medical benefits and time-loss benefits under the claim.

What is the Risk of Prolonged Work Disability?

If your patient is already on work disability, you should assess the probability that she will be disabled for an extended period of time. As a practical matter, it is reasonable to define extended or prolonged work disability as disability that lasts more than 120 days. As we have mentioned, this number takes into account the fact that the recovery curve from a disabling work injury flattens after about 120 days. Thus, if a patient remains disabled at this point, the likelihood is about 50% that she will go on to much more protracted disability.

A considerable amount of research has been devoted to identifying predictors of chronicity among disabled workers. Some of the salient findings are summarized in Table 10-3; the entries are based on two reviews of risk factors for prolonged disability and several individual research papers.

You should be aware, however, that despite much research there is no proven formula that can be applied to assess how likely it is that your patient will slide into protracted work disability. First, data about work disability are found in several sources (10), and researchers have generally not compared these different sources for consistency. For example, in a review of 20 prospective cohort or population-based studies, Turner et al. (11) concluded that the education level of workers did not have a systematic

Table 10-2   Questions to Determine Whether a Patient with a Recent Injury is Likely to Go On Workers' Compensation Disability

Question	Discussion
1. Did you have a job at the time when your low back pain (LBP) started? a. (If patient was out of the work force) Why were you out of the work force? Did that have anything to do with your health?	1. If the patient was out of the work force when he/she developed LBP, he/she cannot file a workers' compensation (WC) claim (although other kinds of disability issues may arise.)
2. What were you doing when your low back pain started? What do you think caused the pain? Did it start because of your work?	2. Be prepared for ambiguity at this point. Sometimes patients report abrupt onset of LBP in the context of an injury stimulus that could plausibly be viewed as traumatic (e.g., the patient may have fallen from a height or been subjected to sudden loading of his/her spine while lifting). Other patients report an abrupt onset of pain during their work but that its onset occurred in the context of ordinary activities. Still others report a gradual onset of LBP, so that it is difficult to say what may have provoked their symptoms. If a patient says that he/she became symptomatic because of work, he/she can file a WC claim. If there was no clear injury stimulus, you can anticipate that the claim will probably be contested.
3. Have you filed a WC claim for your low back pain? What is the status of the claim?	3. If the patient has an open WC claim, you should be concerned about disability issues, even if he/she is still working. If the claim application has been contested or rejected, the situation is less clear. But you should anticipate that in this type of situation the patient may ask you to support an appeal.
4. (If patient is working) Do you believe that your back pain is interfering with your ability to do your job?	4. You should not get lulled into complacency because a patient is working at the time when you do your initial evaluation. If the patient says he/she is barely able to continue working, you should anticipate that he/she will decide to go off work in the near future and will ask you to support this decision.
5. Have you gone off work because of your back pain? Are you getting time-loss benefits? How long have you been off work? Do you think you will be able to return to your job soon?	5. Obviously, a patient is at risk for protracted disability if he/she is already off work at the time of your initial evaluation.

Table 10-3   Factors Associated with High Risk of Prolonged Disability Among Injured Workers

Variable (Reference)	Value Associated with High Risk of Prolonged Work Disability
Sociodemographic Factors	
Age (10,11)	Older workers
Sex (11)	No consistent effect
Education (10,12,13)	Poorly educated
Nature of Injury	
Injury severity (10,11)	Injury required hospitalization
Site of injury (4)	Low back pain, carpal tunnel syndrome
Pain and Functional Status	
Self-rated pain and functional disability (11)	High pain and functional disability at baseline
Psychological Factors	
MMPI hysteria/hypochondriasis scales (10,14)	High hysteria or hypochondriasis
Perceived ability to RTW (10,10a,19)	Worker's perception that he/she will not be able to return to work
History of anxiety or depression (10)	Positive history
Occupational Factors	
Physical demands of job (10,11,15-17)	Physically demanding job
Control over work schedule or sequencing of work activities (10,16)	Low control
Firm size (11)	Small company
Job satisfaction (18)	Low job satisfaction*
Social support at work (10,16,19,20)	Little social support
Economic Factors	
Wage replacement ratio (21)	High wage replacement ratio
Unemployment rate (11)	High unemployment rate

*Research has implicated low job satisfaction as a predictor of onset of work-related low back conditions (18). The evidence is not so clear, however, regarding the effect of job satisfaction on return to work after onset of a disabling back condition (11,16).

effect on chronicity. But data from other sources, such as the SSA (12) and the Census Bureau (13), make it clear that individuals with poor educational backgrounds are much more likely than others to become SSDI beneficiaries and to report that they have a disabling physical condition. In addition, studies of risk factors differ markedly in the populations of injured workers being evaluated (22,23); the relative weights of predictors of prolonged disability have not been assessed; and research on risk factors has focused on variables that are relatively easy to measure, with less attention given to the psychosocial characteristics of patients (24) and the subtleties of the interactions between patients and physicians (22,25).

In light of the above uncertainties, your best strategy is to cast a broad net when you evaluate disability risk in your patients and to combine the information you get informally. You may find useful the list of risk factors given in Table 10-4, which was developed on the basis of consensus among experts in work disability in Washington State.

Assuming Care and Contracting with the Patient

The discussion in this section assumes that you are willing in principle to treat injured workers and manage their disability issues. Even if this is the case, you would be prudent to consider carefully whether to manage a *particular* patient's work injury and, if so, under what terms.

As least three considerations should influence your willingness to assume responsibility for your patient's new low back injury:

1. *Does the patient have a high risk for prolonged disability?* Unless you have significant expertise in managing IWs, you should think twice about accepting responsibility for the treatment of someone who is at high risk.

2. *Do you have an adequate "exit strategy" (i.e., a back-up plan if the patient demonstrates delayed recovery and/or prolonged work disability)?* Typically, this will involve referral to another care provider.

3. *How good is your rapport with the patient?* You should anticipate that some strains will be placed on your relationship as the work injury is treated. If your relationship is already strained, you should be cautious about accepting the role of attending physician for any work injury.

If you are potentially willing to provide care for a patient, you should strongly consider setting up a treatment agreement or at least discussing your approach to the management of IWs. For example, you might emphasize

1. That your goal for an IW is to facilitate RTW, even if the treatment you supervise does not lead to complete resolution of symptoms.

2. That disabling work injuries are typically very stressful for individuals, and that the best way to resolve the stress is for the IW to extricate herself from the WC system as soon as possible.

3. That you expect your patient to be diligent about pursuing all avenues that might help her extricate herself from the WC system. (You should remind her that your responses to the WC questions will at most delay termination of her WC benefits, and that it will be important for her to decide what type of work she

can do, rather than wait for the WC system to come up with a good vocational plan.)

4. That you will agree to manage her LBP for a limited amount of time (perhaps 3 months). If she continues to be disabled at the end of that time, you may insist that her care be transferred to another physician.

Interventions to Reduce the Risk of Prolonged Disability

There is a paucity of literature that you can rely on for guidance as you try to manage disability for an IW. However, there is some evidence that health care systems can reduce disability by following well-designed algorithms for treating IWs (26). There is also evidence that rehabilitative care provided in a structured program by a multidisciplinary team can restore function and reduce disability in patients who have failed other therapies (27). Research indicates that cognitive behavioral therapy provided by psychologists can reduce disability, most likely by helping patients master their fear of activity and promoting goal-directed behavior (28). Some research supports the hypothesis that individual physicians can facilitate the recovery of LBP patients by promoting moderate activity rather than bed rest and by providing educational materials about the nature of non-specific LBP (29-33). The data, however, are by no means unambiguous (22,34-36), and observers have noted that it is exceedingly difficult for studies to capture the subtleties of physician-patient communications and to demonstrate the effects of these communications on patient outcomes (37,38).

Finally, expert opinion and at least some research support the hypothesis that the behavior of employers can make a difference in the rehabilitation of IWs (39-42). The general rule is that if employers take a proactive position vis-à-vis IWs and establish procedures for helping them return to work, then the IWs will in fact demonstrate a higher likelihood of early RTW. For example, companies that permit light-duty work or graduated RTW have better results.

An analysis of disability management strategies is complicated not only by the lack of definitive empirical data but also by the fact that disability management by a physician is always intertwined with medical management. In fact, if effective medical/surgical treatment is available for an IW's condition, the best way to shorten the patient's period of disability is to provide that treatment. Thus one can raise the question of whether effective disability management involves anything over and above effective medical care.

Challenges

One way to think about the issue of disability management is to compare the interventions a physician might make for an IW with LBP to those that she might make for a homemaker with LBP. Experts in the management of

---

Table 10-4   Risk Factors for Prolonged Disability Proposed by Task Force for the Washington State Department of Labor and Industries

---

Group 1: Catastrophic—Cases with catastrophic injuries are very likely to benefit from medical case management.

❑ 1. Catastrophic

Group 2A: High Risk—Cases with any of these factors are likely to benefit from medical case management, unless there is clear evidence the worker is about to return to work.

❑ 1. Hospitalized within 28 days of injury for reasons related to industrial injury

❑ 2. Worker who is 45 years old or older with carpal tunnel syndrome

❑ 3. 90 or more days of time-loss

Group 2B: High Risk—The presence of one or more of the following may indicate an increased likelihood of long-term disability and, therefore, some potential benefit from case management or other intensive services.

A. Medical Factors

❑ 1. Presence of secondary medical condition

❑ 2. Injury to dominant hand

❑ 3. Hospitalized within 28 days of injury for reasons unrelated to industrial injury

❑ 4. Pre-existing psychiatric conditions

B. Injury Descriptions

❑ 1. Non-overt injury: an injury occurring in course of usual work activities

❑ 2. No objective findings on examinations

❑ 3. Diagnosis not consistent with injury description

❑ 4. Time gap in report of injury

❑ 5. Unwitnessed accident

C. Provider/Patient Factors

❑ 1. No identifiable treatment plan or goals

❑ 2. Over-utilization of health care delivery systems and services by either patient or provider, or over-referral by physician; may include frequent changes of attending physician

❑ 3. Misuse of scheduled medications by patient

❑ 4. Physician fostering illness beliefs

❑ 5. Number of surgeries both related and unrelated to work-related problem; may include a number of unsuccessful surgeries in the same area

❑ 6. Spread of diagnosis over time; newly contended diagnosis

❑ 7. No documented medical progress

D. Psychosocial Factors

❑ 1. Exaggerated illness behavior: presence of non-organic signs (Waddell signs); no objective findings

❑ 2. Evidence of abuse of alcohol, illicit drugs, or prescription medication

(Cont'd)

Table 10-4   Risk Factors for Prolonged Disability Proposed by Task Force for the Washington State Department of Labor and Industries *(Cont'd)*

D. Psychosocial Factors *(cont'd)*

❑ 3. Presence of depression or avoidance anxiety, post-traumatic disorder, or other dysphoric affects (e.g., anger at employer or supervisor or L&I)

❑ 4. History of childhood abuse, physical or sexual abuse, substance abuse in caretaker, or family instability

❑ 5. Presence of personality traits or disorders (e.g., presence of specific somatization traits, problematic interpersonal relationships); arrests

E. Demographic Factors

❑ 1. Low educational level, including illiteracy

❑ 2. English not primary language

❑ 3. Age greater than 50 and employed in heavy industry

❑ 4. Back or lower extremity injury with medium or heavy labor employment

❑ 5. Nearing retirement age

F. Job Factors

❑ 1. Anger at employer

❑ 2. Employer anger at worker

❑ 3. Miscellaneous employer factors: seasonal work, strike, plant closure, job becoming obsolete, etc.

❑ 4. Loss of job in which the injury occurred

❑ 5. Singular work history in heavy industry

❑ 6. Complaints of inability to function

❑ 7. History of poor job performance, frequent job change, short duration of employment, job dissatisfaction, or job termination before claims filing

❑ 8. Employer or worker not active in return-to-work efforts

❑ 9. Worker is not clearly headed back to work

❑ 10. Perception of the worker that he/she will be retrained for a better job or other misperceptions of L&I vocational entitlement

G. Administrative Factors

❑ 1. Third-party involvement

❑ 2. Recent claim closures; application for reopening

❑ 3. Employer protest

❑ 4. Current income, including time-loss, compares favorably to net income before to injury

❑ 5. Multiple L&I claims (may include a number of previous claims)

❑ 6. Loss of driver's license or other credentials

❑ 7. Loss of medical insurance

❑ 8. Originally non–time-loss claim that has become time-loss

❑ 9. Non-compliance with medical or vocational treatment

❑ 10. Worker or physician perception that L&I is unresponsive or adversarial

From Attending Doctor's Handbook, rev ed. Olympia, WA: State of Washington Department of Labor and Industries; 1999; with permission.

LBP have articulated several principles of treatment that would apply to both patients; for example, they agree that the needs of both are usually best met by a treatment program that embodies a rehabilitative philosophy (6,42). However, if we compare the situation faced by an IW with LBP to the situation confronting a homemaker with LBP, we do find differences between the two strategies for disability management.

One difference is that the WC system is set up as a temporary benefit system. As noted above, when an IW reaches medical stability, the expectation is that her claim will be closed. Thus, if an IW's functional status is not changing, the WC carrier may move to terminate benefits. The pressure for demonstrable progress is much greater when an individual is receiving time-loss benefits. In this setting, the WC carrier might not close her claim but might declare her employable in some capacity and terminate her time-loss benefits. Other examples of problems that are unique to IWs are shown in Table 10-5.

Strategies

These special considerations suggest strategies for disability management when you are functioning as the attending physician for an IW. Although these strategies are in general not unique to IWs, they may need to be carried out more self-consciously with these patients than with non-WC patients.

Table 10-5   Special Problems Faced by Injured Workers with Regard to Disability Management

---

- Time pressure
  - —Time pressure imposed by the WC system
  - —Disability syndrome (e.g., dysfunctional attitudes and coping strategies more likely to develop with the passage of time)
- Lack of flexibility in work options that impedes return-to-work
- Multiple professionals involved in the claim, with resulting communication problems or conflicts
- WC system is formal and legalistic
- WC system can become adversarial
- IWs may become suspicious of the motives of those involved in the claim. They may also have a strong need to have their LBP "validated"—that is, be shown to have a clearly observable biomechanical lesion:
  - —It is common for pain patients to want the reality of their pain supported by objective data
  - —In addition, the WC demands this validation in order to pay benefits
- Stress due to loss of self-esteem and financial threats

Almost any treatment decision you make is likely to be second-guessed by someone in the WC system. In effect, WC probably intrudes into the doctor-patient relationship more than virtually any other benefit system.

FOCUS ON RETURN-TO-WORK

Make it clear to the patient that you consider RTW to be an important goal. Ask your patient about her progress toward RTW at each office visit.

WATCH THE CLOCK

See the patient frequently, so that she is aware of the need to move through the WC system as briskly as possible. You may end up accelerating the pace at which you provide therapies because of a concern that your patient might slide into a disability syndrome (43).

EDUCATE THE PATIENT

Educate the patient about the injury and the importance of a rehabilitative approach to treating it (see Chapter 2). Although education is important for any patient with LBP, you need to be especially sensitive to the needs of an IW. One reason, mentioned above, is time pressure. Secondly, the WC system demands that an IW have objective evidence of a pathological condition that rationalizes her pain complaints. This demand tends to amplify the already widespread tendency of patients to place excessive emphasis on biomechanical models of LBP (21,44). Thirdly, an IW may eventually confer with several individuals who offer conflicting opinions about her back problem. For example, she might get solicited or unsolicited opinions from her physical therapist, her claims manager, her attorney, and her employer.

Anticipate that your patient will be extremely sensitive to the question of whether her pain is "real", particularly because she will soon understand that her claim may be closed if her symptoms cannot be understood in terms of a biomechanical model. In a general way, also, you need to take the time to give your patient explanations that do not humiliate her, that help her control her anxiety about her condition and its implications, and that encourage her to attempt to expand her physical limitations. There is no single "script" that will work for this, but it is important that your educational message be consistent and genuine.

MAINTAIN CREDIBILITY

There is no dearth of opinions about LBP. Assume that your patient will hear about many miracle cures for her back problem from friends, co-workers, advertisements, and so on. If you are recommending a low technology, rehabilitative treatment program for her, she may well voice skepticism and express the view you are providing suboptimal care. This is always a difficult challenge to confront, but even more so if you are not familiar with the current literature on the various conservative and interventional therapies for nonradicular LBP. It may be appropriate to work in tandem with other professionals (see below).

The patient may also doubt your credibility if she feels that you are representing the interest of the WC carrier rather than her own best interest. However, one way of promoting an open and trusting relationship is by going over the WC form with your patient. By doing so, you make it clear that you will consider her opinions and that you will not communicate crucial information behind her back. (However, it is important to emphasize that you are not her mouthpiece. Although you are interested in her opinions, the answers you give to the WC questions will reflect your best medical judgment.) In addition, your patient may be able to provide important information that you should incorporate into your response to the WC carrier.

GET HELP FROM OTHER PROFESSIONALS
Disabled workers characteristically have multifactorial problems. Develop a network for treating IWs. For example, a team may comprise a physical therapist who is familiar with functional restoration, an orthopedist or physiatrist who specializes in spine problems, and a psychologist. The general rule is: "Don't go one-on-one with a disabled injured worker."

COMMUNICATE WITH OTHERS INVOLVED IN THE CLAIM
When several professionals are involved in a WC claim, there are endless possibilities for communication failures and inconsistencies. You need to make extra efforts to keep the other professionals apprised of your assessment and treatment plan for your patient, and to get notes from their encounters with your patient. It is often helpful to have phone conferences or face-to-face meetings with the other professionals who are involved in the WC claim.

SET GOALS
Develop goals for your patient's medical treatment and vocational rehabilitation, and plan strategies for reaching these goals. You will be able to respond better to requests for information from the WC carrier—and to manage your patient better—if you have developed an overall plan and are working collaboratively with your patient to carry it out.

Should You Order Imaging Studies?
Many observers recommend that when primary providers treat LBP patients who do not have Red Flags for serious disease (6), they should eschew costly diagnostic testing and rely primarily on information, reassurance, and encouragement to patients that they take significant responsibility for managing their back problems (45-47). Reasons for this include, among others, that diagnostic studies function as gateways to interventional therapies; that interventional therapies have at best only modest benefit; and that the combination of diagnostic tests and the promise of interventional therapies undercuts the resolve of patients to take responsibility for their low back problems, to view promises of "quick fixes" with skepticism, and to be willing to accept symptom moderation and ability to function as suitable endpoints of treatment, rather than insisting on a complete cure. This in turn

may start patients on a path that is ultimately more likely to lead to chronic pain and disability than to cure.

The problem when a physician who is following a rehabilitative approach refuses to order imaging studies is that the decision might not be acceptable to the patient. Several factors probably combine to lead patients to over-value imaging studies; for example, they may view abnormalities on X-rays or other imaging studies as providing objective verification that a biomechanical abnormality relevant to their pain exists (21,44), which is combined with a tremendous need to have their pain validated, as mentioned earlier. Patients will often construe a decision to order a test or perform an invasive procedure as evidence that the physician believes they are suffering.

The primary care provider therefore faces a dilemma when considering whether to order imaging for a patient. Providers in one study openly admitted that a major consideration in their decision to order imaging for patients with LBP was reassurance—either for them or for their patients (48). In addition, the demand of the WC system for objective evidence to support an IW's symptoms can pressure a physician into ordering imaging studies. Thus physicians sometimes order imaging tests on IWs more liberally than on other LBP patients.

In light of all these competing goals, there is, unfortunately, no single strategy that will always work when your patient requests imaging studies.

Interfacing with Disability Agencies

The discussion so far has focused on your interactions with your patient—that is, on the approaches you use to evaluate the patient's risk of prolonged disability and to intervene in ways that reduce this risk. But interactions with a patient are only part of the story when you treat an IW; you will also interact with the WC carrier. Of course, if your patient recovers quickly and completely following a work injury, your relations with the WC system will typically be simple and cordial. But they are likely to be complex and ambiguous if your patient complains of ongoing LBP following treatment and asserts that she is unable to return to work. You will then be placed in the position of arbiter between patient and WC system. Both sides will come to you and "plead their case". Often, there will be no objective findings that support your patient's reported activity restrictions, but the WC system will demand that you support your judgments on the basis of such findings.

Frequently, the questions posed by the WC system (see below) will be very difficult to answer. In particular, you will often be uncertain about whether it is realistic for your patient to return to a certain job, or to return to work of any kind. You may well have difficulty getting accurate, detailed information about your patient's physical abilities or the physical demands of the job(s) to which she might return.

To further complicate matters, participants in a WC claim may have hidden agendas. IWs sometimes deliberately exaggerate their incapacitation in order to have their time-loss benefits continued. Employers sometimes use deceptive strategies to get employees' claims refused or closed.

Another factor that makes interacting with the WC system difficult is that it makes assumptions about work injuries that oversimplify complex issues. The LPB patients you will treat will have a wide variety of related problems (e.g., various psychiatric and medical co-morbidities, difficulties reintegrating into the work force). There will be many challenges in trying to forge links between your patients and the "paper" patients in WC policies and procedures.

In order to provide thoughtful, consistent opinions to the WC system about a particular patient, you need to spend some time learning about issues that arise routinely for IWs with pain conditions such as LBP. In particular, you should give some thought to

1. The meaning of the term *objective findings*
2. The significance of patient credibility
3. Questions typically asked by the WC system, especially about causation, need for treatment, physical capacities, and ability to work (Table 10-6)
4. Specific WC policies that affect patient rehabilitation (these differ from one jurisdiction to another, so it is important to become familiar with the WC carriers in your area)

Objective Findings

It is routine for WC carriers to ask physicians to base their opinions on objective findings. This request may seem innocuous, but it has profound implications. As noted above, WC carriers attempt to make decisions based on objectively measurable evidence of incapacitation. But patients with painful conditions typically report incapacitation that goes beyond measurable damage to their organs. Even if you find a patient's pain complaints credible, you will invariably have difficulty stating objective findings that make her activity limitations inevitable. Furthermore, these findings will typically not explain in detail the activity limitations that the patients report. For example, consider a patient with LBP who reports that she can sit for only 20 minutes at a time. There is no objective measure that would make this limitation inevitable.

As a step toward a strategy for dealing with requests for objective findings, it is important to note that the term *objective findings* is not precisely defined. In general it refers to laboratory or physical findings that are objectively measurable and are not subject to voluntary control or manipulation by a patient. Objective findings can be contrasted with *subjective findings* such as patients' reports of pain intensity or activity restrictions caused by pain. However, as shown in Table 10-7, many clinically important examination

---

Table 10-6   Questions from a Workers' Compensation Carrier to an Independent Medical Examiner Regarding a Woman Who Had Sustained a Low Back Injury*

---

1. Are the employee's current complaints supported by objective findings?

2. What are your diagnoses of the conditions found and of the causal relationship, if any, to the above-referenced injury on a more-probable-than-not basis?

3. Is the incident described on the accident report on a more-probable-than-not basis the cause of this condition?

4. Is the present condition due in whole or in part to the accident as described by the patient? If the present condition is due only in part to the accident, or is not due to the accident, please explain fully.

5. Are there any pre-existing or concurrent medical conditions that could be retarding recovery?

6. Is the patient able to return to her work at the time of injury as a nurse's aide without restrictions at this time? (A job analysis for this position has been enclosed for your review.)

7. If the patient is not able to return to full-unrestricted work, is she capable of light or modified duty? If so, please advise what restrictions you feel are appropriate, how long those restrictions would apply, and can the patient work full time on modified duty?

8. Please review the enclosed job analyses for cashier and for merchandiser of potato chips. If the patient is unable to return to her job as a nurse's aide, please indicate whether she is able to perform these jobs. Please base your opinion on objective findings.

9. Are there any medical restrictions due to the residual condition? What are the current physical limitations? Are they permanent or will they improve in time?

10. Are there any other factors affecting the patient's ability to return to full-unrestricted work?

11. Do you feel further active curative treatment measures or diagnostic studies are indicated for the residuals of the patient's condition?

12. If additional treatment is necessary, please submit your recommendations for such, the estimated length of same, and prognosis for recovery afterwards. Please specify what recommendations apply to the work-related condition and what apply to any unrelated conditions.

13. Do you believe that the treatment currently recommended and being provided is reasonably effective and necessary for the purposes of recovery?

14. Is the treatment recommended and being received an acceptable medical option under the particular facts of this case?

15. Do you feel, based on your examination, that the patient is medically stable, as defined in AS 23.39.395 of the Alaska Workers' Compensation Statutes?

16. If you do not feel the patient is medically stable at this time, can you give an estimation of when you feel medical stability will be reached?

17. If you feel the patient is medically stable at this time, do you feel that she has sustained a permanent impairment as a result of her above-referenced injury?

18. If so, please provide us with a permanent partial impairment rating in accordance with the 5th Edition of the AMA's <u>Guides to the Evaluation of Permanent Impairment.</u> Please reference the tables, charts, and pages used to compute your rating and your final rating in a percentage of the whole person.

---

* These questions were actually addressed to a physician who performed an independent medical examination on a patient who was receiving WC benefits in Alaska for a work-related low back injury, but they are similar to those that might be addressed to a treating physician.

Table 10-7   Objective, Subjective, and Semi-Objective Findings in Low Back Pain

---

Objective Findings

1. X-ray abnormalities (e.g., fracture, scoliosis, spondylolisthesis, disk space narrowing, osteophytes)
2. MRI abnormalities (e.g., spinal stenosis, disk herniation)
3. Electromyographic abnormalities (e.g., positive waves and fibrillations, absent H-reflex)

Subjective Findings

1. Patient's reported pain intensity
2. Activity restrictions reported by patient

Semi-Objective Findings

1. Posture (e.g., loss of lumbar lordosis, list)
2. Gait
3. Muscle spasms
4. Soft-tissue hypersensitivity (myofascial pain)
5. Range of motion
6. Abnormal straight-leg raising
7. Some lower extremity deep tendon reflex findings (e.g., reflexes difficult to elicit in patient who is tense)
8. Sensory function in lower extremities
9. Lower extremity strength

---

findings are *semi-objective*. They are objective in the sense that they can be observed and measured, but they are not completely objective, because patients can to some extent voluntarily modify them. Most of the adjudicators who request objective findings are not aware of these subtleties.

There is a fairly simple way to finesse the objective findings issue. If you do not find your patient credible, it would be perfectly reasonable to accept the perspective of the WC system (i.e., to report only those findings that are unequivocally objective and that are plausibly connected to her stated activity limitations). But if your patient has consistent physical findings that you find credible, you can simply list them in the space where you are requested to give objective findings. In most instances, the findings you list will be accepted by the WC system, even if they are only semi-objective or do not necessarily explain the activity restrictions your patient reports. If your findings are challenged, you can indicate that in your clinical judgment they represent valid indices of the patient's condition.

Patient Credibility

As we have shown, assessing the physical capacities of patients with chronic pain is difficult primarily because their statements about activity limitations often cannot be easily rationalized in terms of objectively measurable organ pathology. In this case, the question becomes: Should your patient's statements be accepted as credible?

Table 10-8 lists the factors thought to be relevant to patient credibility. Be aware, however, that the list has not been validated, and that research on deception by medical patients suggests that physicians are not particularly good at assessing patient credibility (49-52). Some guidelines are given in the American Medical Association's *Guides to the Evaluation of Permanent Impairment* (53) and in the follow-up volume, *Master the AMA Guides* (54). These emphasize consistency in a patient's presentation: consistency from one examination to another, consistency between the patient's complaints and the biology of his condition, consistency between the patient's reported activity limitations and information provided by collateral sources, and consistency between these reported limitations and normative data regarding self-reported limitations in patients with musculoskeletal pain problems (55).

It is worth noting that, as a treating physician, you are in a better position than anyone else involved in your patient's WC claim to assess credibility.

Table 10-8   Characteristics Associated with High Patient Credibility

- No pre-existing condition
- No medical comorbidities
- Definite stimulus (e.g., crushed by a tree)
- Definite tissue damage (e.g., fracture)
- Symptoms, signs, activity limitations all fit expectations for the medical problem
- Consistent findings over repeated examinations
- No exaggerated pain behavior
- No inconsistencies between symptoms/signs noted in physician's office and behavior outside the office
- No inconsistencies between activity limitations reported by patient and information gathered from collateral sources (e.g., co-worker, family member, surveillance videotape)
- No chronic psychiatric disorders or long-term psychosocial risk factors
- No reactive psychiatric problems (e.g., anxiety disorder, depression)
- Patient motivated to return to productivity
- Job opportunities exist
- No incentives for disability
- Severity of reported symptoms and activity limitations is consistent with normative data for patients with similar medical problems

From Robinson JP. Psychological aspects of disability. Presented to Employer Advisory Group, Valley Medical Center, Renton, Washington, June 1997; and Turk DC, Robinson JP, Aulet M. The Impairment Impact Inventory: comparison of responses by treatment-seekers and claimants undergoing independent medical examinations. J Pain. 2002;3(Suppl 1):1; with permission.

Because you have the opportunity to observe the patient over an extended period of time, you have the opportunity to observe the consistency of your patient's physical findings over repeated examinations.

Questions Posed by the Workers' Compensation System

A key feature of the WC system is that it requires the attending physician to make a series of judgments about an IW, often over an extended period of time. You will receive a letter asking you questions such as those shown in Table 10-6. This letter represents an attempt by the WC to determine whether to continue providing medical and time-loss benefits to your patient. Although you may be bewildered by the variety of the questions posed to you, there are themes that will come up repeatedly. Basically, most of the questions address five issues: causation, need for further treatment, physical capacities and/or physical restrictions, ability to work, and impairment. One important caveat is that the questions posed to you by a WC carrier are often so specific that they do not give you a chance to communicate an overall perspective on your patient. Thus it is often appropriate for you to write a cover letter in addition to answering the specific questions. In it, you should communicate your overall perspective on the patient and any critical information that was not given when you answered the specific questions. You should bear in mind that the opinions you express to a WC carrier carry great weight.

Causation

The WC system is responsible only for injuries or diseases that arise "out of and in the course of employment". Thus a worker is entitled to WC benefits only if she develops a medical condition that can plausibly be causally connected to her employment. Multiple difficulties arise when physicians attempt to apply this standard.

One problem is that causation of a medical condition is difficult to establish unless a worker who was previously healthy sustains a distinct accident at work that involves an overwhelming injury stimulus and an obvious biologic response (e.g., a worker who sustains a fracture of his ankle in a fall from a roof). But this simple paradigm often does not apply. For example, it is not relevant when workers gradually develop degenerative changes that progress over a period of years (e.g., degenerative arthritis of the knee) or when they develop symptoms as a result of repetitive "trauma" or simply repetitive use of a body part (e.g., "repetitive strain injuries" or carpal tunnel syndrome). WC systems have attempted to address these ambiguous situations but have not come up with consistent solutions.

Other dilemmas regarding causation are discussed by Robinson (7). As a practical matter, issues related to causation are usually raised when a worker initially files a WC claim. When treating a worker with an accepted WC claim, you will generally not have to address issues of causation in detail.

NEED FOR FURTHER TREATMENT

Table 10-9 lists factors to consider in determining whether a patient needs further treatment. It is important to be aware, however, that the determination of whether a patient needs additional treatment is fraught with ambiguity.

Disability agencies generally adopt an idealized model of the course of recovery following an injury (see Fig. 10-1). It embodies the assumption that people show rapid improvement following an injury, but then level off and reach a plateau. Before patients reach this hypothetical plateau, they presumably can benefit from further treatment. When they reach the plateau, they are considered to have achieved maximal medical improvement (MMI). From an administrative perspective, this model is convenient because it provides guidelines for intervention and decision-making. For example, this model assumes that when a patient has reached "Maximal Medical Improvement" the curative treatment should be abandoned and a permanent partial impairment rating should be made.

Table 10-9   Issues to Consider in Determining Maximal Medical Improvement

1. Is patient's condition best construed as:
   a) A distinct injury
   b) A repetitive strain (overuse) syndrome
   c) A disease

2. How long does it usually take for patients with this condition to recover or to reach a stable plateau?
   a) Is there a predictable course?
   b) Is patient's condition likely to get worse?

3. How much time has elapsed since the index condition began?

4. What has been the trend over time with respect to function of the affected organ or body part?
   a) Steady improvement
   b) Steady
   c) Deterioration
   d) Widely fluctuating

5. What has been the trend of time with respect to patient's symptoms?
   a) Steady improvement
   b) Steady
   c) Deterioration
   d) Widely fluctuating

6. Does patient have concurrent medical conditions that obscure recovery curve from the index condition?

7. Has patient had access to treatment approaches that are appropriate for his/her condition?

Unfortunately, patients frequently present with clinical problems that are hard to conceptualize in terms of an idealized recovery. For example, it is not at all clear that patients with repetitive strain injuries should be expected to follow the trajectory shown in Figure 10-1. Another problem is that patients may have comorbidities that complicate recovery and make it difficult to determine when they have reached MMI. An example is a diabetic who has a work-related carpal tunnel syndrome in addition to a peripheral polyneuropathy.

A final complication of the MMI concept is that a patient who has reached maximal benefit from a particular kind of treatment may not have reached maximal benefit from treatment in general. For example, consider a patient who is examined 6 months after a low back injury. Assume that her treatment has consisted entirely of chiropractic care during those 6 months and that she has not shown any measurable improvement during the past 2 months. This patient may be judged to have reached maximal medical benefit from chiropractic care, but an examining physician may believe that she may well benefit from physical therapy, epidural steroids, lumbar surgery, aggressive use of various medications, or other therapies not provided by her chiropractor. This case is not unusual; examiners routinely find that even chronic patients have not had exposure to all possible treatments for their condition.

One other consideration is extremely important for a treating physician. It does not bear on the process of determining MMI, but does bear on the consequences that follow the determination that a patient has reached MMI. The WC system typically takes the position that no further medical treatment should be authorized after a patient has reached MMI. This administrative perspective frequently does not match the clinical needs of patients. For example, a patient may have reached MMI from a low back injury in the sense that a significant period of time has elapsed since the injury and no further curative treatment is available. But the individual may still need *maintenance* treatment for her condition (e.g., ongoing medication). This issue is often ignored by agencies that administer benefits. If you believe that your patient could profit from additional treatment, or that the vocational options offered for her are inappropriate, you should state your rationale for your opinions on the form issued by the WC carrier. It is often best to do this as a narrative rather than to restrict yourself to answering the questions posed to you.

PHYSICAL CAPACITIES

The assessment of physical capacities is a precursor to the determination of a patient's ability to work. Disability agencies typically request detailed physical capacities data and usually provide supplementary forms for this purpose. Figure 10-4 provides an example of a typical physical capacities form.

Table 10-10 outlines issues you should consider in assessing the physical capacities of your patient. In general, a clinical evaluation in your office will not provide the detailed physical capacities information that you will need. You can supplement the information gleaned from your clinical evaluation in a variety of ways.

The simplest way is to ask the patient to estimate her capacities. You should consider filling out a physical capacities form on the basis of a patient's reports if you judge the patient to be highly credible or if you do not have access to objective data. (If you follow this approach, you should indicate this on the form.)

Another way to obtain physical capacities data is to refer a patient for a functional capacities evaluation (FCE) (56-58), which is a formal, standardized assessment typically performed by physical therapists. They typically last from 2 to 5 hours. The therapist gathers information about a patient's strength, mobility, and endurance in tasks related to the work that the patient is expected to do. As noted by King et al. (56), FCEs are popular with insurance carriers and attorneys because they provide objective performance data but there are virtually no data that validate FCEs against actual job performance. If you need this type of information, you should request it in your response to the WC carrier.

Finally, you can get physical capacities data on a patient by referring her to a functional restoration program, a pain center, or a work hardening program (27,59-61). A common feature of these programs is that they all assess physical capacities and provide treatment designed to improve those capacities. The performance data from one of these programs have more face validity than performance data from a FCE, because functional restoration programs, work hardening programs, and pain centers typically observe performance over a few weeks, and indicate what patients can do after they have completed rehabilitative treatment.

ABILITY TO WORK

Ability to work is in many respects the key issue for an IW who has been work disabled for a significant period of time. In essence, the WC system is required to make wage replacement payments to patients if and only if the patients are judged not to be employable because of the work injury. Unfortunately, assessing employability is difficult, and there is no simple set of techniques to apply when a decision about employability is requested. In essence, you need to make a judgment about a patient's employability by balancing the patient's capacities (or limitations) against the demands of jobs for which the patient is being considered. Both sides of the balance involve difficult measurements.

Issues related to assessing physical capacities are discussed above. As far as the demands of jobs are concerned, you will frequently get information from an IW's former employer if there is a reasonable chance for the IW to return to her job. If your patient has been assigned to a vocational rehabilitation counselor (VRC) by the WC carrier, the VRC will often prepare formal job analyses for you to evaluate. A sample job analysis form is

1. In an 8 hour workday, this patient can:

Total at One Time (hrs)	**Total During 8-Hour Day (hrs)**
A) Sit 0 ½ 1 2 3 4 5 6 7 8	0 ½ 1 2 3 4 5 6 7 8
B) Stand 0 ½ 1 2 3 4 5 6 7 8	0 ½ 1 2 3 4 5 6 7 8
C) Walk 0 ½ 1 2 3 4 5 6 7 8	0 ½ 1 2 3 4 5 6 7 8

2. Patient can lift:

	Never	Occasionally	Frequently	Continuously
Up to 5 lbs				
5 - 10 lbs				
11 - 20 lbs				
21 - 25 lbs				
26 - 50 lbs				
51 - 100 lbs				

3. Patient can carry:

	Never	Occasionally	Frequently	Continuously
Up to 5 lbs				
5 - 10 lbs				
11 - 20 lbs				
21 - 25 lbs				
26 - 50 lbs				
51 - 100 lbs				

4. Patient is able to:

	Never	Occasionally	Frequently	Continuously
Bend				
Squat				
Crawl				
Climb				
Crouch				
Kneel				
Stoop				
Reach overhead				

Figure 10-4   Sample physical capacities form (*continues on page 261*).

5. Patient can use hands for repetitive actions such as:

	Simple Grasp	Push/Pull	Fine Manipulation
Right:	__Yes __No	__Yes __No	__Yes __No
Left:	__Yes __No	__Yes __No	__Yes __No

6. Patient can use feet for repetitive movements as in operating foot controls:

Right	Left	Both
__Yes __No	__Yes __No	__Yes __No

KEY: Occasionally = 1% - 33% of an 8-hour workday
    Frequently = 34% - 66% of an 8-hour workday
    Continuously = 67% - 100% of an 8-hour workday

Figure 10-4   Sample physical capacities form. *(Cont'd)*

Table 10-10   Issues to Consider in Determining Physical Capacities

1. What physical capacities issues need to be addressed to determine the patient's eligibility for disability benefits? (*Example:* Most jobs do not require employees to run. Therefore the ability of a patient to run is usually irrelevant to an evaluation of his/her disability.)

2. Does the patient have a clear diagnosis?

3. Does this diagnosis provide clear information about the nature and severity of the activity restrictions the patient is likely to have?

4. Are the patient's symptoms and physical findings consistent over time? Consistent with his/her diagnosis?

5. Does the patient describe activity limitations that are plausible, given the medical information you have on him/her?

6. Do you have reports or behavioral data on the patient's activities outside your medical office?
   a) Data from day-to-day life (e.g., reports from spouse or employer; surveillance tapes)
   b) Data from a Functional Capacities Evaluation
   c) Data from a rehabilitation program (e.g., a work hardening program) or a pain center

7. What is your overall assessment of the patient's credibility?

---

shown in Figure 10-5. Note that the form includes a section in which you are asked whether you believe your patient can perform the job.

A detailed job analysis can be extremely helpful in the assessment of the work demands that a patient is likely to face. However, if the job analysis describes work your patient has done in the past, you need to check with the patient to see if she agrees with the physical requirements listed in the analysis. If the patient vigorously disputes it, attempt to reconcile the discrepancies.

JOB TITLE: **Taxi Dispatcher**   GOE: 07.04.05
DOT: 913.367-010   SVP: 3

JOB DESCRIPTION: Dispatches taxicabs in response to telephone requests for service by entering client name and pick-up and drop-off locations into the computer. Directs calls to dispatch supervisor if necessary.

JOB QUALIFICATIONS: Good customer service skills; ability to type and learn computer program.

TYPES OF MACHINES, TOOLS, SPECIAL EQUIPMENT USED: Telephone with headset; computer.

WORK SCHEDULE: Full-time, 8-hour shifts.

PHYSICAL DEMANDS

1. Stand: Occasionally. Daily total = 0.5 hours
2. Walk: Occasionally. Daily total = 0.5 hours
3. Sit: Constantly with option to stand. Daily total = 7 hours
4. Lift/carry: Occasionally lift/carry
5. Push/pull: Occasionally with minimum force to open file drawers and keyboard trays
6. Controls: Frequently use controls on telephone. Most calls are incoming.
7. Climb: Not required
8. Balance: Not required
9. Bend/stoop: Rarely-to-occasionally
10. Crouch: Not required
11. Twist: Occasionally at the neck while answering the phones
12. Kneel: Not required
13. Crawl: Not required
14. Handle/grasp: Occasionally handle/grasp office supplies and handset
15. Fine manipulation/Fingering: Frequent-to-constant typing is involved during workday. Fingering to dial telephone.
16. Feeling: Not required
17. Reach: Occasionally at mid-waist level, ¾ to full arm extension
18. Vision: Correctable vision is desirable.
19. Talk/Hear: Speech and hearing are mandatory.
20. Taste/Smell: Not required
21. Environmental Factors: Office environment. Floors are carpeted.
22. Work Environment Access: On-site parking available

PHYSICIAN'S JUDGMENT (Check and complete)

❑ The injured worker can perform this job without restrictions and can return to work on
_____.

❑ The injured worker can perform this job without restrictions, but only on a part-time basis for _____ hours per day, _____ days per week. The worker can be expected to return to full-time in _____ days/weeks.

❑ The injured worker can perform this job, but only with the following modifications:
_____. Modifications are needed on a
____permanent ____ temporary basis.

❑ The injured worker temporarily cannot perform this job based on the following physical limitations: _____.
Anticipated release date: _____

❑ The injured worker permanently cannot perform this job based on the following physical limitations: _____.

COMMENTS:

_____   _____
Signature of Physician   Date

Figure 10-5   Sample job analysis form.

Sometimes you will be provided with only a job analysis; in other situations, you will be asked further questions For example, you may be asked to rate the general category of work for which the patient is suited. Broad work categories are defined in several references (57,62,63): *sedentary, light, medium, heavy,* and *very heavy.* The problem with these work categories is that they might not capture specific requirements of jobs for which your patient might be considered. When you are asked to place your patient in a general work category, probably the best approach is to obtain the physical capacities data and then use them to assign the patient.

You may also be given trick questions dealing with employability. For example, you are treating a patient with chronic LBP who has failed multiple spine surgeries and continues to complain of relentless pain despite the implantation of an intrathecal opiate delivery system. You do not believe it is realistic for this patient to return to competitive employment. A disability agency asks whether your patient can work as a telephone solicitor. This question poses a dilemma. If you indicate "Yes", your patient will probably have his disability benefits terminated. If you say "No", you are implicitly saying that the patient's LBP prevents him from doing a job that has essentially no physical demands. The "trick" in this type of situation is that disability adjudicators or vocational rehabilitation counselors sometimes concoct jobs specifically because they demand essentially nothing in the way of physical capacities. When asked a question like this one, you have good reason to be suspicious that the disability system is maneuvering to terminate the patient's benefits. In this situation, it is appropriate to protect your patient and to demand details regarding the proposed job. Ask the adjudicator whether there is an opening for the job and whether the patient would have to commute to an office in order to perform it.

Some patients drag their feet and emphasize the severity of their incapacitation. These behaviors should make you suspicious of their agendas. In such a situation, it is reasonable to stick closely to objective data regarding the patient's capacities, rather than to be influenced strongly by the patient's subjective assessments.

*   *   *

It is important to make an employability determination that is acceptable to your patient whenever this is possible. Physicians sometimes feel that they have resolved a difficult disability claim when they say a patient is capable of employment. If the patient strongly disagrees with this conclusion, she may simply go to another physician or retain an attorney. In many instances, the anticipated resolution of the claim turns out to be ephemeral. The recommendation here is *not* to let the patient dictate what you say on a disability form. Nevertheless, listen carefully to your patient's concerns about employment and look for an employment plan that is both medically sensible and acceptable to the patient and the disability system.

It is worth noting that you can sometimes use disability evaluations as springboards to mobilize patients to take an active role in their vocational rehabilitation. Some chronically disabled patients passively wait for "the system" to solve their vocational dilemmas. When they see the jobs that are proposed during disability evaluations, they are often appalled. In this setting, you can encourage your patient to become more active in seeking vocational options on her own.

Impairment

Permanent partial impairment (PPI) from a work injury may be awarded when a WC claim is closed. Detailed systems have been developed to determine how WC systems will make PPI awards. For example, the fifth edition of the AMA's *Guides to the Evaluation of Permanent Impairment* (53) is 613 pages long and is devoted entirely to procedures that physicians should use to determine PPI awards.

It is important to note that although PPI awards are important financially to an IW, a decision about a PPI award does not affect the rest of the management of a claim. In particular, decisions about medical treatment and vocational rehabilitation are generally independent of the decision that is ultimately made about the amount of permanent impairment compensation a worker should be awarded.

Unless a major part of your practice is devoted to the treatment of IWs, it is probably inefficient for you to learn the subtleties involved in rating permanent partial impairment. It is appropriate to identify a colleague who can help you when a claim is about to be closed and the question of PPI arises.

Follow-Up

Your responses to a disability form may have ongoing consequences for your relationship with your patient. Some patients will object if your statements on a disability form suggest that they are capable of working. In other situations, you and your patient may agree about the information you put on a disability form, but the WC carrier to which the form is submitted may reach a decision that is adverse to the patient's interests. The patient may then feel that you have incompetently or wrongly filled out the form. The best way to avoid such recriminations is to tell your patient at the outset that disability decisions are made by adjudicators rather by physicians, and that you cannot provide information that will guarantee a favorable outcome.

Responses to a disability form may have consequences for your relationship with your patient even if they do not cause any overt conflict. For example, if the WC carrier closes your patient's claim after they have processed the information you have provided, she may experience an increase in the financial obligation she faces when she gets care from you. In an extreme case, an IW may have no health coverage at all after her claim is closed. This is particularly likely if she has lost both the job she had at the time of injury and the medical insurance that came with the job. Before the WC carrier responds to the information you provide about your patient's status, you should talk with her about whether she wants to continue treatment after the claim has been closed and, if so, how she will pay for the treatment.

* * *

A case study of an injured worker with low back pain and a discussion of his disability management are given in the Appendix (page 331).

Conclusion

Disability management is challenging and involves expertise that is almost never taught to physicians during their training. The challenges are particularly great when patients have medical conditions in which pain plays a major role. This chapter has focused on the management of patients with workers' compensation claims. There are many disability systems other than workers' compensation, but none of them is as complex and demanding of your time and energy. As a rule of thumb, if you can manage disability in injured workers, you can probably manage disability in patients applying for Social Security disability or other kinds of disability programs.

Given the fact that millions of Americans seek work disability benefits every year, the medical literature on disability evaluation and management is surprisingly sparse. But as the above discussion indicates, there are some practical steps you can take to facilitate interactions with your patients who have work injuries, including developing strategies for assessing their risk of prolonged disability, contracting with them, and making interventions that are widely believed to reduce their risk of prolonged disability.

Interfacing between your patient and the WC carrier will undoubtedly test your skills in communication and diplomacy. Learn about the laws and regulations that govern the WC carriers with which you interact regularly, familiarize yourself with the main questions that the WC system will ask you to address, and develop strategies for answering them. As outlined above, the administrative needs of WC systems often conflict with the realities of patients, especially when patients have chronic pain. Thus you will have the challenge of finding a reasonable middle ground between the demands of your patients and the demands of the WC system.

After considering all the difficulties involved in disability management, you may well say "Why bother?" and decide that you will simply not treat work injuries. There are two rejoinders to that question. First, it is difficult to separate disability management from medical management in an injured worker. You will often find that as an IW slides into the morass of chronic disability, she will become progressively less responsive to medical or surgical management of her work injury. Thus, when you ignore disability issues, you jeopardize the outcome of your medical/surgical interventions. Second, disability is vitally important to our patients. As physicians, we go to great lengths to address the medical needs of our patients, because we want to make a difference in their lives. Disability management takes us out of our traditional role as physicians, but the emotional, financial, and often physical well-being of our patients depend on the success of their efforts to reintegrate into society and resume meaningful roles after work injuries. We can make a significant difference in their lives if we help them in these efforts.

REFERENCES

1. **Williams CA.** An International Comparison of Workers' Compensation. Boston: Kluwer Academic Publishers; 1991.
2. Analysis of Workers' Compensation Laws. Washington, DC: U.S. Chamber of Commerce; 1998.
3. **Osterweis M, Kleinman A, Mechanic D, eds.** Pain and Disability. Washington, DC: National Academy Press; 1987.
4. **Cheadle A, Franklin G, Wolfhagen C, et al.** Factors influencing the duration of work-related disability: a population-based study of Washington State workers' compensation. Am J Public Health. 1994;84:190-6.
5. Attending Doctor's Handbook, rev ed. Olympia, WA: State of Washington Department of Labor and Industries; 1999.
6. Acute Low-Back Problems in Adults. Clinical Practice Guideline No. 14/AHCPR Publication No. 95-0642. Rockville, MD: Department of Health and Human Services; 1994.
7. **Robinson JP.** Disability evaluation in painful conditions. In: Turk DC, Melzack R, eds. Handbook of Pain Assessment. New York: Guilford Press; 2001.
8. **Robinson JP.** Evaluation of function and disability. In: Loeser JD, ed. Bonica's Management of Pain, 3rd ed. Philadelphia: Lippincott Williams & Wilkins; 2001.
9. **Tousignant M, Rossignol M, Goulet L, Dassa C.** Occupational disability related to back pain: application of a theoretical model of work disability using prospective cohorts of manual workers. Am J Ind Med. 2000;37:410-22.
10. **Krause N, Frank JW, Dasinger LK et al.** Determinants of duration of disability and return-to-work after work-related injury and illness: challenges for future research. Am J Ind Med. 2001;40:464-84.
10a. **Fishbain DA, Cutler RB, Rosomoff HL, et al.** Impact of chronic pain patients' job perception variables on actual return to work. J Pain. 1997;13:197-206.
11. **Turner JA, Franklin G, Turk DC.** Predictors of chronic disability in injured workers: a systematic literature synthesis. Am J Ind Med. 2000;38:707-22.
12. **Committee on Ways and Means, U.S. House of Representatives.** 1996 Green Book. Washington, DC: U.S. Government Printing Office.
13. **LaPlante M, Carlson D.** Disability in the United States: Prevalence and Causes, 1992. Disability Statistics Report No. 7. Washington, DC: Department of Education, National Institute on Disability and Rehabilitation Research; 1996.

14. **Robinson JP, Fulton-Kehoe D, Wu R, Franklin G.** Predictors of response to pain center treatment (unpublished, 2000).

15. **Dasinger LK, Krause N, Deegan LJ, et al.** Physical workplace factors and return-to-work after compensated low back injury: a disability phase-specific analysis. J Occup Environ Med. 2000;42:323-33.

16. **Krause N, Dasinger LK, Deegan LJ, et al.** Psychosocial job factors and return-to-work after compensated low back injury: a disability phase-specific analysis. Am J Ind Med. 2001;40:374-92.

17. **MacKenzie EJ, Morris JA, Jurkovich GJ, et al.** Return-to-work following injury: the role of economic, social and job-related factors. Am J Public Health. 1998; 88:1630-7.

18. **Bigos SJ, Battie MC, Spengler DM, et al.** A longitudinal, prospective study of industrial back injury reporting. Clin Orthop. 1992;Jun(279):21-34.

19. **Marhold C, Linton SJ, Melin L.** Identification of obstacles for chronic pain patients to return to work: evaluation of a questionnaire. J Occup Rehabil. 2002;12:65-75.

20. **Shaw WS, Pransky G, Fitzgerald TE.** Early prognosis for low back disability: intervention strategies for health care providers. Disabil Rehabil. 2001;23:815-28.

21. **Rhodes LA, McPhillips-Tangum CA, Markham C, Klenk R.** The power of the visible: the meaning of diagnostic tests in chronic back pain. Soc Sci Med. 1999;48: 1189-203.

22. **Dasinger LK, Krause N, Thompson PJ, et al.** Doctor proactive communication, return-to-work recommendations, and duration of disability after a workers' compensation low back injury. J Occup Environ Med. 2001;43:515-25.

23. **Krause N, Ragland DR.** Occupational disability due to low back pain: a new interdisciplinary classification based on a phase model of disability. Spine. 1994;19:1011-20.

24. **Kendall NAS.** Psychosocial approaches to the prevention of chronic pain: the low back paradigm. Bailliere's Best Pract Res Clin Rheumatol. 1999;13:545-54.

25. **Loeser JD.** Mitigating the dangers of pursuing cure. In: Cohen MJM, Campbell JN (eds). Pain Treatment Centers at a Crossroads. Seattle: IASP Press; 1996.

26. **Wiesel SW, Feffer HL, Rothman RH.** Industrial low-back pain: a prospective evaluation of a standardized diagnostic and treatment protocol. Spine. 1984;9:199-203.

27. **Guzman J, Esmail R, Karjalainen K, et al.** Multidisciplinary rehabilitation for chronic low back pain: systematic review. BMJ. 2001;322:1511-6.

28. **van Tulder MW, Ostelo R, Vlaeyen JW, et al.** Behavioral treatment for chronic low back pain: a systematic review within the framework of the Cochrane Back Review Group. Spine. 2001;26:270-81.

29. **Burton AK, Waddell G, Tillotson KM, Summerton N.** Information and advice to patients with back pain can have a positive effect: a randomized controlled trial of a novel educational booklet in primary care. Spine. 1999;24:2484-91.

30. **Hagen EM, Eriksen HR, Ursin H.** Does early intervention with a light mobilization program reduce long-term sick leave for low back pain? Spine. 2000;25:1973-6.

31. **Hilde G, Hagen KB, Jamtvedt G, Winnem M.** Advice to stay active as a single treatment for low back pain and sciatica. Cochrane Database Syst Rev. 2002;(2): CD003632.

32. **Indahl A, Haldorsen EH, Holm S, et al.** Five-year follow-up study of a controlled clinical trial using light mobilization and an informative approach to low back pain. Spine. 1998;23:2625-30.

33. **Von Korff M, Barlow W, Cherkin D, Deyo RA.** Effects of practice style in managing back pain. An Intern Med. 1994;121:187-95.

34. **Cherkin DC, Deyo RA, Street JH, et al.** Pitfalls of patient education: limited success of a program for back pain in primary care. Spine. 1996;21:345-55.

35. **Hazard RG, Haugh LD, Reid S, et al.** Early physician notification of patient disability risk and clinical guidelines after low back injury: a randomized, controlled trial. Spine. 1997;22:2951-8.

36. **Hazard RG, Reid S, Haugh LD, McFarlane G.** A controlled trial of an educational pamphlet to prevent disability after occupational low back injury. Spine. 2000;25: 1419-23.

37. **Cedraschi C, Nordin M, Nachemson AL, Vischer TL.** Health care providers should use a common language in relation to low back pain patients. Baillieres Best Pract Res Clin Rheumatol. 1998;12:1-15.

38. **Nordin M, Cedraschi C, Skovron ML.** Patient-health care provider relationship in patients with non-specific low back pain: a review of some problem situations. Baillieres Best Pract Res Clin Rheumatol. 1998;12:75-92.

39. **Frank JW, Brooker A, Demaio SE, et al.** Disability resulting from occupational low back pain. Part II: What do we know about secondary prevention? A review of the scientific evidence on prevention after disability begins. Spine.1996;21:2918-29.

40. **Hunt HA, Habeck, Habeck RV.** The Michigan disability prevention study: research highlights. Kalamazoo, MI: WE Upjohn Institute for Employment Research; 1993.

41. **Volinn E.** Do workplace interventions prevent low-back disorders? If so, why? A methodologic commentary. Ergonomics. 1999;42:258-72.

42. **Waddell G, Burton AK.** Occupational health guidelines for the management of low back pain at work: evidence review. Occup Med. 2001;51:124-35.

43. **Robinson JP, Rondinelli RD, Scheer SJ.** Industrial rehabilitation medicine. 1: Why is industrial rehabilitation medicine unique? Arch Phys Med Rehabil. 1997; 78:S3-S9.

44. **Breslau J, Seidenwurm D.** Socioeconomic aspects of spinal imaging: impact of radiological diagnosis on lumbar spine-related disability. Top Magn Reson Imaging. 2000;11:218-23.

45. **Atlas SJ, Deyo RA.** Evaluating and managing acute low back pain in the primary care setting. J Gen Intern Med. 2001;16:120-31.

46. **Borkan J, Van Tulder M, Reis S, et al.** Advances in the field of low back pain in primary care. Spine. 2002;27:E128-32.

47. **Deyo RA, Phillips WR.** Low back pain: a primary care challenge. Spine. 1996;21: 2826-32.

48. **Owen JP, Rutt G, Keir MJ, et al.** Survey of general practitioners' opinions on the role of radiology in patients with low back pain. Br J Gen Pract. 1990;40:98-101.

49. **Faust D.** The detection of deception. Neuroimaging Clin N Am. 1995;13:255-65.

50. **Hadjistavropoulos T, Craig KD.** A theoretical framework for understanding self-report and observational measures of pain: a communications model. Behav Res Ther. 2002;40:551-70.

51. **Hall HV, Pritchard DA.** Detecting Malingering and Deception. Delray Beach, FL: St. Lucie Press; 1996.

52. **Hill ML, Craig KD.** Detecting deception in pain expressions: the structure of genuine and deceptive facial displays. Pain. 2002;98:135-44.

53. **Cocchiarella L, Andersson GBJ, eds.** Guides to the Evaluation of Permanent Impairment, 5th ed. Chicago: American Medical Association; 2001.

54. **Cocchiarella L, Lord SJ.** Master the AMA Guides, 5th ed. Chicago: American Medical Association; 2001.

55. **Turk DC, Robinson JP, Aulet, M.** The Impairment Impact Inventory: comparison of responses by treatment-seekers and claimants undergoing independent medical examinations. J Pain. 2002;3(Suppl 1):1.

56. **King PM, Tuckwell N, Barrett TE.** A critical review of functional capacity evaluations. Phys Ther. 1998;78:852-66.

57. **Lechner DE.** Functional capacity evaluation. In: King PM, ed. Sourcebook of Occupational Rehabilitation. New York: Plenum Press; 1998.

58. **Rondinelli RD, Katz RT, eds.** Impairment Rating and Disability Evaluation. Philadelphia: WB Saunders; 2000.

59. **Hildebrandt J, Pfingsten M, Saur P, Jansen J.** Prediction of success from a multidisciplinary treatment program for chronic low back pain. Spine. 1997;22:990-1001.

60. **Mayer TG.** Functional Restoration for Spinal Disorders: The Sports Medicine Approach. Philadelphia: Lea & Febiger; 1988.

61. **Niemeyer LO, Jacobs K, Reynolds-Lynch K, et al.** Work hardening: past, present and future. The Work Programs Special Interest Section National Work Hardening Outcome Study. Am J Occup Ther. 1994;48:327-39.

62. **Field JE, Field, TF.** Classification of Jobs. Athens, GA: Elliott & Fitzpatrick; 1992.

63. **Department of Labor Employment and Training Administration.** Dictionary of Occupational Titles, 4th ed. Washington DC: U.S. Government Printing Office; 1977.

11

■ ■ ■

Psychosocial Factors in Chronic Pain Patients: When To Refer

Dennis C. Turk, PhD

ow we think about pain influences the ways in which we evaluate patients who report pain. Clinicians often assume that physical pathology must be present as a necessary and sufficient cause of pain and that the amount of pain reported should be proportional to the extent of the pathology. Consequently, physicians often order laboratory tests and diagnostic imaging procedures in an attempt to identify or confirm the presence of physical pathology that corresponds with the pain report. In the absence of organic pathology or when the objective findings are judged to be inadequate to validate the patient's report of pain, the physician may assume that the patient's report results primarily from emotional factors.

In a case of chronic or recurrent pain, there are a number of perplexing features that do not support the assumption of a simple one-to-one correspondence between the report of pain and underlying physical pathology. For example, the organic etiological basis for two of the most common chronic and recurring acute pain problems (back pain and headache, respectively) is largely unknown. Conversely, there are reports demonstrating that plain radiography, computed tomography scans, and magnetic resonance imaging reveal structural abnormalities such as herniated discs resulting in impingement of neural structures and spinal stenosis in more than 30% of asymptomatic individuals who might be expected to report pain (1,2).

Another conundrum is the observation that the identical surgical procedure, performed after a standard protocol, on patients with the same objective physical pathology may have very different outcomes (3). In one patient the pain may be absent immediately after surgery as anticipated, whereas another patient finds no benefit and may even report the pain is worse. Finally, studies have shown only a modest association between the patients' levels of pain, functional impairment, and degree of tissue pathology (4).

Although factors other than organic pathology have been shown to play a part in these otherwise puzzling observations, further complexities, particularly those of the psychosocial context, may compound the dissociation between pain and physical pathology. Failure to address the complexities of pain may undermine or even mislead our understanding and treatment for chronic and recurrent pain.

Missing from the equation may be a patient's phenomenological representation of pain and the role of contextual factors. Research has implicated the role of the patient's idiosyncratic appraisals of his or her symptoms, expectations regarding the cause of the symptoms, and the meaning of the symptoms, in addition to organic factors, as being essential in understanding the individual's report of pain and subsequent disability (5). Moreover, the patient's mood states, coping resources, and environmental factors may also have a significant effect on modulation of the pain experience (6,7). Consequently, understanding and appropriately treating a patient with pain, particularly chronic and recurrent pain, require an accurate evaluation not only of the underlying organic pathology that may be contributing to the report of pain but also specific psychosocial, behavioral, and psychological factors such as their current mood (e.g., anxiety, depression, anger), interpretation of the symptoms, expectations about the meaning of their symptoms, and responses to the patient's symptoms by significant others, each of which contribute to the subjective presentation (7).

Chronic pain by its very nature extends over long periods of time, often with no end in sight. People will likely continue to experience pain for years, even decades, despite the best efforts of health care providers. The longer pain persists the bigger the impact will be on the pain sufferer's life and the more psychosocial variables will play a role.

The Plight of the Person with Chronic Pain

As with any disease or injury, pain occurs in the context of an individual person, a person with his or her own unique history and one who lives in a social context. Failure to consider the individual and that he or she has a personal history leads to an inadequate understanding and inadequate response to any treatment. Consider a 30-year-old mother of two with migraine headaches who works as a salesperson, a 45-year-old married truck driver with back pain whose wife also works, and a 72-year-old widow living alone with severe osteoarthritis in both of her knees. Although they have pain in common, their unique histories, lives, responsibilities, social supports, and resources vary substantially and will necessarily affect their adaptation to their chronic pain. Because we cannot necessarily eliminate these patients' symptoms, we must bear in mind the myriad of other factors that affect adaptation to pain.

The person who has a chronic pain condition resides in a complex and costly world. The pain condition affects not only the pain sufferer, but also that person's family, health care providers, employers, and third-party payers (insurance companies, government). Family members feel increasingly hopeless and distressed as medical costs, disability, and emotional suffering increase while income and available treatment options decline. Health care providers grow increasingly frustrated as available medical treatment options are exhausted while the pain condition does not abate or worsens. Employers and co-workers grow resentful as productivity declines because the employee frequently is absent from work and others must take over the responsibilities of the absent worker. Government officials are helpless to keep health care costs from soaring with repeated diagnostic testing and growing numbers of unsuccessful treatments, as they are unable to control claims despite repeated efforts at legislation.

In time, those involved may question the legitimacy of the person's pain reports because many times no medical basis of the problem is adequate to substantiate the reported symptoms. Some may suggest that the pain sufferer is attempting to gain attention, avoid undesirable activities, or seek payments for disability compensation. Others may suggest that the pain is not real and is all "psychological." Indeed, psychosocial factors have been shown to be significant predictors of pain, distress, treatment seeking, disability, and response to any treatment (8). These results, however, should not be taken to indicate that psychological factors caused the pain or that the pain is imaginary.

Although people with acute pain often receive relief from primary health care providers, people with persistent pain frequently become enmeshed in the medical community as they travel from doctor to doctor, laboratory test to laboratory test, and imaging procedure to imaging procedure in a continuing pilgrimage to have their pain diagnosed and successfully treated. For many the pain becomes the central focus of their lives. As they withdraw from society, they lose their jobs, alienate family and friends, and become increasingly isolated. The quest for relief often remains elusive. The emotional distress that is commonly observed in chronic pain sufferers may be attributed to a variety of factors, including fear, inadequate or maladaptive support systems and other coping resources, treated-induced (iatrogenic) complications, overuse of potent drugs, inability to work, financial difficulties, prolonged litigation, disruption of usual activities, and sleep disturbance.

Moreover, the experience of "medical limbo" (a painful condition that eludes diagnosis and implies psychiatric causation, malingering, or an undiagnosed life-threatening disease) is itself a source of stress and can initiate psychological distress or aggravate a premorbid psychiatric condition

(Fig. 11-1). In the case of cancer, the stress of pain is superimposed on the general fear of living and possibly dying from a lethal disease.

In contrast to acute pain, persistent pain confronts people not only with the stress created by pain but with a cascade of ongoing stressors that compromise all aspects of their lives. Living with persistent pain conditions requires considerable emotional resilience, tends to deplete people's emotional reserves, and taxes not only the individual sufferer but also the capacity of family, friends, coworkers, and employers to provide support. Thus, it should hardly be surprising that patients become self-preoccupied and experience feelings of anger, demoralization, helplessness, hopelessness, frustration, isolation, depression, and pervasive demoralization.

Research suggests that 40% to 50% of chronic pain patients suffer from depression (9). It is not surprising that chronic pain patients are depressed. Rather, it is interesting to ponder the other side of the coin: Given the nature of the symptoms and the problems created by chronic pain, why are not all sufferers depressed? Turk and colleagues examined this question and determined that two factors appear to mediate the pain-depression relationship: patients' appraisals of the effects of the pain on their lives and

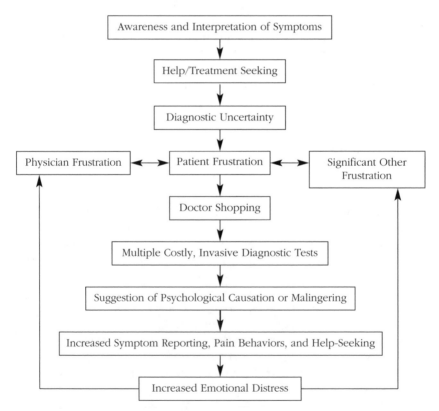

Figure 11-1   Natural history of persistent pain from the patient's perspective.

appraisals of their ability to exert any control over their pain and lives (10,11); that is, those patients who believed that they could continue to function and maintain some control despite their pain were less likely to become depressed.

It becomes obvious that assessing a patient who reports the presence of pain is not solely a matter of attempting to uncover the physical etiology for the symptom. By and large, researchers and clinicians are increasingly adopting the view that every individual who becomes a pain patient has a unique set of circumstances that will affect his or her prognosis. Thus, our assessments of pain patients need to encompass a wide range of psychosocial variables.

Psychosocial Assessment of Chronic Pain Sufferers

The sheer number of psychosocial factors that need to be considered and their complex relationship to pain may very well discourage the primary care provider. Given limited resources, time, and education about assessment of psychosocial factors, how can most primary care providers be expected to manage patients with chronic pain?

The initial psychosocial assessment can be relatively brief. When appropriate, a referral may be indicated for a more thorough evaluation. The objectives of the initial screening and a more comprehensive assessment are to determine the extent to which cognitive, emotional, or behavioral factors are amplifying the pain experience, interfering with functioning, or impeding rehabilitation. Table 11-1 gives three central questions that can guide assessment of people who report chronic pain (12).

Initial Psychosocial Screening

A brief psychosocial screening should be a standard component of the assessment of any patient with chronic pain. Patients should be asked how pain affects their activities (e.g., socializing, eating, ambulating), current and

Table 11-1   Three Central Questions That Should Guide Chronic Pain Assessment

1. What is the extent of the patient's disease or injury (physical impairment)?

2. What is the magnitude of the illness? That is, to what extent is the patient suffering, disabled, and unable to function and enjoy usual activities?

3. How do environmental and behavioral factors influence, and how are they influenced by, the patient's pain? [e.g., What is the patient doing or no longer doing because of pain? How do others respond to the patient's communications regarding pain? How do these responses influence the patient's reports of pain? How does the patient try to cope with pain?]

and past treatments for pain, and their own expectations for pain relief. In addition, behavioral manifestations of pain, "pain behaviors," should be observed (e.g., limping, protective body postures, moaning), and changes should be noted.

Under ideal circumstances, psychological screenings can take as little as 15 minutes, particularly if patients complete paper-and-pencil questionnaires ahead of time. The use of surveys, inventories, and questionnaires will be covered in a later section.

Physicians and other health care providers should conduct a brief screening with all chronic pain patients to determine whether they require a more comprehensive psychological evaluation. Table 11-2 includes areas that should be examined and some sample questions. When a patient demonstrates problems in response to 9 of the 16 areas included in the inquiry or shows a particularly extreme or worrisome response to any one of the questions, we recommend referral for a comprehensive psychological assessment. Table 11-3 lists the topics covered in such an assessment; we expand on several of the areas below to provide additional clarification.

Inappropriate Medication Use/Substance Abuse

A particular concern is that of substance abuse. When patients make frequent requests for increased or stronger medications, rely solely on medications for relief, or when there are indications that the patient may be over-medicated (e.g., the patient can no longer do his job because he is too sedated), a thorough psychological evaluation may be warranted. Patients seeking pain relief may inadvertently become dependent on prescription medications. They may also make use of alcohol and illicit drugs to palliate their symptoms. Patients with histories of substance abuse may be at particular risk for becoming dependent on pain medications. Reviewing the chart and conducting a detailed history of previous and current prescription and substance use may help ascertain whether this area warrants further inquiry.

Excessive Physical, Work, Family, or Social Dysfunction

Patients who abandon most physical activities and who greatly reduce family responsibilities and social activities are at greater risk for problems associated with persistent pain. Lack of physical activity can lead to weakened and more vulnerable muscles, which are more susceptible to exacerbation of pain. Physical deconditioning can further reduce activity, leading to even greater loss of muscle strength, flexibility, and endurance.

Disengagement from family, social activities, or employment can have a number of repercussions, such as leading the patient to greater isolation and diminished self-esteem, and ultimately greater disability. If pain patients demonstrate poor social and physical functioning, particularly in light of the fact that there is little of evidence of physical pathology, a comprehensive evaluation may clarify their situation and help to identify issues to be addressed in a comprehensive treatment plan. One way to assess patient

Table 11-2   Screening Questions for Chronic Pain

If there is a combination of six or more "Yes" answers to the first 14 questions and all "No" answers to Questions 15 to 17, or if there are general concerns in any one area, consider referral for psychological assessment.

1. Has the patient's pain persisted for 3 months or longer despite appropriate interventions and in the absence of progressive disease? [Yes]

2. Does the patient repeatedly and excessively use the health care system, persist in seeking invasive investigations or treatments after being informed they are inappropriate, or use opioid or sedative-hypnotic medications or alcohol in a pattern of concern (i.e., escalating use)? [Yes]

3. Does the patient request specific opioid medication (e.g., dilaudid, oxycontin)? [Yes]

4. Does the patient have unrealistic expectations of the health care providers or the treatment offered ("Total elimination of pain and related symptoms")? [Yes]

5. Does the patient have a history of substance abuse or is he/she currently abusing mind-altering substances? [Yes] Patients can be asked, "Have you ever found yourself taking more medication than was prescribed or have you used alcohol because your pain was so bad?" or "Is anyone in your family concerned about the amount of medication you take?"

6. Does the patient display a large number of pain behaviors that appear exaggerated (e.g., grimacing, rigid or guarded posture)? [Yes]

7. Does the patient have litigation pending? [Yes]

8. Is the patient seeking or receiving disability compensation? [Yes]

9. Does the patient have any other family members who have had or currently suffer from chronic pain conditions? [Yes]

10. Does the patient demonstrate excessive depression or anxiety? [Yes] Straightforward questions such as "Have you been feeling down?" or "What effect has your pain had on your mood?" can clarify whether this area is in need of detailed evaluation.

11. Can the patient identify a significant or several stressful life events (e.g., death of a family member, divorce, loss of a job) prior to symptom onset or exacerbation? [Yes]

12. If married or living with a partner, does the patient indicate a high degree of interpersonal conflict? [Yes]

13. Does pain have a significant impact on the patient's life? [Yes] Ask the patient how much pain has affected different daily activities (e.g., physical, social, recreational, sleep) or provide the patient with a list of functional activities (see, for example, the Impairment Impact Inventory [34]).

14. Has the patient given up many activities (recreational, social, familial, in addition to occupational and work activities) due to pain? [Yes]

15. Does the patient have any plans for renewed or increased activities if pain is reduced? [No]

16. Was the patient employed prior to pain onset? [No] If "Yes," does he or she wish to return to that job or any job? [No]

17. Does the patient believe that he or she will ever be able to resume normal life and normal functioning? [No]

Table 11-3   Topics Covered in Comprehensive Interview with Patient with Chronic Pain

Experience of Pain and Related Symptoms

- Location and description of pain (e.g., sharp, burning)
- Onset and progression
- Perception of cause (e.g., trauma, virus, stress)
- What has the patient been told about his/her symptoms and condition? Do they believe that what they have been told is accurate?
- Exacerbating and relieving factors (e.g., exercise, relaxation, stress, massage). For example: "What makes your pain worse?" and "What makes your pain better?"
- Pattern of symptoms (e.g., symptoms worse certain times of day or after activity or stress).
- Sleep habits (e.g., difficulty falling asleep or maintaining sleep, sleep hygiene).
- Thoughts, feelings, and behaviors that proceed, accompany, and follow fluctuations in symptoms.

Previous and Current Treatments

- Medication (prescribed and over-the-counter). How helpful have these been?
- Pattern of medication use (prn, time-contingent), changes in quantity or schedule.
- Physical modalities (e.g., physical therapy). How helpful have these been?
- Exercise (e.g., Does patient participate in a regular exercise routine? Is there evidence of deactivation and avoidance of activity due to fear of pain or exacerbation of injury?). Has the exercise pattern changed (increased, decreased)?
- Complementary and alternative (e.g., chiropractic manipulation, relaxation training). How helpful have these been?
- Which treatments has the patient found most helpful?
- Compliance/adherence with recommendations of health care providers.
- Attitudes towards previous health care providers.

Compensation/Litigation

- Current disability status (e.g., receiving or seeking disability, amount, percent of former job income, expected duration of support).
- Current or planned litigation (e.g., "Have you hired an attorney?").

Responses by Patient and Significant Others

- Typical daily routine ("How much time do you spend sitting, standing, lying down?").
- Changes in activities and responsibilities (both positive and obligatory) due to symptoms ("What activities did you use to engage in prior to your symptoms?" "How has this changed since your symptoms began?").
- Changes in significant other's activities and responsibilities due to patient's symptoms.
- Patient's behavior when pain increases or flares up ("What do you do when your pain is bothering you?" "Can others tell when your pain is bothering you?" "How do they know?").

(Cont'd)

Table 11-3   Topics Covered in Comprehensive Interview with Patient with Chronic Pain *(Cont'd)*

Responses by Patient and Significant Others

- Significant other's responses to behavioral expressions of pain ("How can your significant other tell when your pain is bad?" "What does your significant other do when he/she can tell your pain is bothering you?" "Are you satisfied with his/her responses?").
- What does the patient do when pain is not bothering him/her (uptime activities)?
- Significant other's response when patient is active ("How does your significant other respond to your engaging in activities?").
- Impact of symptoms on interpersonal, family, marital, and sexual relations (e.g., changes in desire, frequency, or enjoyment).
- Activities that patient avoids because of symptoms.
- Activities that continue despite symptoms.
- Pattern of activity and pacing of activity. Patients can record in a diary their daily activities (time spent sitting, standing, walking, reclining) for several days or weeks.

Coping

- How does the patient try to cope with his/her symptoms? (e.g., "What do you do when your pain worsens?" "How helpful are these efforts?").
- Does the patient view himself/herself as having any role in symptom management? What role?
- Current life stresses.
- Pleasant activities ("What do you enjoy doing?").

Educational and Vocational History

- Level of education completed (and any special training).
- Work history.
- Years at most recent job.
- How satisfied is the patient with most recent job and supervisor?
- What does the patient like least about his or her most recent job?
- Would the patient like to return to most recent job? If not, what type of work would he/she like?
- Current work status (including homemaking activities).
- Vocational and avocational plans.

Social History

- Relationships with family of origin.
- History of pain or disability in family members.
- History of substance abuse in family members.
- History of, or current, physical, emotional, and sexual abuse. Was the patient a witness to abuse of someone else?
- Marital history and current status.
- Quality of current marital and family relations.

(Cont'd)

Table 11-3   Topics Covered in Comprehensive Interview with Patient with Chronic Pain *(Cont'd)*

Alcohol and Substance Use

• Current and history of alcohol use (quantity, frequency).

• History and current use of illicit psychoactive drugs.

• History and current use of prescribed psychoactive medications.

• Consider the CAGE questions as a quick screen for alcohol dependence (35). Depending on response, consider other instruments for alcohol and substance abuse (36).

Psychological Dysfunction

• Current psychological symptoms/diagnosis (depression, including suicidal ideation, anxiety disorders, somatization, post-traumatic stress disorder). Depending on response, consider conducting formal Structured Clinical Interview (SCID) (37).

• Is the patient currently receiving treatment for psychological symptoms? If "Yes," what treatments (e.g., psychotherapy, psychiatric medications). How helpful are they?

• History of psychiatric disorders and treatment including family counseling.

• Family history of psychiatric disorders.

Concerns and Expectations

• Patient concerns/fears (e.g., Does the patient believe he/she has serious physical problems that have not been identified? Or that those symptoms will become progressively worse and patient will become more disabled and more dependent? Does the patient worry that he/she will be told that the symptoms are "only" psychological?)

• Explanatory models ("What have you been told is the cause of your symptoms?" "Does this explanation make sense?" "What do you think is the cause of your pain now?").

• Expectations regarding the future and regarding treatment (will get better, worse, never change).

• Attitude toward rehabilitation versus "cure".

• Treatment goals.

---

functioning is to inquire, "Are there things that you used to do that you no longer do because of your pain?"

Involvement in Litigation/Disability Compensation

Financial compensation from disability payments can serve as positive reinforcement for reports of pain. Financial compensation, especially when combined with other factors, such as those listed above, may contribute to disability. In order to briefly address this area, patients can be asked direct questions such as "Have you hired an attorney to assist you?" "What are your monthly disability payments?" and "What percent of your previous salary is covered by disability payments?" Ongoing litigation can also be an impediment to improvement. It is appropriate to ask patients whether they are currently involved in litigation related to their pain or have retained the services of an attorney and are considering litigation. Affirmative responses regarding litigation and compensation are not by themselves sufficient to warrant referral for a psychological evaluation but are worthy of note, and when combined with the other areas listed in Table 11-2 may suggest that a more comprehensive psychosocial assessment is warranted.

Beliefs About Current and Future Pain and Functioning

When patients have catastrophic beliefs about their situation or express hopelessness about their future, a referral for a psychological assessment is appropriate. Clinicians can ask patients questions about their beliefs such as "What do you believe is the cause of your pain?" and "Do you believe that your pain will improve?"

In addition to gathering information through an interview, health care professionals can administer any of a number of standardized self-report measures (see below and Table 11-3). These instruments are efficient means for obtaining relevant detailed information. Some of these measures require psychological expertise for interpretation; however, a number of instruments require little training (13). Many of these instruments were not developed specifically for chronic pain patients. As a result, it is always best to corroborate information gathered from these instruments with other sources such as chart review and interviews with the patient and significant others. [*Caution:* The results of such brief screening should not be used to diagnose but rather to assist the physician in determining whether a more comprehensive psychological evaluation is appropriate.]

Observation of Behavior

Observation of patients' behaviors (ambulation, body postures, facial expressions) should be made while they are being escorted to interview, during the interview, and when exiting interview. Dramatic, unusual, or any behaviors that communicate the presence and severity of pain should be noted. Observation of significant others' responses to patients can occur at the same time.

Pain behaviors are overt expressions that communicate pain and distress to others. They include verbal or motor behaviors that are almost automatic, such as limping and wincing, or they can be higher-order behavioral patterns such as taking medication or help seeking. Pain behaviors may result from reflexive avoidance of aversive experience or defense response to protect oneself. This is particularly evident in the case of acute pain. For example, we have all seen a person with a sprained ankle limp in an attempt to protect the injured area. In this case, pain behaviors serve to protect a person from exacerbating the pathology and exacerbating the pain. However, there are cases where some patients acquire and maintain pain behaviors because of environmental contingencies that provide reinforcement for the behaviors

(6). For example, if pain leads to limping and limping elicits attention from family members (a contingency pattern of limping), positive reinforcement may become established. Once such a contingency is established, pain may no longer be necessary to maintain limping behavior. Pain behaviors cease to serve as a protective mechanism; rather, their functions become a way to ensure the reinforcements. Several checklists are available to assist in assessing pain behaviors; a sample is provided in Table 11-4 (14).

In addition to quantifying pain behaviors, interviews with patients and their significant others can help identify the controlling factors that reinforce and perpetuate the maladaptive pain behaviors. During an interview, the physician can observe the nonverbal behavior between patients and significant others and identify the topics that are consistently associated with the behavior. For example, the physician should attend to whether pain behaviors are displayed more frequently when the spouse is present. If the significant other is present when pain behaviors occur, the physician should note the following:

- How does he or she respond?
- How do others know when the patient has increased pain, and how do they respond? How does the significant other infer presence of pain, and what does he or she do?
- How do others respond to well behaviors? That is, are behaviors incompatible with disability?
- Are there inconsistencies between patient or spouse report or between interviewer observation of pain behaviors and spouse response?

Table 11-4   Pain Behavior Checklist

Pain behaviors have been characterized as interpersonal communications of pain, distress, or suffering. Place a check in the box next to each behavior you either observe or infer from the patient's comments.

- ❏ Facial grimacing
- ❏ Holding or supporting affected body area
- ❏ Limping or distorted gait
- ❏ Frequent shifting of posture or position
- ❏ Moving extremely slowly
- ❏ Sitting with a rigid posture
- ❏ Moving in a guarded or protective fashion
- ❏ Moaning
- ❏ Using a cane, cervical collar, or other prosthetic device
- ❏ Stopping frequently while walking

Reported use of the health care system and analgesic medication are other ways to assess pain behaviors. Patients can complete diaries in which they record the times when they take medication over a specified interval such as a week. Diaries not only provide information about the frequency and quantity of medication but may permit identification of the antecedent and consequent events of medication use. For example, a patient might note that he took medication after an argument with his wife and that when she saw him taking the medication she expressed sympathy. Antecedent events might include stress, negative thoughts, or activity.

Examination of antecedent is useful in identifying patterns of medication use that may be associated with factors other than pain per se. Similarly, patterns of response to the use of analgesic may be identified. Does the patient receive attention and sympathy whenever he or she is observed by significant others taking medication? That is, do significant others provide positive reinforcement for the taking of analgesic medication and thereby unwittingly increase medication use?

Standardized Self-Report Instruments

A large number of psychological instruments have been used to assess domains relevant to patients with chronic pain (13). A word of caution about psychological measures is in order: Many of these instruments were not developed on patients with medical problems.

Data gathered from measures not specifically developed or standardized on a chronic pain sample should be interpreted with caution because the medical condition may influence some of the responses. Items such as "I have few or no pains" "I am in just as good physical health as my friends" and "I am about as able to work as I ever was" (from the frequently used Minnesota Multiphasic Personality Inventory [MMPI]) illustrate the concern (15). It is reasonable to assume that the sensitivity of these measures may be relatively low and there may be a tendency to "over-pathologize" patients.

Cut-offs for depression on standard measures, such as the Beck Depression Inventory (16), do not apply to chronic pain patients. In addition, it is unclear how pain medications might affect the way patients respond to psychological instruments. As mentioned earlier, it is best to corroborate findings from psychological measures with other sources of information such as the patient or significant other interview or medical records. In some cases, it will not be possible to corroborate information, and interpretations should be made cautiously. Decisions regarding which self-report measures to select will depend, at least to some extent, upon the information obtained during the interview and data derived from the initial psychological screening instruments. Still, standardized assessment measures can provide another source of information about areas that appear to be influencing patients' adaptation to their pain and their response to treatment.

For example, if a high level of marital distress was identified during the interview, the psychologist may request that a patient and his or her spouse both complete a marital adjustment inventory to identify areas of conflict and congruence between the two partners (17). If a patient demonstrates a high degree of defensiveness and unusual personality characteristics during the interview, the examiner may request that he or she complete the MMPI/MMPI-2 to corroborate the clinical impression obtained during the interview (15,18). Patients' perceptions of the impact of pain on their lives can be directly assessed using measures, such as the Multidimensional Pain Inventory (MPI), that have been developed specifically for use with pain sufferers and permit comparisons of any individual patient with groups of other pain patients (19).

Self-Report of Functional Activities

Traditional physical and laboratory measures do not provide direct assessment of symptoms (i.e., subjective interpretations) or functional activities in everyday life; rather, they are proxies. Commonly used physical tests of muscle strength and range of motion correlate poorly with actual patient behavior (20). Similarly, radiographic indicators are only weak predictors of long-term functional capacity, and the validity of direct measures of physical performance such as trunk strength using computerized apparatus has been seriously challenged (21,22). In contrast, self-report functional status instruments quantify symptoms, function, and behavior more directly (23).

Several self-report measures assess patients' ability to engage in functional activities such as walking up stairs, sitting for a specific time, lifting specific weights, performing activities of daily living, and the severity of pain during these activities. Although the validity of self-reports of ability to perform activities is questionable, studies have found good correspondence among self-reports, disease characteristics, physicians' or physical therapists' ratings of functional abilities, and objective functional performance (24,25). Moreover, self-report instruments are economical and efficient. They enable the assessment of a wide range of relevant behaviors and permit social and mental functions to be evaluated.

Additionally, there are a number of brief functional assessment scales such as the Roland-Morris Disability Scale, the Functional Status Index, and the Oswestry Disability Scale (25-27). The measures require no more than 5 to 10 minutes to complete. Mikail, DeBreuil, and D'Eon attempted to delineate a core assessment battery for use with chronic pain patients (28). They factor analyzed nine self-report measures commonly used to assess chronic pain patients and concluded that a core assessment should evaluate general affective distress, social support, pain descriptions, and functional capacities. De Gagne, Mikail, and D'Eon followed up on the Mikail et al study and suggested that a set of measures including the MPI, BDI, and McGill Pain Questionnaire would be adequate to cover the four domains and this set should form the core assessment. I suggest substituting the short-form of the MPQ because it is simpler to use and score (29-31).

Purposes of a Comprehensive Psychosocial Evaluation

When health care professionals suspect that cognitive, emotional, or behavioral factors play a role in patients' suffering (nine or more items identified in Table 11-2 or a particularly concerning area identified during the initial screening), a comprehensive psychological evaluation is appropriate. A thorough psychological evaluation will reveal aspects of the patient's history that are relevant to the current situation. For example, the psychologist will gather information about psychological disorders, substance abuse or dependence, vocational difficulties, and family role models for chronic illness. In terms of current status, topics covered include recent life stresses; vocational, emotional, social, and physical functioning; and sleep patterns. The purpose of the evaluation is to examine whether historical or current factors are influencing the way the patient perceives and copes with pain.

The psychological evaluation cannot provide definitive information about the cause(s) of pain and other symptoms. Moreover, if psychological factors are identified as contributing to pain and disability, this does not preclude the possibility of physical pathology, just as the presence of positive physical findings does not necessarily preclude the possibility that psychological factors are contributing to the patient's pain.

Preparation of Patients for Psychosocial Evaluation

Many patients with persistent pain may not see the relevance of a psychological evaluation. They tend to view their symptoms as physical and are not accustomed to a biopsychosocial approach. Many believe that identification and treatment of the physical cause of their pain is the only road toward finding relief for their symptoms. When compensation or litigation issues are involved, patients may be particularly sensitive to the implications of a psychological evaluation. They may wonder, "Is this psychologist trying to figure out if I am exaggerating my symptoms?" Another concern they may have is that their health care providers believe they are "crazy" or that their pain is "all in their head".

When health care providers refer patients for a psychological evaluation, they can save the patient considerable grief and enhance patient co-operation by engaging in a brief discussion about why they were referred for such an evaluation. Specifically, the provider can inform the patient that an evaluation helps providers ensure that factors in the person's life, such as stress, are not interfering with treatment and not contributing to suffering. Patients can then be told that, used in conjunction with other treatments, those with persistent pain have found that psychological techniques can reduce their symptoms and help them better manage their pain and their lives (Table 11-5).

Table 11-5   Preparing a Patient with Chronic Pain for Psychological Evaluation Referral

---

- Acknowledge that you believe that the patient's experience of pain is real.

- Inform the patient that referral to a psychologist is necessary when pain begins to affect all aspects of life.

- Note that the purpose of the referral is to help formulate a comprehensive treatment plan that addresses both the physical factors involved with pain and the impact of pain on the patient's life.

- Inform the patient that information provided to a psychologist will be confidential and shared only with other health care professionals. If third-party payers are to obtain information, the patient will be alerted to this. Limitations of confidentiality, as required by law, need to be stated.

Although it is not ideal, when referral agents do not prepare patients for psychological evaluations, pain psychologists can provide the rationale for the evaluation themselves. One way for pain psychologists to establish rapport with these patients is to begin the evaluation as less "psychological charged," instead asking patients to describe their pain and its onset.

Ongoing Assessment

Once areas of concern are identified from the evaluation, it is important to develop a plan for how to assess progress. Because conducting repeat comprehensive evaluations will often not be feasible, one way to re-assess patients is to use the psychological screening described earlier. The screening should be supplemented with questions about the particular areas of concern that were detected in the prior comprehensive evaluation. In general, primary care physicians should look for signs that the patient's psychosocial, physical, and behavioral functioning have improved or declined. Several brief measures have been developed that may be used during process ratings (e.g., Pain Disability Index, 8 questions; Brief Pain Inventory-Short Form, 15 questions; and Impairment Impact Inventory, 26 questions [32-37]).

Patients may also be asked to complete diaries in which they report (daily, several times a day) the activities they performed (e.g., number of hours sitting, standing, walking), their mood (e.g., fear, anxiety, depression), thoughts, use of coping strategies, and sleep quality. Be advised that patients may not comply with the requested frequency. For example, instead of completing ratings three times a day, they may fill in all ratings at the end of the day or fill in the data that was supposed to be recorded daily at the end of the week.

There are more reasons to be cautious, however, in the selection of measures. If too little time has elapsed since the original evaluation, results of the measures may not be valid. Also, some psychological measures, such as the MMPI were not designed to assess mood state variables. Instead, most personality inventories are designed to measure traits, and traits should not be expected to change over the course of pain treatment. Hence, they should not be used as indicators of progress. Finally, frequent recording may draw attention to pain and emotional distress when one aspect of treatment may be encouraging distraction from symptoms.

Conclusion

Symptoms of chronic pain are extremely distressing and many times there is no cure or treatment capable of substantially reducing all symptoms. At the present time, rehabilitation, including improvement in emotional functioning, physical functioning, and quality of life, is the goal. Rehabilitation in spite of pain is a daunting task even for patients with ample coping skills.

The high levels of emotional distress, disability, and reduced quality of life noted in many chronic pain patients suggests that psychological screening is essential; in the majority of cases, a thorough psychological evaluation is called for. Biopsychosocial assessment allows health care professionals to tailor treatment to meet individual needs and preferences. A comprehensive assessment is a complex task, involving an exploration of a broad range of areas, and should be administered by an experienced health psychologist.

In contrast to acute pain where the focus of assessment and treatment is on cure, in chronic pain the focus is often on self-management. However, self-management requires many skills. A thorough psychological assessment allows health care professionals to examine what factors in a patient's history and current situation, including emotional well-being, social support, and behavioral factors, might interfere with their functioning. The information obtained should help treatment planning, specifically the matching of treatment components to the needs of individual patients. Once the whole person is evaluated, treatment can focus on the individual's unique needs.

REFERENCES

1. **Boden S, Davis D, Dina T, et al.** Abnormal magnetic-resonance scans of the lumbar spine in asymptomatic subjects: a prospective investigation. J Bone Joint Surg. 1990;72:403-8.
2. **Jensen M, Brant-Zawadski M, Obuchowski N, et al.** Magnetic resonance imaging of the lumbar spine in people with back pain. N Engl J Med. 1994;331:69-73.
3. **North RB, Campbell JN, James CS, et al.** Failed back surgery syndrome: 5-year follow-up in 102 patients undergoing repeated operation. Neurosurgery. 1991;28:685-90.
4. **Waddell G.** A new clinical model for the treatment of low back pain. Spine. 1987;12:632-44.
5. **Flor H, Turk DC.** Chronic back pain and rheumatoid arthritis: predicting pain and disability from cognitive variables. J Behav Med. 1988;11:251-65.

6. **Fordyce W.** Behavioral Methods in Chronic Pain and Illness. St. Louis: CV Mosby; 1976.

7. **Turk DC, Okifuji A.** Psychological factors in chronic pain: evolution and revolution. J Consult Clin Psychol. 2002;70:678-90.

8. **Boothby JL, Thorn BE, Stroud MW, Jensen MP.** Coping with pain. In: Gatchel RJ, Turk DC, eds. Psychosocial Factors in Pain: Critical Perspectives. New York: Guilford Press; 1999:343-59.

9. **Banks SM, Kerns RD.** Explaining high rates of depression in chronic pain: a diathesis-stress framework. Psychol Bull. 1996;119:95-110.

10. **Rudy TE, Kerns RD, Turk DC.** Chronic pain and depression: toward a cognitive-behavioral mediation model. Pain. 1988;35:129-40.

11. **Turk DC, Okifuji A, Scharff L.** Chronic pain and depression: role of perceived impact and perceived control in different age cohorts. Pain. 1995;61:93-101.

12. **Turk DC, Meichenbaum D.** Cognitive-behavioral approach to the management of chronic pain. In: Wall P, Melzack R, eds. Textbook of Pain, 3rd ed. London: Churchill Livingstone; 1994:1337-48.

13. **Turk DC, Melzack R, eds.** Handbook of Pain Assessment, 2nd ed. New York: Guilford Press; 2001.

14. **Keefe FJ, Williams DA, Smith, SJ.** Assessment of pain behaviors. In: Turk DC, Melzack R (eds). Handbook of Pain Assessment, 2nd ed. New York: Guilford Press; 2001:170-90.

15. **Hathaway SR, McKinley JC.** The Minnesota Multiphasic Personality Inventory Manual. New York: Psychological Corporation; 1967.

16. **Beck AT, Ward CH, Mendelson M, et al.** An inventory for measuring depression. Arch Gen Psychiatr. 1961;4:561-71.

17. **Spanier GB.** Measuring dyadic adjustment: new scales for assessing the quality of marriage and similar dyads. J Marriage Family. 1976;38:15-28.

18. **Hathaway SR, McKinley JC, Butcher JN.** The Minnesota Multiphasic Personality-2: Manual for Administration. Minneapolis: University of Minnesota Press; 1989.

19. **Kerns RD, Turk DC, Rudy TE.** The West Haven-Yale Multidimensional Pain Inventory (WHYMPI). Pain. 1985;23:345-56.

20. **Mellin G.** Correlations of spinal mobility with degree of chronic low back pain after correction for age and anthropometric factors. Spine. 1987;12:464-8.

21. **Frymoyer J, Hanley E, Howe J, et al.** Disc excision and spine fusion in the management of lumbar disc disease: a minimum ten-year follow-up. Spine. 1978; 3:1-6.

22. **Newton M, Waddell G.** Trunk strength testing with iso-machines. Part 1: review of a decade of scientific evidence. Spine. 1995;18:801-11.

23. **Deyo RA.** Measuring the functional status of patients with low back pain. Arch Phys Med Rehabil. 1988;69:1044-53.

24. **Deyo RA, Diehl AK.** Measuring physical and psychosocial function in patients with low back pain. Spine. 1983;8:635-42.

25. **Jette A.** The Functional Status Index: reliability and validity of a self-report functional disability measure. J Rheumatol. 1987;14(Suppl 15):15-21.

26. **Roland M, Morris R.** A study of the natural history of back pain. Part I: development of a reliable and sensitive measure of disability in low-back pain. Spine. 1983;8:141-4.

27. **Fairbank JCT, Couper J, Davies JB, O'Brien JP.** The Oswestry Low Back Pain Disability Questionnaire. Physiotherapy. 1980;66:271-73.

28. **Mikail SF, DuBreuil S, D'Eon JL.** A comparative analysis of measures used in the assessment of chronic pain patients. Psychol Assess: J Consult Clin Psychol. 1993;5: 111-20.

29. **De Gagne TA, Mikail SF, D'Eon JL.** Confirmatory factor analysis of a 4-factor model of chronic pain evaluation. Pain. 1995;60:195-202.

30. **Melzack R.** The McGill Pain Questionnaire: Major properties and scoring methods. Pain. 1975;1:277-99.

31. **Melzack R.** The Short-Form McGill Pain Questionnaire. Pain. 1987;30:191-7.

32. **Tait RC, Chibnall JT, Krause S.** The Pain Disability Index: psychometric properties. Pain. 1990;40:171-82.

33. **Cleeland CS.** Measurement of pain by subjective report. In: CR Chapman, JD Loeser, eds. Issues in Pain Assessment. New York: Raven Press; 1989:391-403.

34. **Turk DC, Robinson JR, Loeser JD, et al.** Pain. In: Cocchiarella L, Lord S, eds. Master the AMA Guides: A Medical and Legal Transition to the Guides to the Evaluation of Permanent Impairment, 5th ed. Chicago: AMA Press; 2001:277-325.

35. **Mayfield D, McLead G, Hall P.** The CAGE Questionnaire. Am J Psychiatry. 1987; 131:1121-3.

36. **Allen JP, Litten RZ.** Screening instruments and biochemical screening. In: Graham AW, Schultz TK, Wilford BB, eds. Principles of Addiction Medicine. Chevy Chase, MD: American Society of Addiction Medicine; 1998:263-72.

37. **American Psychiatric Association.** User's Guide for the Structured Clinical Interview for DSM-IV Axis I Disorders (SCID-1): Clinician Version. Washington, DC: American Psychiatric Press; 1997.

12

■ ■ ■

Addiction in Pain Management

Steven D. Passik, PhD

Kenneth L. Kirsh, PhD

remendous progress has been made in the study and treatment of pain in the past two decades (1,2). Efforts have been undertaken to make pain assessment and treatment a priority of medical care and to utilize all of the weapons in our armamentarium to bring relief to the millions of people with chronic pain, including opioid therapy for nonmalignant pain (3,4). Hundreds of thousands of pain patients have benefited from increased willingness to prescribe opioids. Unfortunately, the rhetoric of the pain community has tended to trivialize the complexities of treatment (5). The growing problem of prescription drug abuse has forced the field to take a new look at opioid prescribing and to seek balance in its risks and benefits. Although the rhetoric should be replaced with scientifically based approaches to clinical management, we should not abandon use of opioids: the dramatically expanded use of opioids was undertaken with a paucity of long-term data to justify it, but complete avoidance of opioids is equally unsupported.

When the president of the American Medical Association wrote famously in a 1941 editorial that "the use of narcotics in the terminal cancer [patient] is to be condemned if it can possibly be avoided...[because one] of the unfortunate [side] effects is addiction," he was voicing an extreme view on opioids with little basis in science (6). Today, all practitioners involved in pain management have the dual mission of relieving suffering without contributing to drug abuse. By understanding the principles of addiction medicine as they apply to pain management, health care providers can safely provide pain management to all who need it. Adequate assessment of aberrant behavior is key to mastering these principles.

Although initial reports were optimistic that the increasing production and use of opioids was not accompanied by increased abuse and diversion of these drugs, during the past 10 years the problem has become obvious (7). The media spectacle that accompanied the misuse of sustained-release oxycodone was only the most visible of a multitude of opioid abuses by well-known celebrities and other public figures (8). There is no doubt that much reporting of prescription drug abuse in the popular press has been inaccurate, sensationalized, unbalanced, and distasteful. As a result, many physicians were initially dismissive of the problem because its seriousness was actually obscured for them by the media circus. However, it has become abundantly clear, regardless of what index one uses to gauge the problem (e.g., the Drug Awareness Warning Network, the Household Survey), that prescription drug abuse is on the rise (9-11).

The national problem of prescription drug abuse is only part of the issue, however. Prescribers must also know what drugs are being abused locally, be aware of local trends, and prescribe specific medications carefully, especially if they happen to be locally "hot." For example, in a retrospective and ongoing prospective study in central and southeastern Kentucky, where the vast majority of our patients reside, we have learned a great deal about abuse of "hot" pain medications such as oxycodone and less popular ones such as fentanyl, and which patients are at particular risk for abuse or diversion (12). This understanding affects our work with fellow physicians when deciding which drugs to prescribe and strategies for prescribing the riskier agents. We have a duty to assess and treat our patients as individuals, but we must also assess and treat them in the context of existing drug abuse in their community.

Treatment and Good Practice

As physicians identify and treat patients with pain and comorbid aberrant drug-taking behaviors, they must remember the basic tenets of good chronic pain management, which will aide the care of complicated patients. For instance, any medications chosen to treat the patient should be titrated to effect or toxicity, following the "start low, go slow" principle. Also, patient self-report should be respected, even if the patient has been found to be a questionable source. We must not naively accept completely the patient's words, but neither should we dismiss them out of hand. Furthermore, any pain patient must abide by the rules of therapy and make a good faith effort to achieve a successful outcome. Finally, it is important for the clinician to have an ongoing assessment and thorough documentation of the patient's functioning according to several key domains.

The Four A's

Passik and Weinreb described the "4 A's" of pain management outcomes: analgesia (pain relief), activities of daily living (psychosocial functioning), adverse side effects (side effects), and aberrant drug-taking behaviors (addiction-related outcomes), as a shorthand for the domains that should be assessed and discussed at every return visit for patients on chronic opioid therapy (13). Doing so in a detailed manner is time consuming, and a tool would certainly help to upgrade most physicians' documentation.

Differential Diagnosis

Various definitions of abuse that include the phenomena related to physical dependence or tolerance are not applicable to patients who receive potentially abusable drugs for legitimate medical purposes (14). A differential diagnosis should be explored if questionable behaviors occur during pain treatment (Table 12-1). A true addiction is only one of several possible explanations but is more likely when behaviors such as multiple unsanctioned dose escalations and obtaining opioids from multiple prescribers occur.

The diagnosis of pseudoaddiction must also be considered if the patient is reporting distress related to unrelieved symptoms. Behaviors such as aggressively complaining about the need for higher doses or occasional unilateral drug escalations that appear to be addiction on the surface may be indications that the patient's pain is under-medicated. Indeed, one of the most perplexing aspects of differential diagnosis is the distinction between addiction (the behavior is out of control, continues despite harm)

Table 12-1   Differential Diagnosis Considerations for Assessing Aberrant Drug-Taking Behaviors

Differential Diagnoses	Patient Behavior
Addiction	Out-of-control behavior; compulsive, harmful drug use
Pseudoaddiction	Under-treated pain leads to desperate acting out; patients may turn to alcohol, street drugs, or doctor-shopping; these behaviors subside once pain is adequately treated
Organic mental syndrome	Patients often confused and have stereotyped drug-taking behavior
Personality disorder	Patients impulsive, have sense of entitlement, and may engage in chemical-coping behaviors
Chemical coping	Patients place excessive emphasis on meaning of their medications and are overly drug focused
Depression, anxiety, and situational stressors	Patients marked by desire to self-medicate their mood disorder or current life stress
Criminal intent	Subset of criminals intent on diverting medications for profit

and pseudoaddiction (the behavior is driven by inadequate analgesia, resolves when analgesia is improved) (15). No behavior is universally linked to addiction or pseudoaddiction, despite how aberrant it might appear (we have reported, for example, a case of prescription forgery that was linked to anxiety related to the caregiver's vacation and had nothing to do with abuse/diversion) (16). Generally, patients will describe uncontrolled pain rather than loss of control. Thus, before clinching a diagnosis, clinicians often have to "walk the line" between the two possibilities by imposing limits while titrating drugs upward until the behavior comes under control or escalates further. There is no doubt that the notion of pseudoaddiction was an important step forward in pain management: a recognition of the desperation set in motion by unrelieved pain and a somber realization that patients can be pushed to uncharacteristic ways of behaving driven by our failure to optimally treat them. However, it is also crucial to recognize that pseudoaddiction is not an empirically validated notion. The initial paper on the subject was a small case series (15).

Impulsive drug use may also indicate the existence of another psychiatric disorder, diagnosis of which may have therapeutic implications. For example, patients with borderline personality disorder may be categorized as exhibiting aberrant drug-taking behaviors if utilizing prescription medications to express fear and anger or to relieve chronic boredom. Similarly, patients who use opioids to self-medicate symptoms of anxiety or depression, insomnia, or problems of adjustment may be classified as aberrant drug takers. Occasionally, aberrant drug-related behaviors appear to be causally related to mild encephalopathy, with confusion regarding the appropriate therapeutic regimen. Problematic behaviors rarely imply criminal intent, such as when patients report pain but intend to sell or divert medications. These diagnoses are not mutually exclusive, and a thorough psychiatric assessment is vitally important in categorizing questionable behaviors properly in the population without a prior history of substance abuse and in the population of known substance abusers who have a higher incidence of psychiatric comorbidity (17,18).

Understanding Street Values

It is important for clinicians who treat chronic pain patients to be aware of the street value of the medications they prescribe. National trends exist, but local and practice-specific variations are significant. To learn about the street values of various opioid analgesics, Brookoff asked 130 hospital patients who admitted to abusing medications about their behaviors (19). He discovered that, in general, controlled-release preparations of opioids had less value than other opioids and even some non-opioid formulations. For example, hydromorphone, a short-acting opioid, had a mean value of $47 per pill (4 mg strength) compared with $3 per pill for slow-release morphine.

More recently, our team has undertaken a prospective study of addicts entering a treatment facility for prescription opioid abuse. Designed as a follow-up to an earlier chart review to explore OxyContin abuse in rural Appalachia, addicts are questioned about their prescription opioids of choice, how they abuse the medication, and how much they paid for the medication (12). Patients seeking drug rehabilitation for prescription opioids in our rural Appalachian sample still prefer OxyContin (64% abused it), followed by Lortab (35%) and Percocet (15%) (not mutually exclusive). All of these medications were purchased for roughly $1 per milligram. Interestingly, related to the Brookoff study, hydromorphone was valued at approximately $10 per milligram (19). This shows initial evidence that street pricing for drugs has some stability regionally and during more than a decade.

The Drug Abuse Warning Network provides national data on overdoses in emergency rooms, which reveal that hydrocodone combinations are accountable for most overdoses, followed closely by oxycodone combinations (20). Methadone and fentanyl combinations are typically lower but have occasional fluctuations. Clearly then, it is important to monitor national and local trends in street drugs.

Tailoring the Approach

Clinicians should plan treatment according to their assessment results and diagnoses. Categories of patients (Uncomplicated Patient, Patient with Comorbid Psychiatric and Coping Difficulties, and Patient with Addiction) and recommendations for providers qualified to treat them are listed in Table 12-2. Hubris about the ability to treat anyone under any circumstances needs to be replaced by a sober assessment of who a particular practitioner can treat in his or her practice setting given the practitioner's time, expertise in complex psychiatric issues, and resources. Learning which patients to treat independently, which patients to treat with help, and which patients to refer is crucial for safe pain management. Therefore, health care providers should obtain consultations as needed. Furthermore, drug therapy should be based on informed consent of the risks and benefits of all medicines prescribed. Health care providers should discuss with their patients realistic expectations and functional goals for rational pharmacology. Helping the patient understand how success or failure is to be measured, in terms of pain control (hopefully a meaningful reduction in pain intensity), in terms of function (stabilized or improved), toxicities (manageable or none), and regarding aberrant behaviors (few or none) is crucial for compliance and understanding of therapy goals.

When prescribing, the health care provider must be consistent with state and federal regulations. With this in mind, what does the physician owe the patient/community where initiation of an opioid trial is concerned? The physician must perform a thorough assessment of the patient's risk for

Table 12-2   Categories of Chronic Pain Patients and Treatment Requirements

Patient Category	Treatment Requirements
Uncomplicated patient (has no documented comorbid psychiatric problems or connections to drug subculture)	• Minimally monitored drug-only therapy • Routine medical management • 30-day supply of medications with liberal rescue-dose policy • Monthly follow-ups • Monitoring by primary care physician
Patient with comorbid psychiatric and coping difficulties (addictive behavior with central focus on obtaining drugs)	• Structure, psychiatric input, and drug treatments that decentralize pain medication from patient coping techniques • Decentralization/reduction of meaning of medications and of conditioning and socialization surrounding drug • Pain-related psychotherapy • Monitoring by primary care physician in conjunction with physical therapist, occupational therapist, social worker, and/or psychologist/psychiatrist
Patient with addiction (active abuser; in drug-free recovery or in methadone maintenance)	• High-level structure that includes frequent visits • Limited supply of medications • Long-acting opioids with little street value • Judiciously offered rescues only • Urine toxicology screening and follow-up • Active recovery programs or psychotherapy • Monitoring by specialists (unless primary care physician has training in treating addiction)

aberrant behavior and match it to a level of appropriate opioid treatment. If a patient is at high risk, multiple precautions can be employed to mitigate risk without categorically denying opioid therapy to the patient. However, if a given practice cannot provide the appropriate structured therapy, referral to a more specialized setting may be necessary.

Interdisciplinary Treatment

A multidisciplinary team approach with an interdisciplinary focus (i.e., collaborative, holistic, and embodying tenets of biopsychosocial model) is recommended for the management of substance abuse and misuse in the medical setting (21-24). Mental health professionals with specialization in the area of addiction are usually instrumental given their expertise in developing and executing strategies for behavioral management and treatment compliance. Unfortunately, they are not often readily available to clinicians working in private practice or other medical agencies. Therefore, clinicians in independent practice should establish a collective of complementary practitioners in their area to whom they can refer patients for supplementary pain control services and team-based support.

Clinicians practicing in isolation can quickly become angry, defensive, and frustrated when treating patients with chronic pain, which can unintentionally compromise quality of care and cause the patient to feel alienated, hopeless, and rejected. Structured, interdisciplinary treatment (addiction and behavioral medicine, rehabilitation, social work, and/or psychiatry) is the most effective way to facilitate staff understanding of patient needs. It provides a forum for necessary venting and strategizing and helps develop and administer efficacious, empathetic pain control and substance abuse therapy. Regular staff meetings can also help establish patient-specific and team-based treatment goals, facilitate consistency and confidence in treatment, foster patient compliance, and maximize potential for meeting clinical goals.

Conclusion

The health care provider involved in pain management must recognize that prescription drug misuse is not simply media hype and that it is not confined to remote areas (12). The particular sociology of such locations may have made places like Appalachia especially vulnerable, but prescription drug misuse is a widespread problem.

Before prescribing a controlled substance, the health care provider should medically evaluate the patient for pain and for vulnerability to misuse and aberrant drug-related behavior: understanding of risk factors for chemical dependency and psychiatric co-morbidities, social and familial situation, genetic loadings, and spirituality must be reached. The results of this assessment should not be used to categorically exclude patients from opioid therapy but can guide agreed-upon boundaries required to effectively manage an at-risk patient.

REFERENCES

1. **Berry PH, Dahl JL.** The new JCAHO pain standards: implications for pain management nurses. Pain Manag Nurs. 2000;1:3-12.

2. **SUPPORT Study Principal Investigators.** A controlled trial to improve care for seriously ill hospitalized patients. Study to Understand Prognoses and Preferences for Outcomes and Risks of Treatment (SUPPORT). JAMA. 1995;274:1591.

3. **Osterweis M, Kleinman A, Mechanic D, eds.** Pain and Disability: Clinical, Behavioral, and Public Policy Perspectives. Washington, DC: National Academy Press; 1987.

4. **Verhaak PFM, Kerssens JJ, Dekker J, et al.** Prevalence of chronic benign pain disorder among adults: a review of the literature. Pain. 1998;77:231-9.

5. **Porter J, Jick H.** Addiction rare in patients treated with narcotics. N Engl J Med. 1980;302:123.

6. **Lee LE Jr.** Medications in the control of pain in terminal cancer, with reference to the study of newer synthetic analgesics. JAMA. 1941;116:217.

7. **Joranson D, Ryan K, Gilson A, Dahl J.** Trends in medicaid use and abuse of opioid analgesics. JAMA. 2000;283:1710-4.

8. **Hancock CM.** OxyContin use and abuse. Clin J Oncol Nursing. 2002;6:109.

9. **Colliver JD, Kopstein AN.** Trends in cocaine abuse reflected in emergency room episodes reported to DAWN. Publ Health Rep. 1991;106:59-68.

10. **Groerer J, Brodsky M.** The incidence of illicit drug use in the United States, 1962-1989. Br J Addiction. 1992;87:1345.

11. **Regier DA, Meyers JK, Dramer M.** The NIMH epidemiologic catchment area program. Arch Gen Psychiatry. 1984;41:934-41.

12. **Hays L, Kirsh KL, Passik SD.** Seeking drug treatment for oxycontin abuse: a chart review of consecutive admissions to a substance abuse treatment facility in the bluegrass region of Kentucky. J National Comprehensive Cancer Network. 2003;1:423-8.

13. **Passik SD, Weinreb HJ.** Managing chronic nonmalignant pain: overcoming obstacles to the use of opioids. Advances Ther. 2000;17:70-80.

14. **Rinaldi RC, Steindler EM, Wilford BB, Goodwin D.** Clarification and standardization of substance abuse terminology. JAMA. 1988;259:555.

15. **Weissman DE, Haddox JD.** Opioid pseudoaddiction: an iatrogenic syndrome. Pain. 1989;36:363-6.

16. **Hay JL, Passik SD.** The cancer patient with borderline personality disorder: suggestions for symptom-focused management in the medical setting. Psycho-oncology. 2000;9:91-100.

17. **Passik SD, Portenoy RK, Ricketts PL.** Substance abuse issues in cancer patients. Part 1: prevalence and diagnosis. Oncology. 1998;12:517-21.

18. **Passik SD, Portenoy RK.** Substance abuse issues in palliative care. In: Berger AM, Portenoy RK, Weissman DE, eds. Principles and Practice of Supportive Oncology. Philadelphia: Lippincott Williams & Wilkins; 1998:513-30.

19. **Brookoff D.** Abuse potential of various opioid medications. J Gen Intern Med. 1993;8:688-90.

20. **U.S. Department of Health and Human Services.** Emergency department trends from the drug abuse warning network: final estimates, 1994-2001. Publication D-21; August 2002.

21. **Engel GL.** The need for a new medical model: a challenge for biomedicine. Science. 1977;196:129-36.

22. **Engel GL.** The clinical applicaton of the biopsychosocial model. Am J Psychiatry. 1980;137:535-44.

23. **Orchard WH.** Memoriam to Dr George Engel. Aust N Z J Psychiatry. 2003;37:112.

24. **Sweet JJ, Tovian SM, Suchy Y.** Psychological assessment in medical settings. In: Graham JR, Naglieri, JA, eds. Handbook of Psychology: Assessment Psychology. New York: John Wiley; 2003:291-315.

13

■ ■ ■

Protecting Your Practice: Appropriate Documentation for Pain Management

Steven D. Passik, PhD

Kenneth L. Kirsh, PhD

The use of long-term opioid therapy to treat chronic nonmalignant pain is growing, spurred by evidence from clinical trials and an evolving consensus among pain specialists (1-4). The appropriate use of these drugs requires skills in opioid prescribing, knowledge of addiction medicine principles, and a commitment to perform and document a comprehensive assessment repeatedly over time. Inadequate assessment can lead to undertreatment, compromise the effectiveness of therapy when implemented, and prevent an appropriate response when problematic drug-related behaviors occur (5-7). The failure to perceive and address problematic behaviors, in turn, can have both regulatory and medical-legal consequences for the clinician.

Physicians who adequately assess patients before and during opioid therapy may still encounter problems as a result of poor documentation. In a chart review of 300 patients with chronic pain, 61% had no documentation of a treatment plan (8). Similarly, a review of the initial consultation notes of 513 patients with acute musculoskeletal pain revealed that only 43% of historical findings and 28% of physical examination findings were documented (9). In a review of 520 randomly selected visits at an outpatient oncology practice, quantitative assessment of pain scores was virtually absent (less than 1%), and qualitative assessment of pain occurred in only 60% of cases (10). Finally, a review of medical records of 111 randomly selected patients who underwent urine toxicology screens in a cancer center found that documentation was infrequent: 37.8% of physicians failed to list a reason for the test, and 89% of the charts did not include the results of the test (11).

According to model guidelines for opioid therapy developed by the Federation of State Medical Boards, the medical record should document the nature and intensity of the pain, current and past treatments for pain, underlying or coexisting diseases or conditions, the effect of the pain on physical and psychological function, and history of substance abuse (12). To assess the appropriateness, course, and outcome of therapy, information should be available concerning the patient evaluation, treatment plan, informed consent and agreement for treatment, monitoring approach, consultation requests, medical record keeping, and compliance with the controlled substances laws and regulations (12). Recent standards promulgated by the Joint Commission on the Accreditation of Healthcare Organizations also recommend that physicians record the results of their pain assessment in a way that facilitates regular reassessment and follow-up (5).

With the pressure of regulatory scrutiny and our duty to treat pain but contain abuse or diversion, clinicians often feel that they must avoid being duped by those abusing prescription pain medications at all costs. Thus, while the differential diagnosis of aberrant drug-related behavior is complex, clinicians will tend to simplify the assessment of this issue to either addiction or not addiction. It is important to note, however, that the clinician attempting to diagnose the meaning of aberrant drug-related behaviors during pain management need not be correct in their final assessment regarding addiction. The fear of regulatory oversight makes practitioners feel as if they must be right; that if the aberrant behavior presents even the possibility of drug diversion or abuse, that they have to see through the patient's or family's denials to guard against the possibility of being duped. Under-treatment and avoidance of prescribing is often the result, yet that is not what the existing laws or guidelines on prescribing opioids were intended to accomplish. The clinician has an obligation to be thorough, thoughtful, logically consistent, and careful (not to mention humane and caring), but not necessarily right in the diagnosis of addiction. Indeed there are multiple possibilities in the differential diagnosis of aberrant drug-taking behaviors, with criminal intent and diversion being only one of the more remote possibilities.

Domains of Interest for Documentation

Clearly, strategies are needed to translate these recommendations for patient assessment during long-term opioid therapy to front-line practice. This effort would certainly benefit from the availability of a consistent method of documentation. As a framework, it is important to consider four main domains in assessing pain outcomes and to better protect your practice for those patients you maintain on an opioid regimen: 1) pain relief, 2) functional outcomes,

3) side effects, and 4) drug-related behaviors. These domains have been labeled the "Four A's" (Analgesia, Activities of daily living, Adverse effects, and Aberrant drug-related behaviors) for teaching purposes (13). To that purpose, we describe the Pain Assessment and Documentation Tool (PADT) herein, a simple charting device that is intended to focus on key outcomes and provide a consistent way to document progress in pain management therapy over time (Fig. 13-1).

Pain Assessment and Documentation Tool Origins

Twenty-seven clinicians completed the preliminary version of the PADT for 388 opioid-treated patients (14). Nineteen clinicians (17 physicians, 1 nurse, and 1 psychologist) participated in a debriefing phase. Twelve of the 19 clinicians had participated in the field trial before the debriefing. The debriefing interview for these clinicians used the same standard questions to evaluate the original and revised PADT. Seven clinicians who participated in the development of the PADT, but not in the field trial, reviewed only the revised PADT.

The result of this work is a brief, two-sided chart note that can be readily included in the patient's medical record. It was designed to be intuitive, pragmatic, and adaptable to clinical situations. In the field trial, it took clinicians between 10 and 20 minutes to complete the tool. The revised PADT is substantially shorter and should require a few minutes to complete.

By addressing the need for documentation, the PADT can assist clinicians in meeting their obligations for ongoing assessment and documentation. Although the PADT is not intended to replace a progress note, it is well suited to complement existing documentation with a focused evaluation of outcomes that are clinically relevant and address the need for evidence of appropriate monitoring.

The decision to assess the four domains subsumed under the shorthand designation, the "Four A's," was based on clinical experience, the positive comments received by the investigators during educational programs on opioid pharmacotherapy for nonmalignant pain, and an evolving national movement that recognizes the need to approach opioid therapy with a "balanced" response. This response recognizes both the legitimate need to provide optimal therapy to appropriate patients and the need to acknowledge the potential for abuse, diversion, and addiction (13). The value of assessing pain relief, side effects, and aspects of functioning has been emphasized repeatedly in the literature (8,15-19). Documentation of drug-related behaviors is a relatively new concept that is being explored for the first time in the PADT.

Potential aberrant drug-related behavior has a complex differential diagnosis, including addiction, inadequate analgesia (pseudoaddiction), self-medication of psychiatric and physical symptoms other than pain (encephalopathy,

ANALGESIA

Scale of 0–10 (0 = no pain; 10 = worst pain imaginable) rank:

1. What was your pain level on average during the past week? _____

2. What was your pain level at its worst during the past week? _____

3. Compare your average pain during the past week with the average pain you had before you were treated with your current pain relievers. What percentage of your pain has been relieved? _____

4. Is the amount of pain relief you are now obtaining from your current pain relievers enough to make a real difference in your life?

   Yes____   No____

5. *Doctor:* Is the pain relief clinically significant?

   Yes____   No____   Unsure____

ADVERSE EVENTS

Is patient able to tolerate current pain relievers?

Yes____   No____

Is patient experiencing any side effects from current pain relievers?

Yes____   No____   Detail:

Severity of side effects:

N = None   M = Mild   Mod = Moderate
S = Severe

Constipation:	N	M	Mod	S
Itching:	N	M	Mod	S
Nausea:	N	M	Mod	S
Mental clouding:	N	M	Mod	S
Other:	N	M	Mod	S
	N	M	Mod	S

ACTIVITIES OF DAILY LIVING

Physician observation comparing usual functioning during the past month with usual functioning before being treated with current pain reliever(s):

B = Better   S = Same   W = Worse

Physical functioning: _____

Family relationships: _____

Social relationships: _____

Sleep patterns: _____

POTENTIALLY ABERRANT DRUG-RELATED BEHAVIOR

Frequency of behavior: 1, 2, 3, >4

Purposeful over-sedation _____

Negative mood change _____

Appears intoxicated _____

Increasingly unkempt or impaired _____

Involvement in car or other accident _____

Requests frequent early renewals _____

Increased dose without authorization _____

Reports lost or stolen prescriptions _____

Attempts to obtain prescriptions from other doctors _____

Changes route of administration _____

Asks for meds by name _____

Reports no effects of other medications _____

Contact with street culture _____

Hoarding of medication _____

Victim of abuse _____

Abusing alcohol & drugs _____

Arrested by police _____

Figure 13-1   Questionnaires for charting the four main domains of function.

borderline personality disorder, depression, anxiety), situational stressors, family dysfunction, and diversion (20). The challenge to the clinician is to recognize the occurrence of these behaviors, undertake actions to limit them, and determine the most appropriate management based on the diagnosis. The PADT assesses 17 aberrant behaviors. Some of the items in the checklist are directly observable (e.g., "Appears intoxicated") and others require some probing. The availability of this checklist may improve the ability of clinicians to capture problematic behaviors and implement appropriate actions in response because the relevant questions can be asked consistently over time.

The PADT is in development, and current limitations must be acknowledged. The PADT is a descriptive tool intended to assist clinicians to better organize and document their chart notes. Although measures of internal consistency, which are based on a single administration of the instrument, were completed, measures of "stability" were not done; these measures are intended to provide evidence on how a tool performs on different occasions. Inter-observer reliability or the degree of agreement between different observers and intra-observer reliability (the degree of agreement between observations made by the same observer) were not done. Furthermore, observations on the same subject at two different times were not done. Further studies are needed to confirm its reliability and the validity of the individual items and sections. Predictive validity through the longitudinal use of the tool must be confirmed, and studies are needed to clarify the interval of assessment that optimally balances the need to minimize clinician burden with the need to validly assess and document outcomes that may change continually over time. Finally, the PADT does not capture many characteristics of pain or domains that may be affected by pain or its treatment, and it is not meant to substitute for a comprehensive clinical assessment.

Overall, the results of our study on the PADT were enlightening. Cross-sectional results suggest that the majority of patients with chronic pain achieve relatively positive outcomes in the eyes of their prescribing physicians, in all four relevant domains with opioid therapy. Analgesia was modest but meaningful, functionality generally stabilized or improved and side effects were tolerable. Potentially aberrant behaviors were common (44.6% of the sample engaged in at least one aberrant behavior) but only viewed as an indicator of a problem (e.g., addiction or diversion) in approximately 10% of cases. Thus, there is a clear need to document and assess the intricacies of aberrant drug-taking behaviors (and not just their presence or absence) in chronic pain patients.

Assessing Aberrant Drug-Taking

The aberrant behavior concept was first put forward by Portenoy and then expanded upon by Passik and Portenoy (21-23). While the pain community has been correctly teaching that physiological dependence and tolerance are not to be mistaken for signs of addiction, nor are they particularly related to aberrant drug-taking behavior, pain clinicians have still been in need of a model for understanding what addiction might be, that is, a description of signs of addiction that coincides with the phenomenology of the pain clinician. The aberrant behavior concept suggests that pain clinicians who prescribe opioids are likely to see a wide range of noncompliance behaviors, some of which are relatively rare but very aberrant, some of which are common and more ambiguous in their meaning. Having to ignore certain hallmark signs of addiction because they are misleading in the understanding of potential addiction in cancer patients, clinicians must develop a vocabulary for discussing noncompliance with their patients. Some of these behaviors are so rare and serious, if not illegal, that one occurrence is likely to be grounds for referral to substance abuse treatment if not discharge (e.g., forging prescriptions).

Our work suggests that there is some community consensus among pain doctors about the seriousness of such behaviors and reactions to them (24). On the other hand, much more common, and much less obvious, are behaviors such as occasional unilateral dose escalation, using the drug to treat a symptom other than pain, etc. In such cases, repeated offenses and failure to alter behavior, even in response to efforts at limit-setting, might suggest a behavioral syndrome characterized by loss of control around prescribed opioids that likely maps onto addiction. In our studies, 6%-10% of cancer, AIDS, and chronic pain patients all have the same number of behaviors (5 or more) (14,25).

Assessment of the risk for aberrant behavior and addiction in the context of opioid therapy is complex, though efforts to improve the clinician's ability to perform the assessment have been in development now for some time. The assessment at minimum would focus upon a personal or family history of drug abuse. Given that we know that addiction is a disease with genetic, familial, social, psychiatric, and spiritual determinants, an assessment would touch on each of these areas. There are also several tools under development (WAT, SOAPP, STAR, SISAP), as well as some that have been in the addiction literature for some time and recently altered (e.g., CAGE-AID), which can help the clinician more efficiently perform risk assessment, sometimes in a completely self-report format that can be filled out by the patient before the visit.

Thus, clinicians have the responsibility of assessing the 4 A's and monitoring the patient for aberrant drug-related behavior. Furthermore, when aberrant behaviors are noted the clinician must then consider the differential diagnosis of the behaviors and decide which of several factors might be "driving" the behavior so that a reasoned clinical response can be formulated. However, even if one strives to become an adept "behavioral scientist" of their patients' noncompliance with opioids, there are limitations to what a clinician will be able to ascertain in face-to-face clinical encounters with patients about socially unacceptable behaviors that have grave consequences if they are exposed (e.g., termination of pain medication prescribing). Thus, in certain clinical situations, clinicians have also adopted a variety of techniques for outside corroboration of self-report.

This can take many forms, including: having a patient's spouse or monitor give feedback to the prescriber on the patient's behavior outside of the office (with the patient's consent, of course); the use of urine toxicology screening; and patch and pill counts. In a study by Katz and Fanciullo, 20% of patients without obvious behavioral manifestations of noncompliance were found to have a "positive" urine toxicology screen (presence of illicit drugs or non-prescribed controlled substances or the absence of a drug that had been prescribed and is detectable in urine) (26). This study highlights the need to build in outside monitoring for what is likely to be missed in routine clinical assessment.

Pill counts and patch counts (e.g., for the fentanyl transdermal system) can be another way of monitoring the patient's supply so that one can be reassured that drugs are not being overused and diverted. For patients who live at a distance from the physician, a local pharmacy might be approached about helping to perform pill counts without causing the patient to travel a great distance. Patients can be asked to secure the use of their fentanyl patches by saving used patches, affixing them to colored paper, and bringing them to clinic so that the prescriber can account for the used and intact patches. If these steps are implemented, the findings need to be dictated into the chart to round out all other sources of documentation.

These efforts can help to offer other sources of data to bolster clinician and patient assertions that opioid therapy is proceeding as planned with little or no aberrant behavior. However, with the problem of prescription drug abuse being as widespread as it has become, there are a plethora of companies on the internet offering clean urine samples, devices for producing the faked sample in the doctor's office (even when being observed!), and even for renting pills and patches for counts. While the use of these by pain patients is without doubt rare, it highlights the issue that the savvy clinician, even with the time and resources to carefully monitor patients, cannot completely avoid the possibility of being duped by unscrupulous drug seekers. However, if the clinician is careful, thorough, mindful of guidelines, and takes reasonable steps to secure his prescribing, the person who is lying to the clinician to obtain controlled substances is indeed committing a felony and the onus will be more on their behavior than the clinician's. The physician does not owe it to the patient or the community to be either a branch of law enforcement or a mind reader.

Conclusion

Assessment and documentation are cornerstones for both protecting your practice and obtaining optimal patient outcomes while on opioid therapy.

The Pain Assessment and Documentation Tool (PADT) appears useful in helping clinicians evaluate a group of important outcomes during opioid therapy and provides a simple means of documenting patient care. Besides being an aid to clinical management, the PADT offers a means of documenting the types of practice standards that those in the regulatory and law enforcement communities seek to ensure.

REFERENCES

1. **Collett BJ.** Opioid tolerance: the clinical perspective. Br J Anaesth. 1998;81:58-68.

2. **Portenoy RK.** Opioid therapy for chronic nonmalignant pain: a review of critical issues. J Pain Symptom Manage. 1996;11:203-17.

3. **Urban BJ, France RD, Steinberger EK, et al.** Long-term use of narcotic/antidepressant medication in the management of phantom limb pain. Pain. 1986;24:191-6.

4. **Zenz M, Strumpf M, Tryba M.** Long-term oral opioid therapy in patients with chronic nonmalignant pain. J Pain Symptom Manage. 1992;7:69-77.

5. **Joint Commission on the Accreditation of Healthcare Organizations.** Patient Rights and Organization Ethics. Referenced from the Comprehensive Accreditation Manual for Hospitals, Update 3; 1999. www.jcaho.org/standards_frm.html.

6. **Max MB, Payne R, Edwards WT, et al.** Principles of Analgesic Use in the Treatment of Acute Pain and Cancer Pain, 4th ed. Glenview, IL: American Pain Society; 1999.

7. **Katz N.** The impact of pain management on quality of life. J Pain Symptom Manage. 2002;24(Suppl 1):S38-S47.

8. **Clark JD.** Chronic pain prevalence and analgesic prescribing in a general medical population. J Pain Symptom Manage. 2002;23:131-7.

9. **Solomon DH, Schaffer JL, Katz JN, et al.** Can history and physical examination be used as markers of quality? An analysis of the initial visit note in musculoskeletal care. Med Care. 2000;38:383-91.

10. **Rhodes DJ, Koshy RC, Waterfield WC, et al.** Feasibility of quantitative pain assessment in outpatient oncology practice. J Clin Oncol. 2001;19:501-8.

11. **Passik SD, Schreiber J, Kirsh KL, Portenoy RK.** A chart review of the ordering and documentation of urine toxicology screens in a cancer center: do they influence patient management? J Pain Symptom Manage. 2000;19:40-4.

12. **Federation of State Medical Boards of United States.** Model Guidelines for the Use of Controlled Substances for the Treatment of Pain. May 1998. Available at www.fsmb.org. Accessed 10 April 2003.

13. **Passik SD, Weinreb HJ.** Managing chronic nonmalignant pain: overcoming obstacles to the use of opioids. Adv Ther. 2000;17:70-83.

14. **Passik SD, Kirsh KL, Whitcomb LA, et al.** A new tool to assess and document pain outcomes in chronic pain patients receiving opioid therapy. Clin Ther. 2004;26:552-61.

15. **Daut RL, Cleeland CS, Flanery RC.** Development of the Wisconsin Brief Pain Questionnaire to assess pain in cancer and other diseases. Pain. 1983;17:197-210.

16. **Cleeland CS, Ryan KM.** Pain assessment: global use of the Brief Pain Inventory. Ann Acad Med Singapore. 1994;23:129-38.

17. **Melzack R.** The McGill Pain Questionnaire: major properties and scoring methods. Pain. 1975;1:277-99.

18. **McCarberg BH, Barkin RL.** Long-acting opioids for chronic pain: pharmacotherapeutic opportunities to enhance compliance, quality of life, and analgesia. Am J Ther. 2001;8:181-6.

19. **Portenoy RK.** Opioid analgesics. In: Portenoy RK, Kanner RM, eds. Pain Management: Theory and Practice. Philadelphia: FA Davis; 1996:248-76.

20. **Portenoy RK, Payne R.** Acute and chronic pain. In: Lowinson JH, Ruiz P, Millman RB, eds. Comprehensive Textbook of Substance Abuse, 3rd ed. Baltimore: Williams & Wilkins; 1997:563-89.

21. **Portenoy RK.** Chronic opioid therapy in nonmalignant pain. J Pain Symptom Manage. 1990;5(1 Suppl):S46-62.

22. **Portenoy RK.** Opioid therapy for chronic nonmalignant pain and current status. In: Fields HL, Liebeskind JC, eds. Pain Research and Management. Vol 1. Seattle: IASP Press; 1994:247-87.

23. **Passik SD, Portenoy RK.** Substance abuse issues in palliative care. In: Berger AM, Portenoy RK, Weissman DE, eds. Principles and Practice of Supportive Oncology. Philadelphia: Lippincott Williams & Wilkins; 1998:513-30.

24. **Passik SD, Kirsh KL, Whitcomb LA, et al.** Pain clinicians' rankings of aberrant drug-taking behaviors. J Pain Pall Care Pharmacotherapy. 2002;16:39-49.

25. **Passik SD, Kirsh KL, McDonald MV, et al.** A pilot survey of aberrant drug-taking attitudes and behaviors in samples of cancer and AIDS patients. J Pain Sympt Manage. 2000;19:274-86.

26. **Katz N, Fanciullo GJ.** Role of urine toxicology testing in the management of chronic opioid therapy. Clin J Pain. 2002;18(4 Suppl):S76-82.

14

■　■　■

Medical Board and Drug Enforcement Administration Investigations: How to Handle an Inquiry

Mary Baluss, JD

nevitably, physicians who prescribe opioids worry that some aspect of their practice will draw critical attention. How should you respond? If it is a local pharmacy, with patience and grace. But what if inquiries come from a state medical board or, more unnervingly, from the Drug Enforcement Administration (DEA) and its state counterpart, or both? In that case, how should you respond, and what can you expect? How nervous should you be?

This chapter should help you answer those questions. It is an overview, however, not a manual. It assumes that you pay attention to documentation and practice management and are treating in good faith. It does not try to deal with the exceptions and vagaries that arise under individual state laws and the facts of any particular case. Its purpose is to establish a framework for handling an inquiry and to furnish some caveats. In addition, the chapter provides advice on when to consult a lawyer and how to educate him or her to be an effective advocate in this corner where law, medicine, ethics, and societal pressures dance a complicated reel.

Primary Questions

How Often Do Investigations Occur?

The short answer is that we do not know. There are no data on medical board investigations that do not lead to sanctions or on DEA investigations that do not lead to indictment. However, they substantially exceed the number of sanctions or indictment. Medical boards accounted for 8100 of the 207,000 actions reported to the National Practitioner Data Base in 2000-2003. We do not have data that break down the total reports into the nature of the complaint, and therefore we cannot tell how many of these relate to prescription of opioids. Best information indicates that board actions vary from state to state, with some state boards being highly suspicious of practitioners who treat chronic pain with opioids and other boards being quite accepting.

The data base also records 917 felony drug conviction reports for the period. These, however, do not provide detail that allows us to tell how many of these convictions are related to prescribing for patients rather than to diversion by a practitioner for his or her own or family use. No data are available on investigations that did not eventually result in an indictment. Nor do we know what the percentages would be as a function of prescribers who treat chronic pain.

"Why Am I Being Investigated?"

Investigations often come out of the blue and involve prescribers with no history of medical board complaints or malpractice actions. Frequent categories of complaints include former patients, pharmacists, family members, or ex-family members/partners.

Pharmacists often originate complaints. Many lack up-to-date information about opioids. They may have social prejudices about opioids. More importantly, they know that they could be liable under their "corresponding" duty (with the physician) to maintain the "legitimate medical purpose" standard of DEA regulations (21 CFR 1306.4[a]). For all of these reasons, prescribers should be respectful of pharmacy inquiries. A careful explanation for the prescription done in collegial fashion and consistent with privacy rules functions as a small insurance policy. Rude or dismissive comments may lead the pharmacist to call the medical board or make a comment when diversion control is checking their records.

Anecdotally, insurance carriers who do not want to pay for expensive medications over a long period of time are also frequent complainants. Taking such action is not limited to private companies, however. Workmen's Compensation Boards, Medicaid, and Medicare reviewers do not hesitate to use their fraud-seeking powers to focus on practitioners who are high-level prescribers.

A patient's family can be highly suspicious of opioid therapy. Sometimes this is because they know more about the patient than the patient has been willing to reveal to his physician or because they are more able to observe patient behavior. Sometimes, however, they are reacting to the unrelenting "anti-drug" campaign in the United States and fear their loved one "being on drugs". They also may be frightened by media scare stories; they may honestly believe that the patient will become an instant addict. They may be truly care about the patient and distrust or dislike the physician. A prescriber should include family attitudes and history in his patient's history and, if possible, involve those who live with the patient to share an informed consent discussion.

On the other hand, family members and former spouses and friends of pain patients can be mean and vindictive. Telephone calls, letters, or e-mails from ex-anyone—spouse, friend, "boy or girl friend"—alleging that a patient is misusing or selling his medications present prescribers with a serious ethical and practical dilemma. Common sense dictates that the prescriber document these communications, his subsequent discussion with the patient, and whatever decision results. The physician must not over-react or trust a caller (anonymous or otherwise) above a patient. However, the same individuals who called the physician may complain to the medical board.

The DEA clings to the unsupported belief that licensed physicians are the major source of diverted prescription drugs. Law enforcement frequently and publicly proclaims that it does not want to discourage physicians from prescribing opioids and that volume and amounts alone are not the basis for investigation. Practical experience indicates that numbers and dosages do play a role. High-volume practices in terms of number of patients and amounts prescribed are the most likely to be candidates for the "pill mill" investigation. There is also a persistent belief that "prescribing to an addict" is easily avoided and also clinically unacceptable. Evidence that patients cross county or state lines to seek treatment, which may be only a result of refusals to treat them closer to home, can be viewed as evidence of potential criminality.

Far too often, the DEA has treated the arrest of a drug-diverting patient as the reason to open an investigation of his physician. The most frequent witnesses in doctor prosecutions are former patients who have pled guilty to drug-related offenses and expect downward departures from sentencing guidelines in return for cooperating against their physicians. Law enforcement agencies can view the death of a patient treated with opioids as the potential responsibility of the prescriber. Elected and untrained coroners or outdated, incompetent, or poorly trained medical examiners often have no understanding of tolerance. When a patient dies with blood levels of opioids that would be dangerous for the opiod-naïve, the medical examiner may believe that prescribed medications were the cause.

The foregoing comments may well open the question of "Why take the risk of prescribing opioids?" There are several answers: Because ethical medicine does not abandon patients or refuse to treat pain unless the patient has given significant reason to the contrary. Because there are more decent and needy patients than there are criminals. Furthermore, a well-managed and up-to-date clinical practice that documents the rationale for using opioids, the social history of the patient, all treatments, and the functional changes that occur as a result of treatment has a markedly reduced chance that an investigation will find physician culpability.

Finally, prescribers have the support of clinical guidelines and professional society policy statements that emphasize the importance of treating pain and the role of opioids in that endeavor. These help establish a standard for clinical practice useful in any investigation. Add also the policies, guidelines, and regulations adopted by 45 state medical boards that assure physicians that as long as they conform to practice parameters that amount to no more than good medical practice they should not fear board sanctions for prescribing opioids to chronic pain patients. In addition, a good number of state legislatures have passed versions of the Intractable Pain Act, which supports the use of opioids to treat chronic pain and states that prescribers should not fear sanctions. A few states have gone further and *require* treating physicians to manage pain or refer the patient to a pain expert.

To the best of the present author's knowledge, no state board or statute forbids prescribing opioids to pain patients with a history of substance abuse, aberrant behaviors, or even active addiction, *so long as caution and judgment are evident in the record.* The American Society of Addiction Medicine has reminded prescribers that pain and addictive disorders can be treated simultaneously.

In short, the fact that investigation and legal prosecution can happen even to well-intentioned physicians is not to say that such events are at all likely. The number of patients undertreated or abandoned by their prescribers out of fear of investigation far exceeds the number of physicians who are investigated, let alone prosecuted and, even rarer, convicted.

Structure of the Investigation

The basic questions when one learns of an investigation are whether it is 1) *state* or *federal,* and 2) whether it is *administrative* or *criminal.* State or federal actions can be either administrative (civil) or criminal. If an investigation is brought under administrative law, it also is important to know whether it is *summary* (accomplished without notice before the fact) or will proceed after administrative investigation and procedural entitlement.

The state's medical board initiates state administrative actions. The DEA uses federal administrative procedures to revoke registrations through administrative procedures. Both state and federal administrative actions employ rules of administrative procedure. They also employ a standard of proof (the level of certainty that the finder of fact must have in order to render a decision), which is most commonly "by the preponderance of the evidence". "Preponderance" means that the outcome is "more likely than not" supported by the facts. In some states a board action that could result in loss of a professional license must be supported by "clear and convincing evidence" as a matter of statute and, in a few cases, state courts have interpreted their constitutions to require this more stringent standard of proof. In most states, however, courts have held that concern for public safety and welfare support the weaker standard of proof in administrative procedures involving physicians.

State medical boards and the DEA acting in its capacity as the issuing (and revoking) authority for registration under the Controlled Substances Act can issue summary suspensions. These may come with or after a show-cause order and are appropriate when the administrative agency considers that the licensee/registrant is a danger to the public health or safety. There seems to be little consistency between states (and sometimes within a state between cases) on the decision to proceed summarily. If the board is not ready to proceed rapidly, it will not bring a summary action because a suspension entitles the licensee to a very rapid resolution of the show-cause order.

State and federal governments may also bring criminal cases. Federal criminal cases rest on alleged violations of the Controlled Substances Act (18 USC 841 et seq). They might also include ancillary charges such as racketeering or money-laundering or conspiracy to commit either of these crimes. State criminal cases, which have been rare, occur under laws punishing reckless homicide (manslaughter) when patient deaths are attributed to gross negligence on the part of the physician. In both state and federal criminal cases, the prosecution must show that each element of a crime occurred "beyond a reasonable doubt". Defendants also have more rights and due process protections than administrative actions offer.

The State Medical Board

Administrative Action

The federal system reserves decisions on medical quality and the standard of care to the states. Every state has a medical practice act (MPA), most of which are patterned on the Federation of State Medical Boards recommended structure. A board has only the powers given to it by the legislature. Boards must follow their state's Administrative Procedures Act, which in almost every case follows the broad outlines of the federal Administrative Procedures Act (5 USC 552[b]["APA"]), but they can make other procedural rules that are not inconsistent with the APA if allowed by the MPA.

Medical licenses are "property" protected by federal and state constitutions; the relevant case is *Schware v. Board of Bar Examiners* (353 U.S. 232, 238-39[1957]). Over time courts have defined what protections must occur to provide constitutional due process. The result is an extensive law of administrative procedure that will affect how and what the board may do. Generally speaking, if procedural requirements are followed, board decisions on matters of fact receive a great deal of deference from reviewing courts. They are also allowed more latitude in admitting evidence than in criminal trials. The differences are based on two aspects of administrative procedure: 1) medical boards are assumed to be able to winnow technical evidence more effectively than a court, and 2) boards have a responsibility to protect public health and welfare that trumps in some ways the procedural rights of respondents. In criminal proceedings the social good weighs the other way, in favor of protecting defendants and the integrity of judicial process.

Each medical board has the power and the duty to investigate every complaint within their broad jurisdictions. Some of the regulations may seem unfairly vague, but courts have consistently upheld the right of boards to define concepts such as "unprofessional conduct" when they see it. Thus the MPA will generally enumerate specific examples of such conduct that the board is able to add to or elaborate on in the context of its proceedings. Some relevant examples of "unprofessional conduct" include

- Commission or conviction of a gross misdemeanor or a felony, "whether or not related to the practice of medicine, or the entry of a guilty or nolo contendere plea to a gross misdemeanor or a felony charge"
- Conduct likely to deceive, defraud, or harm the public
- Negligence in the practice of medicine as determined by the board
- Prescribing, selling, administering, distributing, ordering, or giving any drug legally classified as a controlled substance or recognized as an addictive or dangerous drug for other than medically accepted therapeutic purposes
- Violating any state or federal law or regulation relating to controlled substances
- Improper management of medical records, including failure to maintain timely, legible, accurate, and complete medical records.

Of these examples, the most common is the failure to document. In addition to being a stand-alone violation, it serves as a fall-back in cases where the board wants to act but does not have sufficient evidence to proceed based on prescribing alone. Appropriate documentation is a universal requirement among states that have issued guidelines or regulations concerning opioid prescription for chronic pain. Inadequate documentation is preventable. *If you prescribe opioids, good documentation is essential.* With it you have a dramatically improved chance of success in fighting board or legal action.

The medical board decides whether a particular licensee's practice falls short of the standard of care. Traditionally, the standard of care applied is that of the "community" (state) in which the board sits. Now, however, any practitioner in a jurisdiction that is unfriendly to the use of opioids to treat chronic pain will argue that a national consensus as defined by professional societies or federal administrative entities, such as the Institute of Medicine and health care quality protocols or recommendations, should replace the community standard.

Few medical board members have training or experience in the use of opioids to treat chronic pain. Those who do can provide significant education to other board members. Board members may also be educated through the hearing process itself, or at least their views may be somewhat moderated. If the respondent requests a hearing before an administrative law judge (ALJ), the board may not reject facts that the ALJ has found simply because it does not like them or because they choose to integrate other findings into the proceeding. Reviewing courts will not assume that just because a medical board is composed of doctors it has the specialized medical expertise needed to develop its own facts. If the board rejects facts found by an ALJ, it must be specific about where its disagreement lies and must point to evidence in the record developed by the ALJ to support its rationale.

Board actions begin with an investigation. An attorney, who is usually employed by the state attorney general's office rather than by the board, supervises investigators and decides when there is reason to ask the board to issue a show-cause order to a physician. Investigators are not attorneys and more often than not have no training in the pharmacology or treatment of chronic pain. They may form opinions based on the dosages and number of pills prescribed, no matter what the board's own statements may have been about volume and chronicity of dosing. In one of the author's recent cases, an investigator came into an exceedingly well credentialed physician's office and requested to see a single, beautifully detailed chart. He looked at it for a minute and said, "Well, Doc, how long are you going to prescribe that much methadone for this fellow?"

Requests for Charts

All boards have some form of subpoena power. You may simply get a letter "requesting" particular charts. Or an investigator may well show up with an administrative subpoena and a list of charts he wants. (The investigator is already likely to have pharmacy records.) At this stage the physician will have no real information about what is concerning the board. Physicians should not part with their charts without at least attempting to make copies. Copying allows the physician to make sure that *all* interested parties have the same documents and that office files remain intact while being handled by the board. Physicians are also free to retain any charts until they have been able to contact an attorney.

Files that a physician hands over to the board should be complete and include records from the patient's previous doctor and labs if the patient has provided them. Frequently patient records are in several places within a physician's office. Some may be computer generated and not resident in the paper files. Others may be in storage, or the office filing may be behind. There is often room at this stage for the physician or his attorney to negotiate with the board's attorney about the timing of records turn over, copying, and marking procedures. Make certain that you get on record any requests of yours that the state refuses.

"Investigators Are Not Your Friends"

Frequently physicians hope that they can make the investigation go away by being friendly and forthcoming. This is natural for a physician who is confident in the quality of his care. He knows that he is one of the "good guys" and wants the board to understand that right away. There is no reason not to talk with the investigator and certainly no advantage in being hostile or defensive. However, speculating out loud about what you suppose their concerns to be or verbally second-guessing some aspect of your care can be dangerous. Comments such as "I guess the documentation could be better, but . . ." or "I did have some worries about that guy" are extremely unwise. When you know that the requested charts are for patients who have died or been arrested, saying anything is a risk. This is not to say that a physician cannot describe the course of treatment to an investigator, but every such comment must be objective, professional, and consistent with the medical records.

Consulting an Attorney

With the first intimation of an investigation, consult an attorney. Do not wait. Prescribers are reluctant to take this step. Their concerns include cost, hope that all will blow over, and fear that if an attorney is involved that they will "look guilty". Nonetheless, an immediate discussion with an attorney is both helpful and cost-effective, even in the short run. Most attorneys offer a no-cost consultation. He or she may tell you that there is as yet no role for an attorney but may offer up some general advice about what to expect and when involvement will be necessary. Then, should that time come, you will already have someone who is familiar with you and knows a bit about your practice.

A good attorney who has experience with the medical board can be reassuring. His message may be "Nine times out of ten, these cases blow over." He will be grateful if consulted by a client who has not waived any rights, who has not passed up an opportunity to make an effective informal presentation, and who is not facing an immediate deadline.

Who you retain is important. The attorney who has drawn up business papers for you or who has represented you in personal matters may not have the experience with the board procedures, formal or informal, that is required. For a board case you need someone who is competent in administrative law and procedure. Ideally, your attorney will be accustomed to representing prescribers and be an advocate the board's staff will already respect as legally competent and personally trustworthy.

Do not be reluctant to query the attorney on specific experiences with the board. Ask about previous litigations and settlements. Find out what the attorney knows about pain management. It will probably be very little, but an attorney who understands something about controlled substances and good pain management practices will require less education and therefore fewer hours of preparation. If he is unfamiliar with this topic, make sure he will work with you to learn the salient facts.

Make sure you understand the fee structure. It may be hourly, but it could also be task-specific, one fee for evaluating and attempting to settle the case before an official hearing and another fee for the hearing itself if necessary. If hourly, ask what billing detail you will receive. If the attorney is not a single practitioner, ask how much of the work will be done by him and what work can be delegated to younger attorneys or paralegals with lower billing rates. If there is a retainer fee involved, find out how often you will receive an accounting.

It may well be that you will have little choice in who will represent you. When an insurance company is involved, they will usually be specific about who represents you and them. This does not mean that you cannot ask the insurer to approve a particular attorney who may already be known to you.

Be prepared to educate your attorney. Come to the first meeting prepared. Bring copies of the files in which the board is interested. Ideally, you will have had time to make a short summary of each case. *Be sure to write "privileged and confidential attorney-client materials" on any document you create, particularly if you retain copies or have copies in your computer's hard drive.* Provide the attorney with copies, if you have them, of any board regulations or guidelines on prescribing opioids for chronic pain, as well as the state's Intractable Pain Treatment Act if there is one. Copies of virtually all state laws and regulations involving opioids are available at www.medsch.wisc.edu/painpolicy/matrix.htm. Sometimes, however, relevant and useful material is tucked away in obscure code portions (e.g., Florida's law that requires physicians to treat pain are located in the laws relating to advance medical directives). Therefore ask your attorney to make sure that he has all of the state's provisions.

Provide other relevant documents such as the APS/ASAM guidelines for the prescription of opioids for chronic pain and any pain policies of your specialty. Because many issues between prescribing physicians and boards involve "prescribing to addicts" in one form or another, a respondent facing such charges should also provide the lawyer with ASAM's policy statement regarding opioid treatment for patients who are also substance abusers. No state prohibits treating substance abusers' pain with opioids, although guidelines that express support for this form of treatment often urge caution, liaisons with other professionals, and consideration of heightened practice controls such as a contract.

A prescriber must be candid with his attorney. This is not the place for introspection and keeping oneself to oneself. An attorney must have, or develop, an awareness of the weaknesses and the strengths of the case. Shared information will allow you and your attorney to shape a strategy for defending the case, choose expert witnesses, and structure all settlement negotiations. For example, a respondent may know that his documentation is arguably or clearly below standard but believe that his patient care is appropriate. Armed with that information, the attorney may emphasize the amount of time his client spends with patients that is unrecorded or not apparent from the record and state that the physician has agreed to attend CME programs on documentation. Aggressively defending a weak position will increase the likelihood that strong positions will not be taken seriously.

The Respondent Physician's Rights

Legal Notice of Charges

If the matter progresses, a physician will receive a formal complaint or show-cause order from the board. It explains what the board (read board attorney) believes is deficient in a patient(s) care. This is an important document. Usually it will reflect the advice of the board's expert. Although it can be superceded or amended by a later order, the rules of administrative and criminal law require that a defendant/respondent know the charges against him. It must be sufficiently specific that a physician can defend himself on the charges. In criminal cases a motion for a "bill of particulars" would follow an insufficient indictment. Your attorney must be alert to object to any criticism not reasonably reflected in the show-cause order.

Discovery

Your attorney can file a request pursuant to the board's rules for copies of its expert witness report and the expert witness credential. You can ask for (but may not receive) transcripts of previous testimony of the expert before either your state board or other boards, as well as copies of the expert's publications. Other requests might seek identities of investigators, pharmacy records obtained by the board, and any other material that the board or its expert relies on. These requests, if honored, fulfill the "no surprises" goal of any proceeding. If not honored, they will provide the basis for objections at hearing if new documents appear. Expect the board counsel to give you as little as possible as late as possible. Requesting a scheduling conference with the ALJ may have some hastening effect. If state practice permits, do not hesitate to request the board to issue subpoenas to ensure that reluctant witnesses will attend a hearing.

The Right to Be Heard

Due process requires that a respondent have the right to a hearing if one is desired. A respondent who fails to respond to board deadlines for any appearance or notice of request for appearance may waive the right. Read all board notices carefully and respond in a timely manner. Generally, board deadlines can be extended if necessary by motion (usually but not necessarily with the consent of the board counsel), but they cannot be ignored.

The right to be heard includes the right to representation by an attorney and the right to present evidence, including expert testimony, and to cross-examine witnesses. The show-cause order will itself provide a date by which the respondent can rebut the charges in writing. Take care as you draft these because, with informal representations by your attorney, they may lead to settlement. They could also cause the state's expert witness to amend his report and lead to the reformulation or dropping of some (or even all) elements of the charge.

Settlement

Most board cases settle before hearing. There are a number of junctures at which talking about settling some or all of the charges will occur. In some states, the rules provide for an informal conference before a panel of the full board. Not all states have this procedure, but for those that do this is an opportunity to explain and to hear what at least a sample of the board is thinking. The respondent should submit documents to the panel that flesh out any previous submissions. Treat this "informal" session as a very important opportunity because the state's expert witness is likely to be there. The board panel and the state's attorney are able to ask questions of either the respondent or his witnesses, and there is often a possibility for a direct dialogue among the respondent, the state's expert, and the panel members. The respondent's attorney may also question the opposing expert. At the end of this conference the panel will make a recommendation to the board and provide its findings. These could include recommending that the board not take any action against the respondent.

If the process continues, however, the panel's written recommendations do provide another opportunity to frame a settlement. In fact, when it is provided to the respondent before being sent to the board, the respondent can treat it as an offer of settlement. It is quite possible to negotiate its terms with the board's attorney. If the state does not use the panel-review procedures, the respective attorneys will be in contact and can set up a settlement discussion. These discussions are privileged. Any concessions made in ne-gotiations cannot be used in a subsequent hearing.

Settlement is far preferable to the cost, delay, and risk of a bad out-come inherent in any full-blown contest *if* the terms are agreeable. If docu-mentation is an issue, the respondent might agree to attend a remedial program if the board will drop other charges. Or the respondent may agree to pay a fine if the board will forego any NPBD-reportable action. If loss of license looks like a real risk, the respondent may prefer to negotiate for the ability to continue practicing under supervision for a period, using agreed-upon protocols or standards.

Discussion with your attorney about settlement should be an ongoing process. Attorneys must present any settlement offer to their clients. However, the potential for settlement should not interfere with further preparation of the case. Too often the failure to prepare dictates that there must be a last-minute settlement at some disadvantage to the client. Some attorneys are so accustomed to settling their cases that they may press their clients to accept a settlement or may not function well in an actual hearing.

Before any settlement make sure that you understand *all* of the conse-quences. There will very likely be insurance cost increases. Your name may appear in board records. There may be an NPDB report that will be a part of your permanent record. If the board proposes a training course, make sure that you understand how it will react (and how fast) to a successful conclusion. Understand exactly how the board will respond to any in-quiries about you. If the board proposes that you practice under supervi-sion, make certain of who an acceptable supervisor must be and exactly what constitutes "under supervision". For instance: Will you need to have pre-approval for every prescription, or is there only an obligation to discuss your cases at regular intervals?

Witnesses

The Expert Witness

A well-credentialed expert witness is absolutely essential to defending any case that goes beyond the discovery stage. It is far too important to leave this urgent matter solely to your attorney.

As a practicing physician, the respondent will know far better than an attorney who is active and prominent in the field in his state and who will have the clinical background to serve as a witness. You can check the pain management service in a teaching hospital, provided it has physicians who treat chronic pain as well as trauma and post-surgical pain. The state's af-filiate with the American Cancer Society's State Pain Initiatives may well have physicians on the board or as members who are interested not only in treating pain but in improving the quality of pain management. If the respondent is board-certified, checking with that organization, particularly if it has a policy statement that is favorable to treating chronic pain with opioids, should be useful. The members of the drafting committee who are from your or a near-by state may be potential witnesses or sources of further ideas. A literature search for articles that support your judgments may point you to authors who could serve as experts.

Credentials are important, but an expert must also be a good witness. You will want a witness who is an educator, one who can explain clearly the management of chronic pain. He should ideally be licensed and practicing in your state, although in some states it is difficult to find someone qualified and willing to testify. He should be able to project fairness and integrity. He must also be willing to spend time reviewing records, preparing a report for the hearing, and, if necessary, testifying. He also needs to be able to comply with deadlines. There is nothing worse than finding an expert and then having to hound and beg him for a report that is overdue. You and your attorney will need time to review it and provide details that may have been missed.

The expert witness also has to think on his feet. It is very difficult to anticipate every twist and turn of cross-examination. Ideally, he will have experience testifying or at least the confidence to stand up well to cross-examination (without being either belligerent or pedantic). Beware, however, the "professional" expert witness. Make sure he has current or recent clinical experience. Glib professional experts are readily available for the price of a computer search, but they may do you as much harm as good.

Protect yourself by interviewing (with your attorney) a potential expert witness. Your attorney should ask him to preliminarily review the charts and talk with him about any concerns before he is hired. Ask whether he has had any brushes with the DEA or other investigators, malpractice suits related to competence or prescribing patterns, or any other reportable NPDB event. Read any articles or papers he has written that are relevant to the subject of the show-cause order. If he has previously been a witness before the board, make sure your attorney reads the transcripts of his testimony and cross-examination. If he has testified elsewhere, ask him to provide copies of his testimony. If he is an academician and you practice in a small community with many uninsured patients, make sure he understands the imperfections that may bring in terms of extensive testing and a pressured, but acceptable, practice setting. If you have hundreds of patients and he attends a teaching hospital clinic once a week, educate him on how you nonetheless manage a responsible practice. If he sees primarily tertiary referrals and you are a primary care physician, make sure he understands the differences.

The attorney should plan the meetings with the respondent and the expert. The attorney should retain him on your behalf. Materials prepared by the witness or others at the request of the attorney are legally privileged "attorney work-product" and not discoverable except under extreme circumstances unlikely to be relevant here. The attorney's contacts with the witness are also privileged if disclosing them would tend to reveal defense strategy. Moreover, communicating privileged materials to third parties does not waive the privilege. An attorney can provide privileged materials to his or her agents, other attorneys, consultants, and the like in order to prepare the case. Your attorney can advise you about the precise ramifications of the work-product privilege in the context of your case.

The "attorney-client communications" privilege is narrower, but stronger. Your attorney may not disclose what you say to him or what he says to you. Even a potential attorney whom you do not hire cannot disclose facts that you give him as part of the interviewing process. There are no exceptions relevant to cases under consideration here. Therefore you may talk freely with your attorney and his agents/employees and provide them with documents that will help your case. Be aware, however, that a client can waive the attorney-client privilege if he involves third parties in the discussions. If a client shares his attorney's written advice or analysis with another, he may also waive the privilege as to that document.

Preparing an expert witness for the actual hearing is the attorney's job, but his client should also be involved. Preparation requires much more than a hurried last-minute review of the expert's report and credentials (which the board will already have) and a brief discussion with the expert. Preparation includes making sure that the witness need not fumble through the files before every answer, will not volunteer unhelpful facts or theories, and, above all, will be candid without being dangerous. The attorney should review expected cross-examination with the expert and press the witness to be ready to answer difficult questions that might go to the weaknesses of the case. In addition, the attorney should use the witness's expertise to help him prepare to cross-examine the board's witness. The respondent may have to press the attorney to make sure this preparation is going forward thoroughly and in a timely manner.

At the hearing, the respondent's expert must be able to state with honesty and conviction that the respondent's care is consistent with the standard of care and to back that statement up with references to the record and solid clinical expertise. In the post-Daubert environment he should also, where possible, point to peer-reviewed articles and guidelines to support his opinion. If he can do neither with conviction, the case should not have gone to hearing without a strong effort to settle.

Board Witnesses

The quality of board witnesses in substance abuse/pain management cases is shameful. A recent proceeding involved a highly credentialed respondent who had been a fellow in one of the best pain management programs and had taught medical management of pain in a well-regarded medical school. The state's "expert" was a physician who had not practiced medicine in over a decade, had never had special training or certification in pain management, and had never once prescribed opioids for chronic pain, although he had substantial qualifications in addiction medicine. His main business was testifying against prescribing physicians before multiple state boards and running a program to which medical boards frequently sent physicians to learn how (not) to prescribe.

Absent some limiting statute or regulation, most states permit someone to be qualified as an "expert" if his knowledge is likely to be useful in a legal or quasi-legal setting. The Federation of State Medical Board's guidelines for state medical practice do not address the question of expert witness qualifications. About half of the states have a statute defining broad qualifications for expert witnesses in malpractice proceedings. These should, in all reason, be applicable to board proceedings in which the standard of care is also at issue.

For medical doctors, the AMA has established as one of its ethical rules that a testifying physician is deemed to be practicing medicine when he testifies. He is then governed by the same limitations that apply in clinical practice when a physician steps beyond his qualifications. AMA Policy H-265-994 states that:

> [T] the minimum statutory requirements for qualification as an expert witness should reflect the following: (*i*) that the witness be required to have comparable education, training, and occupational experience in the same field as the defendant; (*ii*) that the occupational experience include active medical practice or teaching experience in the same field as the defendant; and (*iii*) that the active medical practice or teaching experience must have been within five years of the date of the occurrence giving rise to the claim.

Many specialty boards impose similar requirements for testifying experts. In pain management cases, it would be helpful if the standards required an expert not just in that area but in the medical management of chronic pain. Some board-certified anesthesiologists, for example, are experts at procedures but have little or no experience in medical management of chronic pain. By challenging the credentials or professional experience of a board expert or cross-examining him on those topics, an attorney can educate the ALJ about these differences. The author further believes that it is appropriate to notify the witness's credentialing society if the witness testifies without the credentials it requires.

Your attorney must also cross-examine the state's expert on the substance of his opinion. It is not uncommon for states to use witnesses who will testify that the standard of care requires a refusal to treat those with past or present addictive disorders. Or he may opine that physicians should always implement a "one-strike" policy of discharging patients whose behavior is either ambiguous (the Red Flag) or clearly violates the informed consent/opioid contract that the patient signed. He may insist that the opioids prescribed were not necessary, or were too much, too often. An expert should be willing to make concessions when confronted with national and state standards. His testimony is required to address the consensus standard of care, not his own personal opinions. The expert will also agree that he has not examined or treated the particular patient under discussion and is responding to hypothetical questions. How extensively and aggressively an attorney cross-examines the expert depends on the attorney's personal style and the facts of the case.

The Respondent's Role as Witness

In criminal cases, where the burden of proof is on the government and the standard of proof is "beyond a reasonable doubt", it is common for the defendant not to take the stand. In board proceedings, this is virtually impossible. A respondent has to articulate his thought processes and explain his judgments. Above all, he has to be credible. A great deal will rest on the ALJ's assessment of whether the respondent is splitting hairs or obfuscating or skirting the truth. If any of those behaviors are necessary, good sense should dictate a settlement.

In cases where there is any chance that a criminal indictment may be in the offing, deciding whether to testify must be based on advice from a criminal attorney and a careful assessment of the risk. A prescriber can expect that law enforcement personnel will attend the hearing, tape or videotape the proceeding, and will likely use the transcript against him. This is also a prosecutor's opportunity to learn more about the prescriber's practice, the quality of his witnesses and theirs, and other useful information. A good outcome from the board is not binding on the prosecutor, although it should certainly give him serious doubts. The same considerations should also apply if there is a malpractice case arising out of the same set of facts. Expect that the plaintiff's attorney and possibly the plaintiff or his family will be present and may testify.

The key to being a good witness is preparation. The respondent must know the charts and have organized his testimony so that he can support what he says with reference to the record. If documentation is poor, he will have to flesh out his treatment plan, judgment, and functional observations. He will have discussed his testimony with his attorney and should have run through at least one practice session. His attorney will also have practiced both direct and cross-examination with him and will have helped him prepare for tough questions. He will have explained to the respondent how to answer questions directly and to avoid obviously defensive answers. Knowing when to stop talking is of vital importance.

By the time the physician testifies, he will also have heard the board's testimony in its entirety. He will have heard whatever concessions his attorney has been able to wring out of the board's witness. More importantly, he should have some idea of what might concern the ALJ. All of that needs to be woven into his testimony or addressed head on.

For an articulate person, the best way is usually just to tell a story in words not much different than he would use to describe a case to a group of colleagues. With preparation, this should be familiar territory. The attorney can help keep things on track and prompt if something is left out. If the respondent is disorganized, the attorney can help by breaking his testimony down into a series of questions.

Patient Witnesses

Testimony from the respondent's patients who had good outcomes can be extremely powerful witnesses for the defense. These patients testify about the quality of care, the thoroughness of an examination or history, and about functional improvement. If the complaint features lack of physical examination or documentation, consider calling patient witnesses to testify about the quality of informed consent and treatment.

When the board calls patient witnesses, these are almost certainly those whose outcomes have been less good. Such a witness may claim that the practitioner got him "hooked" on drugs. Your attorney should be prepared to cross-examine about previous or contemporaneous drug use or polypharmacy. If the patient deceived the prescriber, that too can be brought out.

Post-Hearing

After the hearing, both parties will file post-hearing briefs. The ALJ will write a recommended decision, findings of fact, and conclusions of law. He may recommend penalties if he finds fault with the respondent's care. In some states, he may have a mandatory deadline to complete his work. In others, this process can drag out disgracefully. Either party may appeal the ALJ's decision to the board, which will either adopt the ALJ's opinion in whole or part, or disagree. If it disagrees, it will have to explain why, using the hearing record as its only source. If the decision goes against the respondent, he may appeal to a state appellate court that will rule on the board's record without further testimony. The appellant's brief will spell out the errors of fact or law that he believes merits reversal of the board's decision.

DEA Registration Proceedings

Everything said about preparing for and defending a state board proceeding applies to DEA proceedings to revoke a prescriber's registration under the Controlled Substances Act. The respondent's rights are the same except that the DEA and federal courts have never obligated the DEA to use a "clear and convincing" evidentiary standard in place of the "more likely than not" standard.

In registration proceedings, the DEA may act summarily if it can convince an ALJ that delaying for a hearing would endanger the public health or safety. In all cases, the DEA must show that continued registration is "inconsistent with the public interest" (21 USC 824[a]). This sounds horribly vague, but in practice it is more limited. The statute requires the DEA to consider any or all of the following to determine the public interest: 1) the registrant's experience in prescribing controlled substances; 2) any violations of state or federal controlled substances law; 3) the registrant's conviction for violating a state or federal controlled substances provision; and 4) the recommendation of the registrant's state board or professional disciplinary proceeding (21 USC 823[f][1]-[4]). In addition or instead, the DEA may take into account "such other conduct as may endanger the public health and safety" (21 USC 823 [f][5]).

DEA proceedings that are not summary also begin with a show-cause order and feature the right to respond in writing, the opportunity for a hearing before an ALJ, and a written opinion along with proposed findings of law and fact. In DEA cases, the latter are forwarded to the DEA Assistant Administrator, who may reject or adopt them in whole or in part under the same basic rules that bind a state board's reaction to its ALJ's opinion (21 CFR 1316.67 [2004]). The Deputy Administrator has never hesitated to overrule an ALJ and has often done so despite a recommendation for revocation. A registrant may appeal the administrator's final order, but in matters of substance and the agency's interpretation of the law it will be given deference by the courts.

Criminal Charges

Federal and State Controlled Substances Acts

The Controlled Substances Act permits registered prescribers to distribute opioids via prescription in the course of medical practice, or as DEA regulations state, "with a legitimate medical purpose and within the scope of professional practice."

Much of what has been said above regarding experts and preparation applies to criminal cases, but there are important distinctions. Some of these are procedural. First and foremost, a prescriber should retain a competent criminal lawyer at the first inkling of an investigation. In the interim, do not meet with or talk to any law enforcement officials. Tell them that you are waiting until you get an attorney's advice. Then seek out an attorney who is experienced in criminal law. Preferably he will also be a specialist in white-collar crime or, even better, have significant experience in the type of case you are involved in. White-collar cases are often complex and involve expert witnesses to prove accounting, corporate management, or tax issues, and these are skills you may need.

Another important difference between criminal and board defense is that in a criminal matter, a private investigator may have to do significant work. This will involve finding and interviewing potential witnesses for or against, as well as developing the background of patients who have pled guilty and are now working with the DEA in the expectation of a more lenient sentence.

There are usually opportunities to head off an indictment. Your attorney will need you and the experts to help him understand where the weaknesses of the case may be before such discussions. If there is an indictment, settlements routinely involve pleading to a lesser offense, possibly a misdemeanor, and/or payment of a fine. Deciding on whether to accept such a bargain is difficult and painful. Before you hire any attorney, try to determine his success in both heading off and bargaining away criminal charges. Experience in heading off an indictment is wonderful. Experience in plea bargaining is easier to come by. You will not want an attorney who effectively limits his practice to guiding his clients into plea bargains. This may not always be in the client's best interests.

The most important thing that a client can do is educate his attorney. The physician must demand that the attorney learn how his practice works and how he handles his patients. Attorneys for opioid-prescribing physicians have learned much about effective strategy and preparation in recent years.

Probably the most important lesson is that the defense must refuse to permit the case to proceed as if it were a malpractice case. The Controlled Substances Act allows only registered physicians to prescribe scheduled drugs and requires that the practitioner is "acting in the course of his professional practice or except as otherwise authorized by [this statute]" (21 USC § 844[a]). The elements of a federal care are 1) proof that the prescriber acted knowingly; 2) proof that a scheduled drug was prescribed; and 3) proof that the prescriber did not have a medical purpose for the prescriptions. Treating chronic pain is indisputably a legitimate medical purpose. Prescribing for the purpose of maintaining addiction is not. Because the first two elements are usually easy to prove, the only real question is whether the physician (even wrongly or incompetently) was trying to relieve a patient's pain.

A former chief counsel of the DEA has put the statutory language in perspective:

> Acts of prescribing or dispensing of controlled substances which are done within the course of the registrant's professional practice are, for purposes of the Controlled Substances Act, lawful. It matters not that such acts might constitute terrible medicine or malpractice. They may reflect the grossest form of medical misconduct or negligence. They are nevertheless legal.

In prosecutions, however, the DEA has strayed from this central distinction. The DEA and federal prosecutors approach their cases as if they were malpractice cases. Bad outcomes, such as a patient death from polypharmacy, being conned by drug-seeking patients, failure to police patients for potential drug abuse, or even poor documentation and sloppy office procedures are treated as evidence of criminality.

Using this approach, much of the evidence they regard as important includes the quality of the physical examination and history, the efforts made to confirm a patient's history through previous medical records, and the extent to which the drugs were appropriate to the physical complaint and in reasonable amounts. They focus also on risk management issues: a prescriber's failure to perform blood or urine tests; the absence or presence of a "patient contract"; the reaction to ambiguous patient behaviors; or outright contract violations. They question whether and how the prescriber responded to information from the patient's family or others. They also look to facts that have nothing to do with whether or not a professional practice is involved by presenting testimony about crowded waiting rooms and the unkempt appearance of patients. They emphasize facts that they believe show that the doctor "knew or should have known" that a patient could not control his use of the medications. They want to know whether the prescriber has steered patients toward or away from a particular pharmacy.

When enough of these factors are put together, the prosecution considers that it has proved criminal intent "beyond a reasonable doubt." In fact, it could be right. However, it could also have shown only that a prescriber is more willing than most to prescribe opioids, trusts his patients, and is less willing than many to discharge patients whose behavior is ambiguous. It may be that the physician has been shown to be negligent or sloppy but still believes that he is treating pain successfully.

The government may prove intent through circumstantial evidence. However, circumstantial evidence must be consistent with all of the facts and inconsistent with reasonable innocent alternatives that may explain the facts. The defense must refuse to concede the legitimacy of quality-of-practice issues, that is for the state medical board. His defense may be that although his practice quality had imperfections, even glaring ones, his intent was to treat pain. He should also educate the jury on the interaction of pain management and substance abuse. Unfortunately, federal pattern jury instructions on the subject of good faith read more like a malpractice charge (Federal pattern jury charge § 54.16). Your attorney should, if it comes to trial, be certain to educate the judge on the statute's actual requirement and ask for this and other "not malpractice" instructions be given to the jury.

Disproving intent presents serious strategic hurdles for the defense. Good faith is an absolute defense for the physician. One way to support a good-faith defense is through the defendant's testimony. However, the good faith has to rest on some reasonable belief that the patient needed the medication to treat pain and not to further a drug habit. Therefore such a defense can be rebutted by proof that the prescriber, ostrich like, refused to look or listen to evidence that the patient was using him and was not in pain. If the physician considered the possibility and, as an exercise of medical judgment, continued opioid therapy as a treatment for pain, he should do well. Expert testimony should support his decision as not inconsistent with a good-faith judgment.

State Charges for Reckless Negligence

A physician can be held responsible for a patient's death if there is proof beyond a reasonable doubt that the physician acted with gross negligence, defined as a quality of treatment significantly below the standard of care. A malpractice standard may not be used.

There have been only a few reported cases in which a reckless negligence action was brought, and even fewer convictions. Most such cases are dropped. The cases were brought after a patient died with significant amounts of opioids in his system and it became known to investigators that the deceased had been prescribed opioids for chronic pain. A pathologist or medical examiner report reported the cause of death to be substance overdose.

In every case that the present author has read or reviewed, the facts are also consistent with suicide, the patient's abuse of his medications in concert with other controlled substances obtained illegally and alcohol, or an idiosyncratic response to medication that could not have been predicted even by a normally competent prescriber. There is little or no evidence the physician knew that the patient was engaging in polypharmacy and abuse or had consciously ignored evident facts without applying any exercise of medical judgment as to practice controls. Without in any way minimizing the tragedy that these deaths represent, the intervening purposeful or suicidal acts of the patient were the cause.

The defense should contest any assertion that there was a causal relationship between the doctor's prescriptions and the patient's death. It should also investigate the circumstances of the death to show polypharmacy and misuse. It would also be advisable to educate the prosecutor and, if necessary, the jury about practice management tools that the physician used in the patient's case and to show that the patient deceived the doctor. The defense should also tell the jury about the medical management of chronic pain, the applicable state statutes and regulations, and professional guidelines.

Conclusion

Any inquiry is, to say the least, unnerving. But physicians who treat pain with opioids, particularly those who treat pain in the substance abuser, must expect that it could occur. If it can be shown that the physician followed all applicable regulations and guidelines, however, results should be favorable. An educating defense based on good faith will help. If medical procedures and documentation need to be improved, it should be the province of the medical board rather than the prosecutor to remedy the situation.

APPENDIX

■   ■   ■

Disability Management Issues for an Injured Worker with Low Back Pain

James P. Robinson, MD, PhD

Chronology and Comments

JANUARY 10

Roger Smith is a 40-year-old auto mechanic who works in Washington State and is eligible for workers' compensation benefits through the Department of Labor and Industries. He sees you on an urgent basis. He indicates that he sustained a low back injury earlier in the day during the course of his work. He was bent over the hood of a car and was lifting out a carburetor when he felt a "pop" in his lower back and had a sudden onset of severe low back pain. Mr Smith denies pain, sensory loss, or motor loss in the lower extremities. He has not noticed any problems with bowel or bladder control.

Past medical history is noteworthy in that the patient had a workers' compensation claim from ages 37 to 39 because of a low back injury that he sustained at work. During that time, Mr Smith underwent L4-5 and L5-S1 discectomies for right lower extremity sciatica, followed by an L4-S1 fusion with Steffee plates. His radicular symptoms resolved, but he has had ongoing low back pain (LBP). His claim was closed after his last surgery, and he returned to the work force 6 months ago. His employer now is different from the one he had when he was injured 3 years ago. The rest of Mr Smith's past medical history is unremarkable.

Social history indicates that the patient is a high school graduate. All of his work experience has been in the area of automobile repair. Mr Smith is married, and he has two children aged 10 and 7.

Physical examination is noteworthy in that Mr Smith stands leaning forward, with complete flattening of the lumbar lordotic curve. He walks very slowly. Palpation reveals diffuse spasms in the lumbar paraspinal muscles, along with significant soft tissue tenderness. The patient demonstrates virtually zero range motion of the lumbar spine in all planes. Straight leg raising is limited by back pain rather than radicular symptoms.

Neurological examination reveals diffuse, bilateral lower extremity weakness that appears to reflect pain inhibition. The only focal sign is a diminished right ankle jerk, which the patient says has been present since his original back injury. He is positive on three of the five Waddell signs.

Mr Smith says he is in too much pain to work. He asks you to fill out a Department of Labor and Industries (DLI) Accident Report (see Fig. 10-3 on page 243). You supply the following information (*in italics*):

#41   Diagnosis = *Lumbosacral strain (847.2)*
#45   Objective findings = *Muscle spasms, severely restricted lumbar range of motion in all planes, diminished right ankle jerk*
#47   Was the diagnosed condition caused by this injury or exposure? *Probably*
#48   Will the condition cause the patient to miss work? *Yes – 10 days*
#49   Is there any pre-existing impairment of the injured area? *Yes*
#50   Has the patient ever been treated for the same or a similar condition? *Yes*

Comments

1. The patient's presentation is a typical one: acute onset of non-radicular low back pain.

2. In filling out the required Accident Report, you are forced to make several judgments about the patient's disability:

A. You must decide whether to conceptualize the patient's problem as a new injury or as an aggravation of the lumbar spine problem he developed at age 37. If the problem is conceptualized as a new injury, claim opening is fairly easy. If it is conceptualized as an aggravation, DLI will ask you to review past records on the patient and indicate whether there is objective evidence that his condition has worsened.

(*i*) The diagnosis of lumbosacral strain embodies the concept that you are conceptualizing the patient's problem as a new injury.

B. Administrative agencies always demand that a physician buttress his/her conclusions with objective findings. This embodies the administrative myth that reports of incapacitation by patients should be closely correlated with objectively measurable signs of tissue injury or organ dysfunction. Any "objectivity" is illusory because there is no clear definition of "objective findings".

(*i*) Most physicians would accept the objectivity of a depressed ankle jerk reflex. In this patient, it is quite likely that the depressed right ankle jerk reflex stems from the back injury 3 years ago. But because DLI insists on objective findings, you should strongly consider listing the abnormal reflex in answer to item #45 above.

(ii) The status of muscle spasms and restricted lumbar range of motion is less clear. They are not completely objective, because patients have some control over the tightness of muscles in their backs and over how much they move when a physician assesses active range of motion.

(iii) What *is* clear is that you need to answer item #45 in some way. As a practical matter, the claims managers who review Accident Reports are likely to accept virtually any answer you give.

3. When a physician gives a diagnosis (#41), states objective findings that support the diagnosis (#45), and says that the diagnosed condition was probably caused by the patient's work (#47), he/she is in effect urging the DLI to accept the patient's problem as a work injury. This is a necessary step on the way to medical or disability benefits (i.e., a worker must have a valid workers' compensation claim before he can get benefits from DLI).

4. When you indicate that Mr Smith's condition will cause him to lose 10 days of work (#48), you are supporting the idea that he is work-disabled and therefore entitled to disability benefits. In the language of workers' compensation law, Mr Smith deserves benefits if he is judged to be temporarily, totally disabled from work.

5. Items #49 and #50 address the issue of previous problems that Mr Smith has had with his lumbar spine. As noted above, his new symptoms can be construed as either an aggravation of an old lumbar spine condition or as a new injury.

6. In a general way, it is important to note that in filling out the required Accident Report, you have made important disability judgments regarding Mr Smith. You have indicated that he has a legitimate musculoskeletal injury, that the injury was probably caused by his work, and that he will be disabled from work because of the injury. These judgments are typically made primarily on the basis of what the patient says; one rarely has completely objective indices of the severity of a patient's incapacitation from low back pain, and one often does not have independent confirmation that the patient became symptomatic because of his work.

7. The DLI system tends to be permissive when it processes Accident Reports (i.e., the accuracy of physician statements is rarely questioned).

FEBRUARY 10

Mr Smith has undergone evaluation by a spine surgeon. He is felt not to be a candidate for further surgery. He receives conservative therapy consisting of physical therapy and medications. He appears to have improved modestly but continues to complain of persistent, localized low back pain that precludes employment. His employer contacts you and requests a conference to discuss Mr Smith's ongoing symptoms and prospects for return to work.

Comments

1. Many experts in workers' compensation emphasize that treating physicians can do a better job if they talk with employers, or even visit

work sites. Aside from the time required for this, you must be aware of the possibility of the employer presenting a distorted picture of the worker or of the job to which the worker might return. Probably the best way to deal with this is to have a conference that includes both the injured worker and a representative of the employer.

MARCH 10

You receive a letter from DLI. It asks whether Mr Smith has reached maximal medical improvement and whether he continues to have impairments that prevent him from working. It insists that you present the objective findings on which your conclusions are based. You respond that Mr Smith's functional capacities as measured by his physical therapist continue to increase, so that he is not yet at maximal medical improvement. You express the view that he is not currently able to return to his job as an auto mechanic. You cite his limited lumbar range of motion and his diminished right ankle jerk reflex as objective findings buttressing your conclusion.

Comments

1. The issue of maximal medical improvement is closely linked to disability issues for an individual with a workers' compensation claim. Typically, compensation systems accept the judgments of treating physicians more-or-less at face value while a worker is recovering from an injury. But when an injured worker has reached maximal medical improvement, compensation law generally requires that some permanent decision be made about the workers' employment capabilities. As a result, claims managers are more likely to challenge the opinions of the attending physician (e.g., by commissioning an independent medical examination).

2. The demand for "objective findings" reflects the myth that work incapacitation can be objectively assessed by a physician. In fact, your conclusion that Mr Smith can not work as an auto mechanic is based largely on the following considerations: (*a*) He has a complex lumbar spine problem that can produce intolerance of physically demanding work; (*b*) He has repeatedly stated that he cannot handle the physical demands of work as an auto mechanic; and (*c*) Having treated him for 2 months, you have formed the clinical judgment that his reports regarding his physical capacities are credible. This is an example of the fundamental dilemma of assessing disability based on pain. The patient reports severe activity restrictions because of his pain; there is nothing you can do in your office to confirm or disconfirm his statements about his activity restrictions. To a large extent, your decision about whether to support his assertions rests on whether you find the assertions credible. But the compensation system insists that you rationalize your disability determination on the basis of objective findings. Probably the best way to address this mismatch is simply to state the patient's physical findings, and disregard the fact that the physical findings do not lead inevitably to a conclusion about the patient's work capacity.

APRIL 10

Mr Smith has now been assigned a vocational rehabilitation counselor by DLI. The counselor has filled out a job analysis for the position that Mr Smith held at the time of his injury. You review the job analysis with Mr Smith at his next visit. He complains that it is grossly inaccurate. For example, whereas the job analysis says that his job requires lifting no more than 35 pounds, Mr Smith insists that before his injury he had to lift objects weighing up to 100 pounds. He also asserts that he is unable to spend long periods of time bent over the hood of a car. You request a formal *physical capacities evaluation* to determine his lifting capacity and ability to work in the postures required by his auto mechanic job.

Based on Mr Smith's statements, the physical exam findings, and the results of the physical capacities evaluation, you indicate that Mr Smith is not able to do the work described in the job analysis.

Comments

1. It is common for injured workers to complain that job analyses provide a distorted picture of what their work actually requires. It is important for you to discuss a job analysis with an injured worker so that you learn whether there is a significant difference between the job as described in the job analysis and his perception of what the job requires.

2. Physical capacities evaluations are usually performed by physical therapists. The purpose of such an evaluation is to provide objective data about what an injured worker actually does in a test situation (e.g., how much he/she lifts, how long he/she sits continuously). A physical capacities evaluation is by no means a foolproof solution to the problem of determining activity limitations in a patient with a chronic pain problem. In fact, a recent review concludes that there is no firm evidence that such evaluations predict work performance (1). They do, however, provide some performance data—more than a physician can glean simply by doing an office examination on a patient.

MAY 10

Mr Smith brings two forms to his scheduled office visit. One is from a company that has financed the purchase of his car. When he arranged financing, he purchased an insurance option; it stipulates that his car payments will be deferred if his treating physician asserts that he is totally disabled from any kind of work and that the disability is likely to continue for more than a year. You agree to support his request for deferment. The second form is from the Department of Motor Vehicles. It is an application for a disabled parking sticker. The patient says he needs to have a disabled parking sticker because his back pain becomes intolerable if he has to walk more than a quarter of a mile. You tell Mr Smith that you will not support his application for a disabled parking sticker.

Comments

1. These two requests have no inherent relation to Mr Smith's DLI claim. But they give a flavor of the types of disability decisions a treating physician is called upon to make. These "extraneous" disability requests can create stress for the treating physician and may well have an impact on a patient's perceptions regarding his work disability. The car insurance form is a problem because it requires you to characterize Mr Smith as having long term, total disability. This message is likely to be incongruent with messages that you expect to give Mr Smith in relation to his DLI claim. A disabled parking sticker may also affect M. Smith's perception of himself as an able-bodied versus a disabled person. Although there is no logical incompatibility between Mr Smith's having a disabled parking sticker and his returning to work, there may well be a psychological inconsistency.

JUNE 10

Mr Smith indicates that his DLI claims manager has strongly urged him to apply for Social Security Disability. He indicates that he has started the SSDI application process and has been told that disability adjudicators for the SSA will soon be asking you to provide information about his medical condition. You urge him to delay the SSDI application process until he has gotten definitive information about whether DLI will provide vocational rehabilitation services for him.

Comments

1. You may well be surprised that a workers' compensation agency, which is nominally devoted to helping individuals return to work, would urge an injured worker to apply for SSDI, a program established for individuals who are totally and permanently disabled. Yet clinicians who treat injured workers see this pattern frequently.

2. In terms of perceptions of disability by an injured worker, an SSDI application represents a "kiss of death". An individual can obtain an SSDI award only if he can convince adjudicators that he is totally and permanently disabled. Long-term studies show that only about 3% of individuals awarded SSDI benefits ever return to the work force on a sustained basis. Although it is theoretically possible for a person to continue to seek employment while he is applying for SSDI, informal observation and the limited data available (2) strongly suggest that an individual's probability of vocational rehabilitation is low once he starts the SSDI application process.

3. The treating physician is often in an uncomfortable position when an individual on workers' compensation starts an SSDI application. On the one hand, the physician will appropriately anticipate that the worker will be more refractory to vocational rehabilitation once he starts the SSDI application process. On the other hand, he/she may well be concerned about time lines and back-up plans for the worker. One issue is that individuals who apply for SSDI on the basis of painful conditions like low back pain

often have their initial claims denied (3). Their claims may be accepted upon appeal, but the process of going through multiple levels of the SSA appeals process can easily take more than a year. In the meantime, the worker faces the risk of having his time-loss benefits abruptly terminated by DLI. From this perspective, an early application for SSDI might be viewed as an "insurance policy" for a worker who is having difficulty returning to work, even if he has not totally given up the goal of returning to work. In an ideal world, workers' compensation agencies would work cooperatively with other agencies to make sure that injured workers do not get caught in the middle between different benefit programs. In fact, this kind of cooperation rarely occurs.

JULY 10

Mr Smith's claims manager schedules an independent medical examination for him. The exam is performed by an orthopedist, a physiatrist, and a psychiatrist. The orthopedist and physiatrist collaborate to generate a medical/surgical report; the psychiatrist submits a separate report. The former states that Mr Smith has reached maximal medical improvement from his lumbar strain of January 10. He is felt to have no permanent partial impairment over and above the 10% impairment that was awarded when his earlier lumbar spine claim was closed. It concludes: "There are no objective findings that would prevent Mr Smith from working on a full-time basis in a job with medium physical requirements." The psychiatrist diagnoses "pain disorder associated with both psychological factors and a general medical condition" (DSM IV #307.89). Both reports indicate that Mr Smith's claim is ready for closure.

A copy of the independent medical examination report is sent to you. You are asked: 1) to indicate your agreement or disagreement with it, and 2) to state the objective findings on which your opinions are based. You respond that Mr Smith probably has reached maximal medical improvement but that you are concerned about his ability to work on a full-time basis. You note that he has shown consistent activity limitations and that his reported activity limitations are credible. You indicate that he needs a careful vocational assessment and identification of specific job options before his claim is closed.

Comments

1. Independent medical examinations routinely perpetuate the myth that impairments and associated work restrictions can be objectively measured by physicians. The statement: "There are no objective findings that would prevent Mr Smith from working on a full-time basis in a job with medium physical requirements" could be made about virtually every patient with low back pain. But the reality is that back pain is the most common cause of disability in working-aged people (4-6). To paraphrase Osterweis et al., back pain disables people not because their backs fail

mechanically but because back problems can create unbearable sensations that limit activities (3). Treating physicians need to avoid falling into the conceptual trap of concluding that disability can be supported only if there are objective findings that make the disability inevitable.

2. Non-psychiatric physicians may well feel intimidated by psychiatric evaluations that purport to say what is "really" underlying an injured worker's pain complaints. Although psychiatric disorders may be major factors underlying the pain complaints of some patients, this is by no means universal. Even if a chronic low back pain patient has a psychiatric condition, the role that this plays in his ongoing pain complaints is often uncertain. Also, while diagnostic criteria for some psychiatric disorders (e.g., major depressive disorder) are well established, the diagnoses given to many chronic pain patients are much less well validated.

3. Attending physicians may feel overwhelmed by a strongly worded independent medical examination report signed by three physicians. It is important to remember that courts have generally taken the position that the opinions of treating physicians should be given great weight (7). Therefore: *If you disagree with the conclusions of an independent medical examination, you should feel free to state your objections.*

AUGUST 10

The DLI claims manager retains a vocational rehabilitation counselor to conduct an employability assessment of Mr Smith (i.e., to see whether Mr Smith's physical capabilities and past work history permit him to work in any field other than auto repair). The vocational rehabilitation counselor notes that at the age of 27 Mr Smith worked for 3 months as a dishwasher while he was taking an extended leave from his work as an automobile mechanic, and was traveling in Europe. The counselor asks you to sign a job analysis for the patient to work as a dishwasher. You meet with Mr Smith to discuss the job analysis. He protests that dishwashing requires more bending, lifting, and standing than he can do. He also notes that he and his family will be impoverished if he is left with no choice other than doing entry-level work. You refuse to sign the job analysis on the ground that the physical demands of dishwashing exceed Mr Smith's capabilities.

Comments

1. The DLI system requires that if an injured worker is unable to return to the job he had at the time of injury, a vocational rehabilitation counselor is assigned to review his entire work history and to determine whether, based on his skills and physical capabilities, he can perform any kind of work. Most workers who go through this kind of vocational assessment are placed in one of three categories:

A. They are judged to be employable based on the basis of work they have done at an earlier time in their lives. (Workers in this category typically have their time-loss benefits terminated.)

B. They are judged to need vocational retraining in order to be employable. (Workers in this category are typically authorized for vocational rehabilitation services.)

C. They are judged to be unemployable under any circumstances. (Workers in this category typically receive a pension.)

2. Injured workers and treating physicians often look at category (A) with some skepticism. One issue is that a worker may be judged employable on the basis of entry-level work he did when he first entered the labor force. Even if a worker is physically able to do such work (e.g., a job at a fast-food restaurant), the remuneration from the work is often very low. Also, some of the jobs that are proposed by vocational rehabilitation counselors seem contrived (e.g., a person with a severe lumbar spine condition is judged to be employable as a telephone solicitor).

OCTOBER 10

Mr Smith is accepted for vocational rehabilitation services. He and his vocational rehabilitation counselor develop a plan for him to work in an auto parts store. It is determined that Mr Smith will need 6 months of training in order to have the skills needed for this kind of work. DLI insists that you review the physical requirements of a salesman in an auto parts store. You review the appropriate job analysis with Mr Smith, then sign it. Mr Smith completes the 6-month training program and shortly thereafter is hired for a full-time position as a salesman in an auto parts store. Although he continues to complain of back pain, he is able to carry out his job responsibilities consistently, with no time lost from work because of back pain. His DLI claim is closed 4 months after his successful return to work.

Comments

1. A formal vocational rehabilitation plan represents the last step in DLI procedures for assisting injured workers to return to the work force. A vocational rehabilitation counselor assigned by DLI works with the injured worker to develop a vocational rehabilitation plan. DLI provides only modest funding (about $3000) for retraining, and it generally insists that the attending physician indicate that the job for which the patient will be trained is within his physical capacities.

2. This case history has a happy ending. Mr Smith makes a successful re-entry into the work force, and his claim is closed. In real-life situations, the likelihood of the outcome described in the example is low for a person who has had multiple spine surgeries and has been disabled for three of the past four years. Moreover, an outcome that is successful from the standpoint of an individual claim may not be generalized to a population of patients with a chronic low back problem (8-10). Long-term follow-up data indicate that an individual such as Mr Smith is at high risk to have still another back injury and file another compensation claim before he reaches retirement age.

Conclusion

The treating physician in this case study included Mr Smith in crucial decision-making and generally paid a great deal of attention to Mr Smith's concerns. Some physicians might take a very different approach to this kind of patient. For example, a physician might focus on the fact that Mr Smith lacked unequivocally objective findings and support early closure of the claim.

Judgments about disability in the workers' compensation system are multi-layered and interwoven. It is rarely the case that a treating physician renders a single judgment about the ability of a patient to work. Instead, as this case study shows, the physician is *repeatedly* asked or required to make judgments that bear on the disability status of his patient.

The questions posed to the physician in the above examples were not explicitly about pain. Pain was central to the entire problem, because Mr Smith's medical condition was one in which activity limitations are created primarily by pain. But the role of pain was constantly obscured by the demand of the DLI to have decisions rationalized in terms of objective findings. In essence, questions were posed to the treating physician in a manner that pressured him or her to construe Mr Smith's limitations in terms of an objective "mechanical failure" model of incapacity. The challenge for a treating physician therefore is to analyze cogently how pain is affecting his patient in the face of ongoing pressure to be "objective".

In this case study, the physician ended up interfacing between the patient and several organizations (i.e., the Department of Labor and Industries, the Social Security Administration, the Department of Motor Vehicles, and Mr Smith's automobile loan credit company). It is not unusual for a treating physician to make disability determinations for two or more agencies at the same time. As this example has shown, the contradictory needs of the various agencies make the difficult task of disability evaluation even more taxing.

REFERENCES

1. **King PM, Tuckwell N, Barrett TE.** A critical review of functional capacity evaluations. Phys Ther. 1998;78:852-66.
2. **Rucker KS, Metzler HM.** Predicting subsequent employment status of SSA disability applicants with chronic pain. Clin J Pain. 1995;11:22-35.
3. **Osterweis M, Kleinman A, Mechanic D (eds).** Pain and Disability. Washington, DC: National Academy Press; 1987.
4. **Cheadle A, Franklin G, Wolfhagen C, et al.** Factors influencing the duration of work-related disability: a population-based study of Washington State workers' compensation. Am J Public Health. 1994;84:190-6.
5. **Dionne CE.** Low back pain. In: Crombie IK, Croft PR, Linton SJ, et al (eds). Epidemiology of Pain. Seattle: IASP Press; 1999.

6. **Lawrence R, Helmick C, Arnett F, et. al.** Estimates of the prevalence of arthritis and selected musculoskeletal disorders in the United States. Arthritis Rheum. 1998;41:778-99.

7. **Ruskell RC.** Social Security Disability Claims, 3rd ed. Norcross, GA: The Harrison Company; 1993.

8. **Robinson JP.** Disability in low back pain: what do the numbers mean? Am Pain Society Bull. 1998;8: 9-13.

9. **Butler RJ, Johnson WG, Baldwin ML.** Managing work disability: why first return-to-work is not a measure of success. Industrial and Labor Relations Review. 1995;48:452-69.

10. **Johnson WG, Baldwin M.** Returns-to-work by Ontario workers with permanent partial disabilities. Report to the Workers' Compensation Board of Ontario. Ottawa: Workers' Compensation Board of Ontario; 1993.

Index